CARE
of the
SURGICAL CARDIOPULMONARY PATIENT

CARE *of the* SURGICAL CARDIOPULMONARY PATIENT

Edited by

WILLIAM E. NEVILLE, M.D.

Professor of Surgery, New Jersey College of Medicine and Dentistry, Newark, New Jersey

YEAR BOOK MEDICAL PUBLISHERS, INC.

35 EAST WACKER DRIVE • CHICAGO

Library of Congress Catalog Card Number: 70-148565

International Standard Book Number: 0-8151- 6361-4

Contributors

WALTER S. BARKER, M.D.
Associate Professor of Surgery, University of Illinois Abraham Lincoln School of Medicine, Chicago, Illinois

RAYMOND A. DIETER, JR., M.D.
Thoracic Surgeon, Glen Ellyn Clinic, Glen Ellyn, Illinois

WILLIAM M. HAMBY, M.D., PH.D.
Chief, Renal Disease—Hemodialysis Section, VA Hospital, Hines, Illinois

HIRAM T. LANGSTON, M.D.
Clinical Professor of Surgery, University of Illinois Abraham Lincoln School of Medicine, Chicago, Illinois

BERNARD J. LEININGER, M.D.
Assistant Professor of Surgery, Loyola University Stritch School of Medicine, Maywood, Illinois

ROBERT D. LYNCH, M.D.
Thoracic Surgeon, Methodist Hospital, Omaha, Nebraska

E. TRIER MÖRCH, M.D., PH.D.
Professor of Anesthesia, Rush-Presbyterian-St. Luke's Medical Center, Chicago, Illinois

WILLIAM E. NEVILLE, B.S., M.D.
Professor of Surgery, New Jersey College of Medicine and Dentistry, Newark, New Jersey

ROBERT M. VANECKO, M.D.
Associate in Surgery, Northwestern University School of Medicine, Chicago, Illinois

MILTON WEINBERG, JR., M.D.
Associate Professor of Surgery, Rush-Presbyterian-St. Luke's Medical Center, Chicago, Illinois

Foreword

THE INGREDIENTS OF SUCCESS in management of the cardiac and pulmonary problems which are submitted to surgery today are skill on the part of the surgeon and anesthesiologist during the operating room phase and the application of an understanding in depth of the massive pathophysiologic changes which appear in the postoperative period. Of these two ingredients, technical skill is most easily taught and far more time is spent in communication between preceptor and trainee in the operating room than in the postoperative care area. The cardiopulmonary operations of today are complicated, but the variety of problems met is absurdly limited as compared to the variations in the response of patients in the early days after their operations.

The derangements produced in function of the major organ systems can be related logically to the surgical trauma by an application of a thorough knowledge of the basic physiologic principles involved. Early recognition of derangement is exceedingly important so that corrections can be made before a complication develops. This volume relates functional derangement to fundamental cause and provides the information upon which early detection is based. In postoperative management it is possible to develop the discipline of a mental checklist for each patient in order to review the data pertinent to the early detection of threatening situations.

This book is the outgrowth of many years spent by the editor in laboratory work having a direct bearing on the alterations of a wide range of body functions produced by cardiopulmonary bypass, pulmonary surgery and trauma. With the enormous development of surgery and of the postoperative care of patients during the past 20 years, it is important to recognize that the information is current. In view of the imposing content it is perhaps somewhat overwhelming to consider that all of it should be at the command of the surgeon responsible for seeing patients through their cardiopulmonary experiences.

ORMAND C. JULIAN, M.D., Ph.D.

Preface

THE INNUMERABLE HOURS SPENT in the Intensive Care Unit ministering to patients following cardiothoracic surgery and the paucity of books devoted exclusively to the immediate treatment of their problems prompted the Editor to organize this treatise. Although several excellent thoracic surgery texts are available, their attention is focused primarily on diagnosis, pathology and surgical expertise. The postoperative guidelines to establish normalcy after a surgical onslaught are either deleted or discussed briefly. How often has the fledgling (and the experienced) thoracic surgeon performed a classic textbook procedure only to be confronted with the dilemma in recognizing, differentiating and properly treating some complex, diverse postsurgical sequelae?

Prior to undertaking this task, the thoracic residents, medical students and even the Intensive Care nurses were surveyed as to the material they considered most beneficial to them. Thus, the book was designed to eliminate the esoteric and to present practical methodology. In order to accomplish this goal, physiologic parameters are included so that the reader will better understand the overt manifestations of postoperative irregularities.

Following this, several of the Editor's clinically oriented, knowledgeable associates were requested to write a chapter on the modus operandi for their specific surgical forte. The contents, therefore, entirely reflect the individual authors' own attitudes. In no way has their style in writing or presentation been altered. Although an attempt has been made to avoid repetition, since this is a multiauthored book, some reiteration has been inevitable and even desirable in order to maintain continuity in discussion of related subjects. For example, in a dissertation on the management of the adult thoracic patient, respiratory insufficiency and artificial ventilation are necessarily alluded to even though there is a separate chapter on mechanical ventilation. Similarly, acid-base disturbances and electrolyte alterations are as germane to the treatment of a patient in hemorrhagic or cardiogenic shock as one in whom primary respiratory failure predominates or where acute renal failure exists.

Admittedly, this text cannot compensate for experience. It can, however, serve as a guide not only for the recognition and treatment of undesirable postsurgical anomalies but also alert the neophyte surgeon as to the possible prevention of these complications. It can even be helpful to the nurse in the Intensive Care Unit who is intimately involved in these problems 24 hours a day.

ACKNOWLEDGMENTS

The onerous burden of typing the Editor's contributions fell on the individuals in the Office of the Associate Chief of Staff for Research and Education, Dr. Y. T. Oester at the VA Hospital, Hines. I am deeply indebted to the secretaries under the direction of the Research Coordinator, Joanna X. Wheeler. These include Miss Karen Nawrocki, Miss Mary Ann Kment, Miss Kathryn Koester, Mrs. Carol Haberman and Mrs. Corrine Veronica Popelka. In addition, Miss Therese Kronkowski, the nurse in charge of open heart surgery, was invaluable in proofreading the manuscript and orienting the references. I also wish to thank the staff of Year Book Medical Publishers for their wise counsel during the drafting of this book.

Lastly, my family should receive accolades for their acceptance of my preoccupation with the manuscript until the mission was accomplished.

Table of Contents

CHAPTER
1

Water, Electrolytes and Acid-Base Balance

WILLIAM E. NEVILLE, M.D.

Distribution of Body Water

WATER IS THE LARGEST single constituent within the body, representing 45–75% of the total body weight (TBW), depending upon the fat content of the body. For purposes of discussion, body water is divided into two main anatomic compartments, the *intracellular fluid* (ICF) compartment (about 50% of the TBW) and the *extracellular fluid* (ECF) compartment (about 18–20% of the TBW).

In the average 70-kg. (154-lb.) man, in whom approximately 60%, or 42 liters, of the TBW consists of water, about 28 liters (30–40% of the TBW) will be in the intracellular compartment and 14 liters (22%) in the extracellular compartment. However, the percentage of ECF is higher in infants and children, in adults who have lost a significant part of their skeletal mass from starvation or trauma or from cancer or other diseases, and in patients with edema due to heart failure or hepatic, renal or nutritional disorders.

The extracellular fluid consists of *interstitial fluid* (16% of the TBW), *plasma* (4.5%) and *lymph* (about 2%). In the average normal 70-kg. man, the interstitial-fluid volume is about 10.5 liters and the plasma volume is 3.5 liters (see Fig. 1–1). The ECF surrounds and invades the body cell mass, bringing materials required for metabolism and growth to the body cells from the gastrointestinal tract, lungs and body depots and transporting the waste products of metabolism to the lungs, liver and kidneys for excretion.

The interstitial fluid is both extracellular and extravascular. It represents the largest subdivision of the ECF compartment and is in intimate contact with the plasma, separated from the plasma only by capillary membranes which allow rapid transfer of all elements

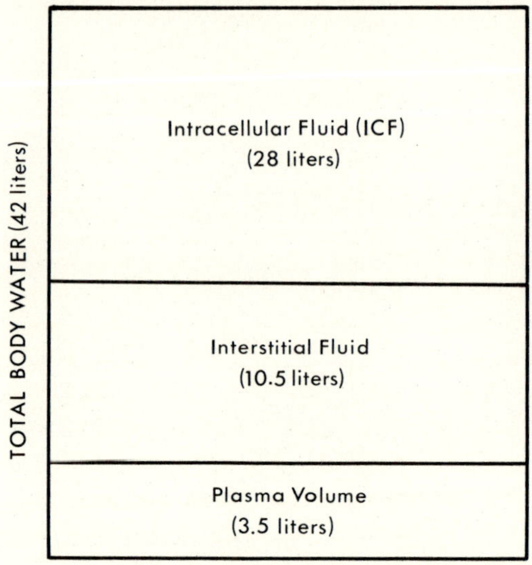

Fig. 1-1.—The distribution of body water. The blood plasma and the interstitial fluid comprise the extracellular fluid (ECF).

except cellular and large protein molecules. The protein content of the plasma component of the ECF is somewhat higher than that of the interstitial-fluid component. Approximately 93% of the plasma is water in which are suspended red cells, white blood cells and platelets.

Transcellular fluids, which pass through or are secreted by the cells, are also extracellular. These fluids include the cerebrospinal (CSF), the joint synovia and secretions into the gastrointestinal tract. As all these represent only about 1% of the TBW, they are usually disregarded for clinical purposes.

Electrolyte Composition of Body Fluids

Electrolytes are distributed in solution throughout all the body fluids. Water and electrolytes both pass freely through the extracellular compartment, in the plasma and around the cells, but potassium ions (K^+) are contained within the cells while sodium ions (Na^+) and magnesium ions (M_3^{++}) are kept out of the cells by an active mechanism. As electrolytes are soluble in water, their concentration in the plasma is 5% lower than in the interstitial fluid.

The average electrolyte values for a healthy person vary within a fairly narrow range. Commonly reported normal values (in mEq. per liter) are:

Cations: sodium (Na^+) 136–145
potassium (K^+) 3.5–5
calcium (Ca^{++}) 4.3–5.3
magnesium (Mg^{++}) 1.5–2.5

Anions: chloride (Cl^-) 100–106
bicarbonate (HCO_3^-) 21–32
phosphate (HPO_4^{--}) 2.6–3.2

In the plasma and in the interstitial fluid, both the cations, or positive-charged ions, and the anions, or negative-charged ions, including also organic acids and proteins, total about 154 mEq. per liter. On the other hand, the electrolyte content of the ICF, which contains an abundance of K^+ but little Na^+ or Mg^{++}, is approximately 205 mEq. per liter for both cations and anions.

While the exact electrolyte values for the ICF are uncertain, due to the difficulties of direct analysis of fluid within the cells, the following values (in mEq. per liter) are generally accepted as normal approximations for the ICF:

Cations:		Anions:	
	K^+:125		HPO_4^{--}:140
	Na^+:10		HCO_3^-:8
	Ca^{++}:15		Cl^-:2
	Mg^{++}:30		SO_4^{--}:15
			Protein (Pr^-):55

Although the composition of the ICF is not known with certainty, electrolyte distribution can be approximated by the study of cell activity and the fact that certain cell constituents are nondiffusible; hence, a Donnan distribution curve is imposed on the diffusible ions.

To summarize, the most important cation in the ECF is Na^+ while in the ICF, K^+ is dominant. In the ECF, Cl^- and HCO_3^- are the predominant anions; in the ICF, protein and organic phosphate (H Org Phos) predominate, the latter including adenosine, mono- , di- and triphosphate, glycerophosphate and creatine phosphate. The total amount of Na^+ and K^+ in the body is reversed as between the two major fluid compartments; about 96% of the exchangeable Na^+ is extracellular and 4% intracellular, while about 98% of the K^+ is intracellular and about 2% extracellular.

Osmotic Disorders of Water and Electrolytes

Water leaves the body through the kidneys, lungs, skin and gastrointestinal tract. In a 24-hour period, the kidneys excrete an average of 1,500 ml. of water, and 1,000 ml. of fluid is removed through the skin and lungs. Following surgery, the loss of fluid through the non-urinary routes will increase from fever and an increase in respiratory rate.

The kidney water loss varies with the solute load and the level of antidiuretic hormone (ADH). With an increase in the solute load, the kidneys must excrete sufficient urine to carry the solutes into the bladder. On the other hand, the ADH controls the resorption of water in the distal convoluted tubules. Following surgery, this hormone is increased, leading to increased resorption of water, which in turn results in a more concentrated urine.

The effects of osmotic changes upon the volume and the distribution of body fluids are paramount in the diagnosis and treatment of body-fluid disorders. Since most of the cellular membranes are permeable to water, the effective osmotic pressure of the fluids in the ECF and ICF compartments is considered equal. Any situation that alters the effective osmotic pressure in either direction or in either compartment must be accompanied by a corresponding redistribution of water in the two compartments.

For example, an increase in the osmotic pressure in the ECF results in a transfer of water from the cell to the extracellular compartment. This increase in osmotic pressure is commonly related to an increase in the concentration of Na^+ and its salts. Hyperglycemia will also increase the effective osmotic pressure, since glucose cannot traverse the cell membranes freely. In either event, such a state is described as hyperosmolality. On the other hand, a low plasma sodium, that is hyponatremia, results in hypo-osmolarity of the plasma, with a transfer of water into the cellular compartment. With a normal amount of Na^+ in the plasma, the osmolality is usually 290–310 milliosmols. This can be estimated to be equal to twice the Na^+ concentration in millimoles plus 6–8 milliosmols for the crystalloids.

The practical importance of osmolality, which is in essence the total number of osmotically active particles, is in the effective changes on cell hydration. Normally the cells and ECF are in osmotic equilibrium. Any alteration in ECF osmolality will produce a compensatory change in cell water and destroy that equilibrium. Thus, if the concentration of Na^+ is above normal, the ECF will be hypertonic and water will be withdrawn from the tissue cells. In addition, the osmol receptors in the posterior pituitary are stimulated to secrete ADH, which results in retention of water in the extracellular compartment. When the extracellular fluid is hypotonic, the tissue cells will take up water and swell, just as erythrocytes do in hypotonic salt solution. With hypotonicity, the ADH is suppressed and a diuresis results in loss of extracellular fluid.

Intravenous fluids can be either hyper- or hypotonic, depending upon whether their osmolality exceeds that of normal extracellular fluid. Five per cent glucose in 0.9% NaCl has an osmolality of 585 milliosmols and is therefore hypertonic. Administration of this fluid at a rate more rapid than the rate at which glucose can be removed results in an increase in the ECF osmolality and a compensatory loss of water from the cells. In addition, plasma glucose levels may be raised by any glucose-containing solution to a level that exceeds the capacity of the renal tubules to resorb glucose, and osmotic diuresis results.

On the other hand, hypotonic solutions cause the cells to take in water. Glucose solutions without isotonic salt are ultimately hypotonic as the glucose is removed and converted into glycogen or burned. The resulting free water is normally excreted in the urine and lost insensibly, but, in the presence of the antidiuretic hormonal effects of trauma, excess amounts result in dilution of the ECF and overhydration of cells. This is the commonest cause of hyponatremia in the surgical patient.

Measuring Water Balance

The simplest and most accurate way to monitor water balance after intracardiac surgery is by means of a platform scale. A weight change of 1 kg. (2.2 lb.) equals a fluid loss or gain of 1 liter. As a rule following operation, there is an initial weight gain due to sequestration of extracellular fluid. Thereafter, the patient on parenteral fluids should lose 150–300 Gm. of weight a day, depending upon the extent of the injury, the amount of fever and the presence or absence of infection. Diuresis will usually begin on the 3d or 4th day after the operation, at which time the sequestered ECF in the area of the trauma is removed and the weight gained during and immediately following surgery will be lost (see Fig. 1-2). Weight continuously gained after surgery is usually due to overhydration or to spreading infection with increasing sequestration of extracellular fluid. Failure to lose weight, accompanied by a fall in urine volume after 48 hours, may be the first evidence of further sequestration of ECF due to infection or tissue necrosis. In selected cases after open-heart surgery, an abnormal loss of water, electrolytes and plasma protein may occur plus temporary functional losses resulting from fluid shifts within the body.

Although not common, excessive losses may occur later in the postoperative period in open-heart surgery patients who develop diarrhea from tube feeding. More commonly, this occurs in the

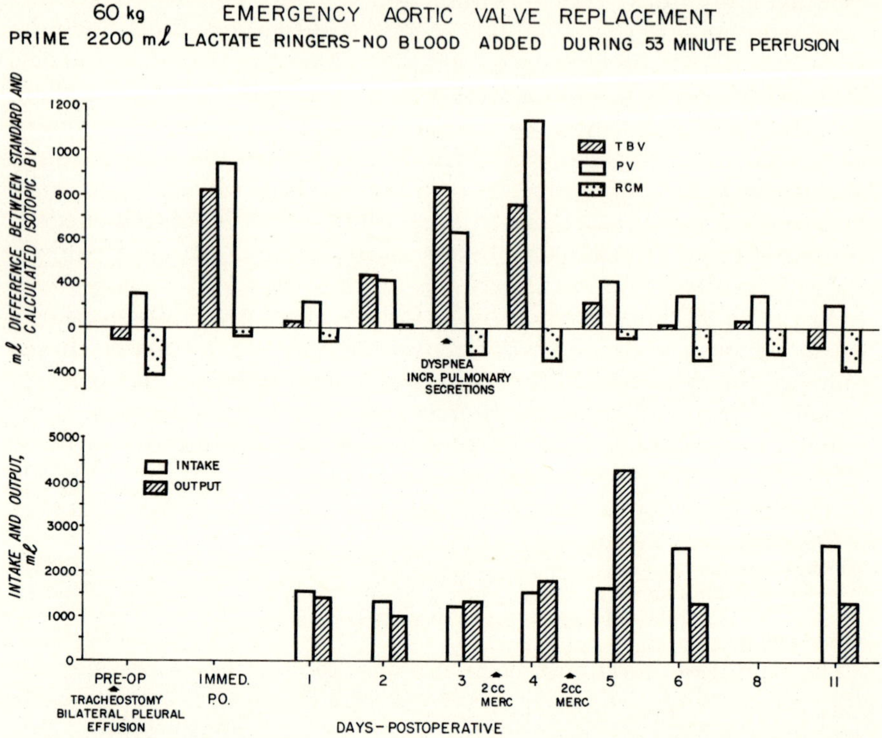

Fig. 1-2.—Diuresis usually begins, as shown here, on the 3d or 4th postoperative day. Note the marked increase in plasma volume on the 4th postoperative day, with incipient pulmonary edema. This occurred despite rigid curtailment of fluids postoperatively. A mercurial diuretic helped to remove the excess fluid, which amounted to 4,500 ml. of urine, between the 4th and 5th postoperative days.

cardio-thoracic patient from vomiting, drainage from nasogastric or long intestinal tubes without adequate replacement, from fistulas and from losses from wounds. In thoracic patients internal fluid shifts occur with pleural effusion and infection, hemorrhage into soft tissues of the chest following fractures or penetrating wounds and from plasma and blood loss after crush injuries. An internal fluid shift, in which large transcellular pools develop, occurs in ileus. These pools may become external losses through vomiting or aspiration with tubes, or they can resolve through resorption as the patient recovers bowel function.

THE "THIRD SPACE."—Two varieties of internal fluid shifts are observed frequently in surgical patients. The one is transcellular and the other involves accumulations of interstitial fluid and plasma in a so-called third space which is sequestered from the normal extracellular fluid. This occurs in crush injury, effusions, infection and particularly in burns. Although the sequestered fluid is in continuity with the normal extracellular fluid, it is unavailable to it. Therefore, it is just as essential to replace this temporary fluid deprivation as it is to replenish an external loss. The differences between external and internal fluid losses are a gain in weight from the sequestered fluid and an eventual return to the circulation of this fluid when the causative factor is removed.

Provisions should be made during the first 24–48 hours after surgery for the development of a third space, particularly in operations involving extensive dissections or for trauma to large muscle masses, where considerable edema may occur. However, it is possible

Fig. 1-3.—Postoperative blood volume determinations, weight gain and fluid intake and output in a patient following mitral valve replacement. Note occurrence of pulmonary and peripheral edema on the 4th postoperative day, at which time the fluid intake far exceeded the urinary output and the blood volume was over 900 ml. in excess of the normal. On the 3d or 4th postoperative day, the sequestered interstitial fluid re-enters the intravascular space and marked increase in edema can occur unless oral fluid intake is curtailed.

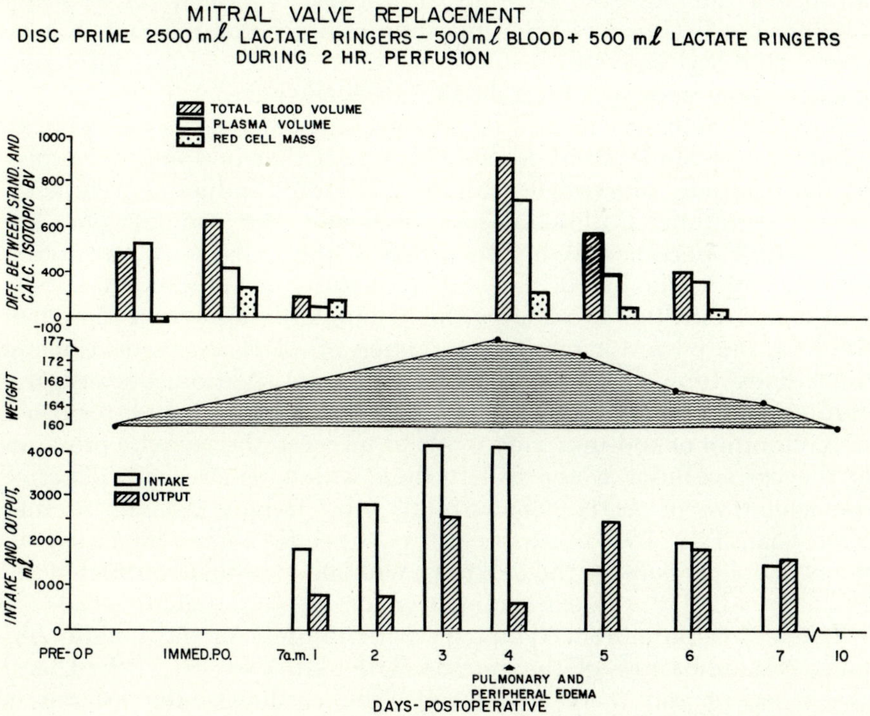

to initially overcompensate for the sequestered fluid, thereby creating a problem when this fluid is mobilized for evacuation on the 3d or 4th postoperative day. Circulatory overloading may occur in patients with decreased renal function and following open-heart surgery using hemodilution technics (see Fig. 1–3).

Following major surgery, it is mandatory to continuously monitor the central venous pressure, measuring fluid intake and urine output and specific gravity every hour until recovery is guaranteed. In addition, serum electrolytes are determined twice daily. In seriously ill individuals during and after open-heart surgery, an indwelling plastic catheter in the radial artery permits frequent withdrawal of blood for determination of acid-base balance, Po_2 and direct measurement of the arterial blood pressure.

Pathophysiology of Water Balance

Water loss (hyperosmolality).—Hyperosmolality is due either to decreased intake or excessive loss of water through the skin, lungs, kidneys or gastrointestinal tract. In the postsurgical period it is often seen in the debilitated, comatose patient, in whom intrinsic kidney disease prevents the conservation of water, or when a solute diuresis occurs from ingestion of high-protein foods. Excessive water loss can also occur from the respiratory tract following tracheostomy because of a reduction in dead space.

Another common cause of postoperative water loss is the replacement of hypotonic fluid losses (vomiting, diarrhea and sweating) by an isotonic electrolyte solution, thereby inducing a relative water depletion. Following loss of water, the osmotic pressure of the ECF becomes higher than that of the cells, with a resultant diffusion of water out of the cells into the extracellular fluid. This will occur until the two compartments are in equilibrium. To offset the loss, the posterior pituitary secretion of ADH increases, causing the kidney tubules to resorb more water. In addition, because the volume of the ECF is decreased, aldosterone is secreted, resulting in a retention of sodium. This tends to increase the osmotic pressure of the extracellular water still further, which negates the effect of the secretion of ADH. Concurrently, the kidney tubules secrete large quantities of K^+ in excess of Na^+. Since K^+ comes from the cell, the osmotic pressure of the cell falls, with more cellular water flowing from the cells into the extracellular water.

Thirst is a prominent symptom, with dryness of the tongue and mucous membranes of the mouth. The skin may be flushed, and sweat, saliva and tears are absent. The cardiovascular system is usually unaltered; however, a tachycardia may develop when fever exists. In fact, hyperosmolality may cause no symptoms until it is far advanced. Then the symptoms are cerebral, varying from lethargy to stupor and finally coma. The blood findings in the early stages may be normal but as water continues to be lost, the hematocrit, the serum sodium and blood urea nitrogen (BUN) begin to rise and the serum osmolality is increased. A concomitant increase in hematocrit and sodium serves to differentiate water loss from sodium loss.

Therapy for water loss alone consists in giving only water. However, sodium usually is lost as well and should be replaced. Since an infusion of pure water causes the red blood cells to swell and hemolyze, the most propitious solution is to give 5% glucose in normal saline solution.

WATER EXCESS (HYPO-OSMOLALITY).—After trauma or surgical operations, water and sodium, regardless of intake, are retained in the body for at least 24 to 48 hours as a result of excessive ADH secretion, whereas normally, when a patient is given excess of water with dilution of the extracellular water, the resultant decrease in osmotic pressure will cause water to diffuse into the cells. This triggers the posterior pituitary gland to stop secreting ADH and water diuresis results. However, if the patient is in an antidiuretic state, the water will be retained, which further decreases the osmotic pressure with more water entering the cells. In addition, sodium is excreted by the kidneys without water which causes the osmotic pressure to decrease further and a vicious cycle is created. The latter is the result of the hemostatic body mechanisms which stop aldosterone secretion when the volume of the extracellular fluid increases. However, normally, water and sodium are concomitantly excreted inappropriately since ADH is not secreted. Oliguric renal failure, prolonged hypotension following surgery and excessive intake of fluid when the kidneys cannot compensate with water diuresis can increase the total body water without a comparable increase in total body sodium. The latter exists after operation when an inordinate amount of antidiuretic hormone is produced, in liver disease with ascites and in congestive heart failure when excessive amounts of sodium are lost in the urine.

TABLE 1-1.—PATIENT'S TISSUE COMPOSITION AFTER CPB WITH RINGER'S LACTATE SOLUTION

Water	—Markedly increased ($p < .05$)
Cl^-	—Increased ($p < .05$)
Na^+	—Increased ($p < .001$)
K^+	—Decreased (not significantly)

TABLE 1-2.—PATIENT'S SERUM AFTER CPB WITH RINGER'S LACTATE SOLUTION	
Water	—Markedly increased ($p < .001$)
Bicarbonate	—Decreased ($p < .05$)
K^+	—Decreased ($p < .001$)
Ca^{++}	—Decreased ($p < .001$)
Mg^{++}	—Decreased ($p < .01$)
pH, Cl^- and osmolality unchanged	

A similar situation is present after cardiopulmonary bypass (CPB) using hemodilution technics. The serum and tissue water are significantly increased due to the necessity of reinfusing the diluted oxygenator contents into the patient to restore hemodynamics (see Tables 1–1 and 1–2). Studies by the author using Ringer's lactate solution to prime the disc oxygenator demonstrate that the excess water immediately after bypass is in the extracellular compartment and not the

Fig. 1-4.—Hematocrit and blood volume determinations following cardiopulmonary bypass using only Ringer's lactate solution to prime the pump oxygenator. Note the marked decrease in plasma volume (PV) 10 hours after surgery, due to diffusion of fluids into the interstitial space, and the gradual return of the fluid to the intravascular space in the subsequent 3–4 days. The decline in hematocrit is due to hemodilution effect of return of fluids into intravascular space. (TBV: total blood volume. RCM: red-cell mass.)

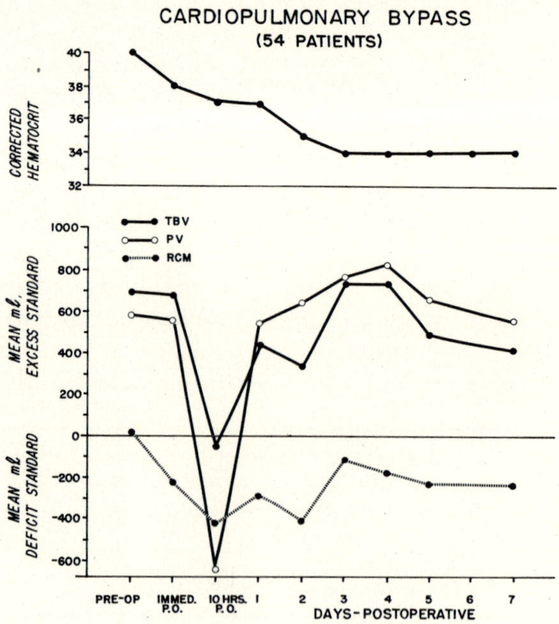

intracellular. Postperfusion determination of the total blood volume using radioactive iodinated serum albumin shows an increase in plasma volume and a decrease in red-cell mass and hematocrit (see Fig. 1–4). However, a symptomatic dilutional syndrome does not occur, since the electrolyte solution used for perfusion is isomolar and, in contrast to water intoxication, diuresis is elicited in the early postoperative period. The latter is even more dramatic when 5% glucose in lactated Ringer's solution is used as the oxygenator perfusate. This hypertonic solution increases the serum osmolality and an intense diuresis occurs in the hours after surgery. Despite this early removal of excess water by the kidneys, a considerable portion enters the interstitial fluid compartment, as judged by a gain in body weight. In addition, there is also a net gain in water from oxidation and catabolism of fat, carbohydrate and protein. For these reasons, it is mandatory to curtail the fluid intake for 2 to 3 days, giving only enough to supplement insensible loss. If intravenous and oral fluids are not limited, a true water intoxication can occur with peripheral and pulmonary edema, even though kidney function is adequate (see Fig. 1–3).

Electrolytes

Cations

Sodium.—Sodium is the principal cation of the extracellular fluid, with approximately 2,000 mEq. being outside the cells. This cation is most important in fluid balance and plays a large part in the therapy of fluid and electrolyte disturbances. Changes in concentration of sodium stimulate an appropriate response by the pituitary through the antidiuretic hormone.

As the concentration of sodium in the extracellular fluid varies between 136–145 mEq. per liter, in a normal 70-kg. (154-lb.) man, the total body content of exchangeable sodium is from 2,700–3,800 mEq. Only a small amount of sodium is within the cells, probably in the neighborhood of 10 mEq. per liter of intracellular water. Normally, most of the ingested sodium appears in the urine. Since the kidneys can conserve sodium, normal requirements are met by the average diet, which usually contains at least 100 mEq. daily.

Under normal conditions and in temperate climates, sodium loss from the skin is negligible. With increased environmental temperature, fever or muscular exercise the loss of sodium may become quite marked. Concentration of sodium in the sweat is usually about 25–30 mEq. per liter, though it may be as high as 100 mEq. per liter. Under abnormal conditions of temperature in the postoperative patient, sodium loss may be considerable. Chief regulation of sodium occurs through the kidneys. Total urinary excretion of sodium for 24 hours approximately equals sodium intake and varies according to sodium levels in the diet. When conservation of body sodium is desirable, the normal kidney is capable of excreting an essentially sodium-free urine.

Sodium balance is influenced by the adrenal secretion of aldosterone, the most potent natural-occurring inhibitor of renal sodium excretion. Also, the antidiuretic hormone of the pituitary promotes water resorption in the distal tubules and thus has an affect on the concentration of extracellular sodium. Not only does sodium pass into and out of the body in a continuous and well-regulated balance, but it is maintained in a constant internal circulation. Large amounts of secretions of varying sodium content are produced in the alimentary tract; according to Gamble, total volume in 24 hours may reach 8,200 ml. In addition, sodium can move rapidly from vascular and interstitial spaces; this exchange is closely related to the fluid exchange between plasma and interstitial fluid. The hydrostatic pressure of the blood inside the capillaries tends to force the intravascular fluid into the tissue spaces. This force is opposed by slightly higher osmotic pressure of the intravascular protein. At the arterial end of the capillary, the hydrostatic pressure exceeds the osmotic pressure and fluid leaves the capillaries.

At the venous end of the capillary, conditions are reversed because the hydrostatic pressure gradient has fallen and the osmotic pressure of the plasma proteins in the capillary has risen with the earlier loss of fluid. Thus, fluid from the tissue space will enter the venous end of the capillary. Since the fluid in both cases contains sodium, there is a relatively rapid exchange of sodium between intravascular and interstitial fluid. Sodium also enters the cells from the extracellular fluid but this shift is very slow. However, the concentration of sodium within the cells may change quickly due to rapid movement of water into and out of the cell. Any interference with the resorption of intestinal secretions will cause profound alterations in fluid and electrolyte balance.

Although not prevalent following open-heart surgery, gastrointestinal disturbances such as vomiting and diarrhea will lower the sodium content, since the gastric mucus has a high sodium concentration. Irritative conditions which cause vomiting will also induce increase in the production of mucus so that considerable amounts of sodium may be lost. As the total daily quantity of all intestinal secretions is double the plasma volume, loss from vomiting or from stools, coupled with little or no intake, can quickly produce dehydration and a sodium deficit. Loss of water and sodium from the plasma is followed by transfer of sodium and water from the interstitial fluid in replacement. If the loss continues, the water will be drawn from the cells. When the plasma volume can no longer be sustained, the circulation will fail.

Sodium deficiency (depletion).—Increased sodium loss in the surgical patient can occur from profuse sweating due to fever or a rise in the external temperature, vomiting, external fistulae, gastric aspiration or diarrhea and in the urine during certain diseases and diuretic therapy. When hemorrhage is uncompensated by whole blood, sodium is lost from the body. On the other hand, a severe sodium deficiency can also occur in patients with pleural effusions, ascites and congestive failure with marked edema, without sodium being actually lost from the body.

Since the concentration of sodium in the extracellular water is so great, its loss can result in a marked decrease in the osmotic pressure of the extracellular water, the hypotonicity of the ECF causing water to flow into the cells to equalize the osmotic pressure. As a result, hemoconcentration occurs which offsets the loss of sodium. In addition, for some inexplicable reason, the plasma proteins are eventually lost from the circulation, which further lowers the osmotic pressure of the blood. As a result, shock occurs from the decreased circulating blood volume.

The clinical picture varies from severe shock which is unresponsive to pressor amines, to weakness, apathy, lassitude and fatigue. Mental confusion, delirium and even coma may occur. The skin loses its turgor and the extremities may be cold with absent peripheral pulses.

The blood picture is one of hemoconcentration with gradually increasing concentration of hemoglobin, hematocrit, plasma proteins and urea. The plasma sodium and chlorides diminish in proportion to the degree of sodium deficiency, as does the urinary excretion of these electrolytes. Hence, serum osmolality measurements can be used to differentiate true sodium loss from other conditions, such as water excess, in which hyponatremia is observed.

Treatment consists in giving sufficient sodium to compensate for the loss. In addition, other electrolytes, such as potassium, chloride and bicarbonate, may have to be replaced. All this can be accomplished with Ringer's lactate solution to which sodium bicarbonate can be added. Although intravenous therapy is recommended, large volumes of isotonic saline or Ringer's lactate solutions can be given by means of a nasogastric tube, rectally, or by hypodermoclysis. When shock predominates, dextran or plasma may be beneficial.

Sodium excess (retention).—Sodium excess occurs in two forms.

In one form edema is seen, in which proportional amounts of both sodium and water are retained so that the osmotic pressure of the extracellular fluid remains essentially normal. In the second variety, only sodium is retained and the osmotic pressure of the ECF is raised. This is characterized by hypernatremia and is usually accompanied by hyperchloremia.

The factors responsible for hypernatremia may be due to either an excessive intake, such as overinfusion with isotonic or hypertonic sodium-containing fluids, or to an inability to excrete sodium. This is observed in primary hyperaldosteronism and Cushing's syndrome and can be seen following excessive therapeutic dosages of corticosteroids. The symptoms vary with the disease, but edema of the lungs may be present and the hyperosmolarity gives rise to confusion, dullness and apathy, and coma. In the blood, the plasma sodium and chloride are raised and the hemoglobin and plasma proteins are normal. The condition can be differentiated from the hypernatremia of water deficiency by the absence of clinical signs of dehydration, by the extremely low concentration of sodium and chloride in the urine, and by the high urine volume.

Cardiac edema with retention of sodium and water is due primarily to failure of the heart, with contributory backward and forward mechanisms. The inability of the heart to pump satisfactorily elevates the venous pressure and causes the cardiac output to fall. The pressure within the great veins reduces the resorption of tissue fluid at the venular end of the capillary, with a resultant slow accumulation of fluid within the tissues. Concurrently, the renal venous pressure is increased, which, combined with a reduction in cardiac output, contributes to a fall in glomerular filtration rate and renal blood flow and to retention of sodium and water. The kidney and the adrenal gland attempt to prevent a depletion in blood volume by retaining sodium and water to replace that being lost from the circulation at the capillary level.

Treatment involves improving the cardiac output with digitalis, lowering the venous pressure, promotion of fluid and sodium loss with diuretics and aldosterone antagonists, plus restriction of sodium and water intake.

Although admittedly oversimplified, the contraction and expansion of body fluids has been conveniently grouped by Welt into six different categories, depending upon whether water or salt is lost singly or in combination. If the gain in volume is due to water alone, all the compartments will be increased in size and proportion. The effective osmotic pressure of the body fluids will be reduced owing to dilution, but the cellular and extracellular fluids will remain isosmotic. The sodium will be reduced in concentration from the increase in plasma volume, the latter being reflected by concomitant *decrease* in the hematocrit, the concentration of hemoglobin, and the total protein. When water without salt is lost from the body, the deficit in volume will be proportionately shared by both the intracellular and extracellular compartments. In this instance, the effective osmotic pressure will be increased in both compartments; this is manifested by an increase in the concentration of sodium and its salts in the serum. The decrease in plasma volume will be reflected by an *increasing* hematocrit and in the concentrations of hemoglobin and total protein in the serum. The increase in volume with water can be spoken of as *hypotonic expansion,* and a decrease in volume on the basis of water alone is referred to as *hypertonic contraction.*

If the volume of body fluids is increased by the administration of fluid whose composition is identical with that in the extracellular compartment, only this one compartment will be expanded. Since the addition of this fluid does not alter the effective osmotic pressure of the extracellular fluid, there is no force promoting the movement of water to and from the cellular compartment. This is referred to as *isotonic expansion.* Conversely, a deficit in volume characterized by loss of water and salts in equal proportion will result in a decrease in volume of the extracellular compartment. No change in intracellular volume would occur since there has been no alteration in effective osmotic pressure of the extracellular fluid. This is categorized as *isotonic contraction.*

When a hypertonic saline is administered, the volume of the extracellular compartment will expand and increase the effective osmotic pressure of this fluid from an increase in the concentration of sodium. This will promote a transfer of water from the cells to the extracellular compartment until the two compartments are in equilibrium. The net result will be an increase in the volume of both components of the extracellular compartments and a decrease in the volume of the intracellular compartment. The expanded plasma volume will be reflected by a decrease in hematocrit and in the concentrations of hemoglobin and total protein. This increase in extracellular volume is referred to as *hypertonic expansion.*

On the other hand, a deficit in volume due to a net loss from the body fluids of sodium salts in excess of water will decrease the extracellular volume and decrease the concentration of sodium in the serum. The decrease in effective osmotic pressure of the extracellular fluids will cause a movement of water from this compartment into the cells in order to equalize the two compartments. At equilibrium, the two major compartments will be isosmotic, but the final effective osmotic pressure would be less than it was prior to the loss of salt in excess of water. Although both components of the extracellular compartment are contracted, the intracellular volume is expanded as a result of the movement of water into the cells from the extracellular fluid. The plasma volume will be contracted and the hematocrit will be increased as well as the concentration of hemoglobin and total protein. The body fluids will be hypotonic as manifested by the hyponatremia. At the same time the blood is hemoconcentrated in terms of red cells, hemoglobin and total protein. This deficit in extracellular volume is referred to as *hypotonic contraction.*

POTASSIUM.—As the principal cation of the intracellular fluid, the potassium balance of the body plays an extremely important role in the therapy of fluid and electrolyte disturbances. A normal 70-kg. man has a total body content of exchangeable potassium of about 3,200 mEq., with approximately 2,300 mEq., or about 125 mEq. per liter, being intracellular. The extracellular potassium in the normal adult ranges between 3.5 and 5 mEq. per liter.

As with sodium, the daily intake and output of potassium is well balanced and in the normal adult averages 50–150 mEq., which represents 1.5–5% of the total potassium content of the body. Almost all foods contain relatively high concentrations of potassium when compared with the small amount present in the plasma. In contrast to sodium, the kidney cannot completely stop the excretion of the potassium when there is potassium deficiency. At least 8 mEq. is lost obligatorily in the urine daily, with approximately 11 mEq. being removed from the body in the feces over a 24-hour period. The gastrointestinal fluids contain up to ten times more potassium than exists in plasma so that their loss involves a proportionately heavier loss of potassium than of sodium or water from the extracellular fluid.

Since kidneys do not conserve potassium as well or as promptly as they conserve sodium, a significant potassium depletion may occur in the normal adult in a week if he fails to receive potassium but continues to receive sodium. Potassium and hydrogen ions compete for exchange with sodium ions in the renal tubules, and the adrenal steroids increase urinary potassium loss when sodium is provided. The patient with normal kidneys undergoing the stress of disease or in the postoperative period may excrete as much as 60–100 mEq. per 24 hours. If extensive tissue injury occurs, the urinary excretion can rise as high as 200 mEq. in 24 hours. Because of the profound effect of open-heart surgery on cardiac function, potassium balance is extremely critical in such procedures.

As is true for other electrolytes, potassium is in a dynamic state. The total amounts and concentration in the body fluids remain relatively constant, but potassium continually moves into and out of the cells. The potassium gradient between intra- and extracellular compartments is influenced by adrenal steroids, testosterone, pH changes, glycogen formation and hyponatremia. The plasma potassium increases about 0.6 mEq. per liter for each 0.1 unit fall in pH. Conversely, plasma potassium falls about 0.6 mEq. per liter for each 0.1 unit rise in blood pH. Thus, in metabolic acidosis, the potassium diffuses from the cell into the fluid, while in alkalosis, potassium reenters the cell, thereby depleting the extracellular concentration of this ion. As a result, the plasma potassium concentration must always be evaluated in terms of the status of acid-base balance of the blood.

For example, in a patient with severe metabolic acidosis and plasma potassium concentration of 4.5 mEq. per liter, the plasma potassium concentration would fall to a level of about 2 mEq. per liter when the blood pH returns to normal.

Hypokalemia.—A subnormal concentration of potassium in the extracellular fluid, as well as usually also in the intracellular fluid, is caused in several ways. A decreased intake due to inability to swallow, such as occurs in coma, debility, cancer or stricture of the esophagus, will deplete the serum potassium. Parenteral therapy with potassium-free fluids or a diet that does not contain potassium will also lower the concentration of this ion in the body. Decreased absorption will lead to potassium deficiency, such as steatorrhea from enteritis or following intestinal stenosis or short-circuiting operations in the gastrointestinal tract. A significant potassium depletion can occur as a result of an increased loss in the urine, in such conditions as hyperaldosteronism, Cushing's syndrome, chronic renal disease and treatment with corticoid steroids or their derivatives. In the cardiac patient, hypokalemia is seen commonly during intensive treatment with mercurial diuretics. Potassium can also be lost from the gastrointestinal tract as a result of vomiting, gastric aspiration, or from external biliary and intestinal fistulas.

With rare exception, potassium is an essential part of the electrolyte replacement regimen following surgery. As many as one third of patients, other than those with total renal failure, exhibit hypokalemia and require supplemental potassium. For this reason, the hospitalized patient receiving intravenous fluids needs potassium daily. The minimum daily requirement is about 40 mEq., but the optimum intake should range between 60 and 120 mEq. where stress or losses from gastrointestinal or biliary secretions call for a greater amount.

Potassium balance in the surgical patient is as important as sodium balance. While the normal intake and turnover of potassium is high, the difference between potassium and sodium is that the body can rigorously conserve its sodium but its potassium is poorly retained, particularly in stressed individuals. Thus, it is important to supplement intravenous fluids with potassium therapy, if sufficient amounts are not included in the original solution.

Because of the profound effect of open-heart surgery on cardiac function, potassium balance is extremely critical in such procedures. Hypokalemia causes an increase in pulse rate with extrasystoles leading to cardiac dilatation and failure as the potassium deficiency becomes more severe. Conversely, hyperkalemia may result in heart block and cardiac arrest. Although the latter is not commonly seen after cardiopulmonary bypass unless severe renal damage occurs, a diminution in serum potassium is frequently observed. Such significant depletion in serum potassium after cardiopulmonary bypass can be attributed to several factors. These include preoperative administration of digitalis and diuretic therapy (see Fig. 1–5), hemo-

Fig. 1–5.—Average serum K^+ excretion in 21 patients, 11 of whom received a preoperative diuretic agent and 10 received no diuretic.

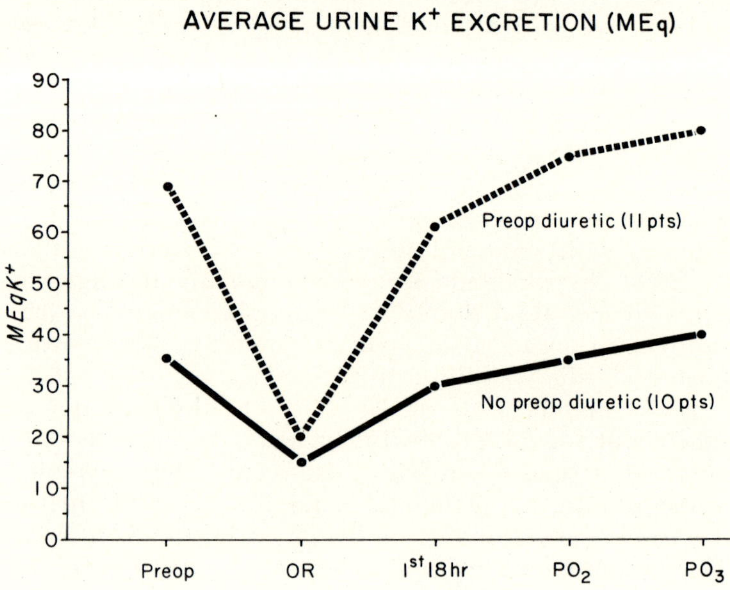

TABLE 1-3.—POSTPERFUSION SERUM K^+ DEPLETION

Preop.	Prolonged diuretic therapy
During Op.	1. Hyperventilation by anesthesiologist (Respiratory alkalosis)
	2. Excretion into urine
	3. Diffusion into cell
	4. Lowered K^+ content of perfusate with hemodilution
Postop.	1. Adrenocortical response to surgery (Hyperaldosteronism)
	2. Mechanical ventilators
	3. Increased Na^+ content of perfusate

dilution technics for priming the heart-lung machine, postoperative respiratory alkalosis, increased mineralocorticoid secretion due to surgical stress, and a continued postsurgical loss of potassium in the urine from a combination of the foregoing (see Table 1–3, Fig. 1–6).

Fig. 1–6.—Marked postoperative excretion of K^+ in the urine and a concomitant decrease in serum K^+ as seen in one patient following a mitral valve replacement.

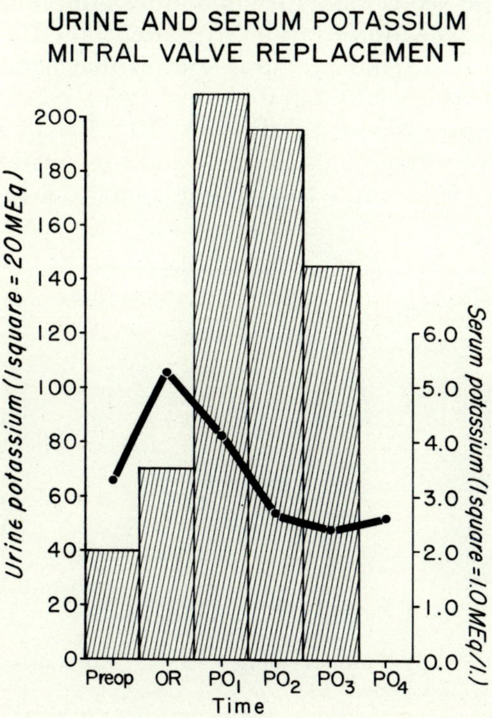

The effects of hypokalemia on the heart can be profound (see Table 1–4). Atrial and ventricular ectopic rhythms can occur from a decrease in the serum potassium and the association of digitalis toxicity. The action of digitalis glucoside changes the potassium concentration of heart-muscle cells. It is believed that digitalization may prevent the return of potassium to the cell following contraction, interfering with cardiac function. Thus, an ordinarily nontoxic amount of digitalis may become toxic in the presence of potassium deficiency. In a recent study of 30 patients following cardiopulmonary bypass by the author and his associates, seven hypokalemic individuals developed cardiac arrhythmias. Of these, four individuals were receiving diuretic agents before therapy and all were taking digitalis preparations.

Because of the seriousness of atrioventricular arrhythmias and the propensity for the development of a postperfusion hypokalemic alkalosis from mechanical ventilation, a policy of discontinuing digitalis and diuretics several days after surgery has been adopted in our hospital. In addition, preoperative supplemental potassium chloride is given to all cardiac patients undergoing cardiopulmonary bypass and, near the end of the perfusion, 30 mEq. of KCl per liter is slowly dripped into the oxygenator. Immediately after bypass, the serum electrolytes are measured in order to guide future therapy. Since it is presumed from these and previous studies that potassium depletion is a distinct possibility after open-heart surgery, especially in patients who do not require blood transfusions, 30 mEq. of KCl is added to each 1,000 ml. of intravenous fluid. In addition, acid-base studies are performed every hour while the patient is on the respirator and when

TABLE 1-4.—SERUM POTASSIUM IN PATIENTS WITH ARRHYTHMIAS

Pt. No.	Preop. Diuretic	Potassium (mEq/l) Preop.	Immediate Postop.	3-Day Average	KCl Postop.	Blood transfusions (# units)
4	No	4.9	3.8	3.7	Yes	4
9	No	4.5	—	3.6	Yes	0
11	Hygroten	4.1	2.8	2.6	Yes	3
19	No	4.3	4.4	3.0	Yes	6
23	Hygroten	4.4	3.4	3.4	Yes	1
26	Hydrodiuril	3.7	2.8	2.8	Yes	3
28	Hygroten	3.5	2.7	2.6	Yes	0
Average		4.2	3.32	3.1	(7)	2.4

Decrease in postoperative serum level in 7 patients with cardiac arrhythmias. These were reversible with intravenous KC1.

TABLE 1-5.—MEASURES USED TO MINIMIZE POSTOPERATIVE HYPOKALEMIA

1. D.C. digitalis and diuretics 3 days before surgery
2. Acid-base balance and electrolyte monitoring
3. Intermittent mechanical ventilation
4. Infusion of KCl (30 mEq.) during bypass and P.O
5. Measurement of 24-hour secretion of K^+ in urine

a respiratory alkalosis develops, the ventilator is temporarily discontinued. Since initiating this regimen, no documented instance of cardiac arrhythmia due to lowered serum potassium has been observed (see Table 1–5).

CALCIUM.—More than 90% of the calcium in the body is found in bone as phosphate and carbonate, so that when the serum calcium falls, the bones act as a ready source of calcium. In addition, the kidneys normally regulate the composition of the extracellular fluid in contact with bone in such a way that bone is constantly being resorbed. The major factors which regulate bone resorption and formation are the presence or absence of vitamin D, the availability of parathyroid hormone, the serum concentrations of calcium and phosphate ions, and the ability of the kidneys to excrete or hold these ions.

Calcium is not required for routine intravenous therapy because of the tremendous reservoir of calcium in the bone. Furthermore, intravenous calcium will not prevent the disused decalcification of bone that occurs when patients are in bed. In addition, there is a practical advantage to the absence of calcium in solutions to be infused. Calcium-containing solutions are not suitable for use when citrated blood is to be transfused via a secondary administration set. If such blood is mixed in the primary bottle with solutions containing calcium, the citrated blood may clot, blocking flow in the chamber.

Hypocalcemia.—Postoperatively, hypocalcemia is observed when the serum calcium concentration is below the normal value of 9 mg./100 ml. (4.5 mEq. per liter). It is usually associated with a loss of calcium in both the extracellular fluid and bone. Hypocalcemia may be associated with retention of phosphate, as in chronic renal disease, or with other factors localized in the extracellular fluid. These include an abnormal increase in citrate, or acute pancreatitis which results in the binding of calcium in the inflammatory exudate and the peritoneal cavity. Following open-heart surgery using hemodilution technics, calcium depletion with resultant tetany has been observed by the author. However, in the majority of patients, the calcium levels in the serum are normal in the postoperative period and supplemental calcium is not usually required.

Hypocalcemia can be induced by chelating agents such as disodium ethylenediamine tetraacetate and also can occur during an exchange transfusion or as a result of a transfusion of a large volume of citrated bank blood. When sodium citrate is infused, it is ordinarily oxidated to sodium bicarbonate with a resultant transfusion alkalosis. However, if a large amount of citrate is infused rapidly, or in the presence of shock or liver damage, the excess citrate may bind calcium, producing hypocalcemia. This may cause tetany and even shock. In addition, banked blood contains an increased amount of potassium, which can cause serious hyperpotassemia, especially in the presence of hypocalcemia.

The most characteristic sign of hypocalcemia is tetany. However, this can be caused by either a depletion in serum calcium concentration or by an increased pH, as in metabolic or respiratory alkalosis. On the other hand, a low pH decreases the tendency to tetany. This is the reason that tetany does not appear in metabolic acidosis due to chronic renal disease, even when the serum calcium concentration is very low. When the pH is increased, as in alkalosis, tetany occurs even if the serum calcium concentration is normal. This may be the reason that tetany has been observed on occasion in patients who are on a respirator, the resulting alkalosis, not a depletion in the serum calcium, causing the tetany. When both the serum calcium and potassium concentrations are low, tetany is inhibited. However, tetany will appear in such a patient if the serum potassium concentration is raised while the serum calcium concentration is allowed to remain low.

The cardinal intrinsic signs of hypocalcemia include carpopedal spasm, Trousseau's and Chvostek's signs, facial muscle spasm, changes in mood, paresthesias, and even convulsions which are often misdiagnosed as epilepsy. Therapy involves either treating the alkalosis or raising the serum calcium concentration. Calcium gluconate can be given intravenously at a daily dose as high as 10 Gm. Calcium lactate can also be given, at a daily dose of 8–12 Gm.

It has been suggested that hypocalcemia due to citrate toxemia can be prevented, if no more than 1,000–1,500 ml. of blood is given per hour to an adult and if 10 ml. of calcium gluconate is given intravenously with each 1,500 ml. of blood. However, others believe that the administration of calcium salts with blood-bank blood transfusions of 2,500 ml. or more may be associated with ventricular fibrillation. It is therefore proposed that calcium salts should not be given with blood bank transfusions.

Hypercalcemia is not often seen following cardiopulmonary surgery. When seen, it is usually the result of hyperparathyroidism and would be of concern when it is necessary to explore the mediastinum for a parathyroid adenoma, when there is marked hypotonicity of the muscles. Increased calcium excretion in the urine may result in the formation of calcium kidney stones. In addition, metastatic calcification can occur in various organs in the body, particularly when the local pH of the body is elevated, as in the lung, gastric mucosa and kidneys. Calcification can also occur in arterial walls, around joints, in the cornea and in the conjunctiva. If hypercalcemia is due to hyperparathyroidism, osteolytic bone lesions may develop when the patient is in a negative calcium balance due to a low-calcium diet. This is due to the direct bone-resorbing effect of parathyroid hormone.

MAGNESIUM.—Magnesium is predominantly an intracellular ion. It is essential in many enzymatic systems involving lipid carbohydrate and protein metabolism. The total body content of magnesium in the average adult is about 2,000 mEq. but only about half of this is rapidly exchangeable. In healthy adults, the plasma magnesium normally ranges between 1.5 to 2.5 mEq. per liter. The intracellular concentration is 5–10 times greater and in that respect is similar to the distribution of potassium. In the normal adult about 5–10 mEq. of magnesium is excreted in the urine each day, but the large majority of ingested magnesium is excreted in the feces. The minimum daily need is about 5 mEq. and the maximum daily tolerance to an acute low is about 400 mEq.

Magnesium deficiency is known to occur in severe malabsorption. The conditions which may lead to magnesium deficiency include prolonged nasogastric suction, acute pancreatitis, primary aldosteronism, diabetic acidosis, and treatment of chronic alcoholism. The clinical picture of magnesium deficiency is often characterized by neuromuscular and central nervous system hyperirritability. Some patients may even have muscle tremor, tetany, convulsions or delirium. The deficiency may occur after prolonged periods of intravenous therapy with magnesium-free solutions; this condition may be avoided by the routine use of intravenous solutions containing 3–5 mEq. per liter of magnesium. Excess magnesium acts as a sedative and extreme excesses may cause cardiac arrest, such as may occur during uremia.

Electrolyte Anions

Chloride.—A chloride loss usually follows loss of sodium, but the proportions will differ since a depletion of chloride can be compensated by an increase in bicarbonate. Such compensatory changes do not occur when sodium is lost, because of the loss of body water. Chloride losses will produce the same effects in intracellular and extracellular compartments as seen with potassium loss, and a deficiency of either chloride or potassium leads to a deficit of the other.

This anion plays an integral role in the buffering action during O_2 and CO_2 exchange in the red blood cells, the so-called chloride shift. When blood is oxygenated, chloride travels from the erythrocytes to the plasma whereas bicarbonate leaves the plasma and enters the red cells. This shift in ratio of cell chloride to plasma chloride also occurs when blood becomes more alkaline. Thus, venous blood will have a lower plasma chloride concentration than will oxygenated arterial blood. Water travels in the same direction as chloride, with the red cells becoming dehydrated when blood is oxygenated.

The normal plasma chloride content is 100–106 mEq. per liter, but the amount of chloride found within the cells is about 1 mEq. per liter of cell water. Even though the intracellular chloride is minimal, it is present within certain specialized cells, the largest amount being found in the interstitial lymph and fluid compartments (see Table 1-6).

Bicarbonate.—Although bicarbonate is always present as a result of the production of CO_2 as an end-product of metabolism, its concentration depends upon kidney function to regulate the amount of cation which as a rule is available to combine with it. The serum values reflect metabolic acidosis or alkalosis; that is, a low serum bicarbonate is seen in metabolic acidosis and a high serum bicarbonate is observed in metabolic alkalosis. However, this relationship does not hold in respiratory acidosis and alkalosis. In respiratory acidosis, the serum bicarbonate concentration is above normal and in respiratory alkalosis, it is below normal. Very little bicarbonate is excreted in acid urine, while bicarbonate is present mainly in alkaline urine. In metabolic alkalosis with a resultant high plasma bicarbonate there is a decrease of intracellular potassium and an increased urinary excretion of potassium.

Other Anions.—The major organic acid found in blood is lactic acid, constituting approximately 20% of the total organic acids. The serum level of lactic acid is 8–17 mg. per 100 mm. or 0.9–1.9 mEq.

TABLE 1-6.—SERUM ELECTROLYTES BEFORE, DURING AND AFTER CARDIOPULMONARY BYPASS USING RINGER'S LACTATE OXYGENATOR PRIME

	HINES NORMAL	PREOP. AVERAGE RANGE	PUMP AVERAGE RANGE	IMM. POSTOP. AVERAGE RANGE	LATE POSTOP. AVERAGE RANGE
Sodium	135–150	139	133	142	145
(mEq./L.)		125–149	126–147	124–176	135–176
Potassium	4.0–5.0	4.4	4.0	4.13	3.5
(mEq./L.)		3.3–6.1	2.5–5.3	2.4–7.7	2.4–4.3
Chloride	100–108	100	104	103	107
(mEq./L.)		80–109	91–130	88–134	94–134
CO_2	24–32	26	20	24	20
(Serum)					
(mEq./L.)		21.5–34.2	12.5–27.5	12.5–38	12.5–27.1
Calcium	9–11	9.6		8.6	8.3
mg./100 ml.		8.3–11		6.6–9.9	6.6–9.2
Phosphorus	2.5–4.5	3.6		3.08	2.3
mg./100 ml.		2.4–4.5		0.8–7.8	0.8–6.8
Zinc	80–160	86.5		67	56
mcg./100 ml.		54–131		24–112	24–91
Magnesium	1.7–2.5	2.06		1.87	1.71
(mEq./L.)		1.6–2.85		1.25–3.3	1.25–2.10

per liter. The other most common organic acids in the blood are citrate, 1.4–3 ml. per 100 ml., acetoacetate, 0.8–2.8 ml. per 100 ml. and pyruvate, 0.4–2 ml. per 100 ml. of blood. Because organic acid is a part of the normal intermediary metabolism of the cells, none is shown to exist as such in the intracellular fluid compartments.

Acid-Base Balance

HYDROGEN ION CONCENTRATION AND pH

The acidity or alkalinity of a solution depends upon the concentration of hydrogen ion (H^+). An increase in the concentration of H^+ shifts the reaction to a lower pH, making the solution more acid. A decrease in H^+ concentration by adding a base to the plasma will increase the pH and the solution will be more alkaline. Thus, the body is able to maintain a stable balance by replacing strong acids and bases—which are highly ionized—with weakly-ionized acids or bases.

The subject of acid-base balance has been confusing because of the terminology involved. For example, some writers have called both a cation, such as sodium, and an anion, such as bicarbonate, "bases," but have called the chloride ion "an acid." Other writers have loosely called all cations "bases" and all anions "acids." This confusion can be eliminated if one accepts the chemical definition: (1) An acid is a hydrogen ion or proton donor. (2) A base is a hydrogen ion or proton acceptor. Thus, carbonic acid (H_2CO_3) is an acid because it can lose an H^+, to become HCO_3, while bicarbonate (HCO_3^-) is a base, since it can accept an H^+, to become H_2CO_3.

The weight of ionized hydrogen water is about 0.0000001 Gm. per liter. This quantity can be expressed mathematically as 10^{-7}; however, this is rather confusing and, for convenience, the H^+ concentration is usually expressed as a negative logarithm, denoted by the symbol pH, introduced by Sorenson in 1909.

Subsequently, Henderson-Hasselbalch devised an equation for the determination of pH in body fluids:

$$pH = 6.1 + \log \frac{\text{proton acceptor (base) } Na^+, K^+ \text{ bicarbonate (27)}}{\text{proton donor (acid) } H_2CO_3 + CO_2 \text{ (135)}}$$

The acid-base changes thus involve increases or decreases in either the numerator or denominator of this equation. When the bicarbonate concentration rises or carbonic acid falls, the pH becomes greater than normal, since the bicarbonate-carbonic acid ratio increases. Conversely, when the bicarbonate falls or the carbonic acid increases, the pH becomes less than the normal value of 7.34–7.45.

Three factors help to maintain an optimal pH: (1) chemical buffers that can neutralize strong acids in the body fluids and cells, and bases produced within the body or that enter the body; (2) respiratory mechanisms that help eliminate and regulate the concentration of carbonic acid, the major acid end product of metabolism; and (3) the kidneys, which also help to eliminate excess acids or bases. Because the kidneys are able to compensate for any deficiencies in the action of buffer salts or respiration, they are the most important of the three factors.

THE BUFFER SYSTEM.—In the ECF and the ICF, certain combinations of chemicals act as a "buffer" against sudden changes in H^+ concentration. These substances maintain the body fluids at a relatively constant pH when a strong acid or base is added. A buffer system always consists of two parts: a weak ionized acid (H^+ donor) and a salt of that acid. Thus, when a strong acid is added to the solution, the liberated protons (H^+) are usurped by the proton acceptors (base) to form molecules of undissociated (weak) acid. Similarly, when a strong base, i.e., OH^-, is added to the solution, it appropriates protons from the weakly ionized acid to form H_2O, thus minimizing the changes in H^+. Four main buffer systems in the body help maintain a constant pH: (1) The bicarbonate-carbonic acid system; (2) phosphates; (3) proteins; and (4) hemoglobin of the RBC.

For practical purposes, the chief buffers in the ECF are: (1) carbonic acid (H_2CO_3)-bicarbonate ion (HCO_3^-); (2) plasma protein (HPr)-proteinic anion (Pr^-); and (3) organic phosphate (H Org Phos)—organic phosphate anion (Org $Phos^-$).

The intracellular buffers, in order of importance, are: (1) protein (HPr)—proteinic anion (Pr^-); (2) carbonic acid ($H_2CO_3^-$); and (3) organic phosphate—organic phosphate anion.

Although the bicarbonate-carbonic acid buffer provides 90% of the buffering of plasma, it assumes less importance inside the cell. The hemoglobin in the red cells, in terms of the intracellular protein, plays the predominant role in buffering in this locale. This system is responsible for the transport from the tissues and release from the lung of CO_2 formed during cellular metabolism. As the concentration of CO_2 increases in the plasma, it diffuses into the red blood cells, where it is converted by the enzyme, carbonic anhydrase, to carbonic acid ($CO_2 + H_2O = H_2CO_3$). This dissociates into H^+, which unites with reduced hemoglobin (HHb) ($H^+ + Hb^- = HHb$) and bicarbonate (HCO_3^-), which combines with K^+ to form $KHCO_3$ within the red blood cell. With an increase in intracellular HCO_3^-, the bicarbonate ion diffuses into the plasma and is replaced by a chloride ion to form KCl:

$$\text{RBC}: KHCO_3 \rightarrow K^+ + HCO_3^- \rightarrow \text{to plasma}$$
$$\text{Plasma}: Cl^- \rightarrow \text{RBC} \rightarrow KCl$$

In the lungs, the reduced hemoglobin, HHb, accepts O_2 and becomes $HHbO_2$. This in turn reacts with bicarbonate salts from which carbonic acid is formed ($HHbO_2 + KHCO_3 \rightarrow H_2CO_3 + KHbO_2$). As the carbonic acid is formed, the Cl^- in the cells re-enters the plasma and the K^+ reunites with oxyhemoglobin to again form $KHCO_3$. The newly formed carbonic acid is converted into CO_2 and H_2O by carbonic hydrase. The CO_2 passes from the red blood cell into the plasma and into the alveolar capillaries, from which it is eliminated.

The phosphate buffer system is important in red blood cells and, particularly, in the kidney tubules, where it facilitates the excretion of H^+. For example, if HCl is added to the body fluids, it is converted to a neutral salt, NaCl, by a phosphate buffer which is changed into a mildly acid form: $HCl + Na_2HPO_4 \rightarrow NaCl + NaH_2PO_4$. Similarly, a strong base such as NaOH is converted into water (H_2O) by a phosphate buffer salt, which is concomitantly changed from a mildly acid to a mildly basic form.

Normally, a ratio of 1 part carbonic acid to 20 parts of bicarbonate is present in the extracellular fluid. The total amount of carbonic acid or bicarbonate need not be stationary, only the ratios must remain the same to maintain acid-base balance. Addition of H^+ (acid) will result in the formation of more carbonic acid (H_2CO_3). For example, $H^+ + Cl^- + Na^+ + HCO_3^- = NaCl + H_2CO_3$. Thus, the buffering of the HCl is brought about by the formation of carbonic acid. This in turn is broken down into CO_2 and H_2O through the action of the enzyme, carbonic anhydrase, with the CO_2 being eliminated by the lungs. The ratio of bicarbonate to carbonic acid is altered, with the numerator being decreased proportionately more than the denominator, and the absolute value of the ratio falls, resulting in an acid pH. The bicarbonate is replaced by renal mechanisms and the urine is acidified with the excretion of the fixed anion (Cl^-). If these processes occur, the buffer ratio returns to its original value of 1:20. When such chemical reactions do not occur, the result is an acid shift in pH arising from a gain of acid, or an alkaline shift in pH when there is a loss of acid.

BICARBONATE.—The diagnosis of metabolic acidosis and metabolic alkalosis can be made from the bicarbonate level in the plasma, the normal being 22–26 mEq. for arterial blood and 24–48 mEq. for venous blood. The concentration of bicarbonate in the plasma is regulated by the kidney through acidification of the urine, in which case there is a relative or absolute deficit of the bicarbonate, or by alkalinization of the urine, which gives a relative or absolute excess of bicarbonate. In the first instance, the kidney makes new bicarbonate by reverse action of carbonic anhydrase, thereby sending hydrogen ions into urine and HCO_3^- back into the body fluids. In the second instance, HCO_3^- is excreted in the urine with Na^+ and K^+. In respiratory acidosis and alkalosis, primary changes in carbonic acid are reflected by secondary changes in bicarbonate. Respiratory acidosis is characterized by accumulation of CO_2 due to *hypo*ventilation. Carbonic acid is increased, so that the normal ratio of 1:20 is decreased and the pH falls. Conversely, in respiratory alkalosis, there is a deficit in H_2CO_3 due to *hyper*ventilation. The result is an increase in the ratio 1:20 with bicarbonate, and a rise in pH is observed.

Acidosis and Alkalosis (Tables 1–7 and 1–8)

Four types of disturbances may occur in acid-base equilibrium: 1. Respiratory acidosis; 2. Respiratory alkalosis; 3. Metabolic acidosis; 4. Metabolic alkalosis.

1. Respiratory acidosis (carbonic acid excess) (Fig. 1–7).—This is associated with an increase in plasma P_{CO_2} due to a decrease in ventilation. The latter may be due to pneumothorax, pleural ef-

TABLE 1-7.—Summary of Etiologic Factors Involved in Respiratory and Metabolic Acidosis

Respiratory			Metabolic	
			Acid Increase	Base Reduction
1. Depression of Respiratory Center	1. Drug Overdosage, e.g. Morphia, Barbiturates, Anesthetics 2. Raised Intracranial Pressure 3. Bulbar Poliomyelitis		1. Renal Failure A. H_2SO_4 B. H_3PO_4	Diarrhea Duodenal, Pancreatic or Bilary Fistulae
2. Interference with Respiratory Muscles	1. Motor Neurone Disease 2. Myasthenia Gravis	Fixed Acid	2. NH_4Cl Administration 3. $CaCl_2$ Administration	Renal Tubular Acidosis
3. Disorders of Thoracic Cage	1. Kyphoscoliosis 2. Spondylitis 3. Extreme Obesity		1. Diabetes Mellitus	(A) Beta-Hydroxybutyric (B) Aceto-Acetic
4. Disease of Lungs	1. Emphysema 2. Bronchitis 3. Asthma	Volatile Acid	2. Anoxia	Lactic Acid
			3. Exercise	Lactic Acid
			4. Starvation	Keto Acids
5. Circulatory Disorder	1. Profound Hypotension 2. Pulmonary Edema		5. Spontaneous	Lactic Acid
			6. Low Cardiac Output Syndrome	Lactic Acid
			7. Low Flow Pump Oxygenator Perfusion	Lactic Acid
			8. Rewarming Following Profound Hypothermia Extracorporeal Perfusion	Lactic Acid

fusion, atelectasis or airway obstruction. In the chronic form it is caused by obstructive emphysema, asthma, bronchitis, suppression or injury of the respiratory center, certain diseases of the chest wall or disorders of the muscles involved in respiration. Under these circumstances, the lungs withhold CO_2 and breathing is suppressed, thus upsetting the normal 1:20 ratio of carbonic acid to base bicarbonate. In the early stages, the base bicarbonate remains normal; however, due to the increase in CO_2, the carbonic acid increases so that the ratio may be 2:20. Compensatory mechanisms are set up

Fig. 1-7.—Diagrammatic representation of respiratory acidosis. Note increase in carbonic acid and action of compensatory mechanisms involved in increase of base bicarbonate.

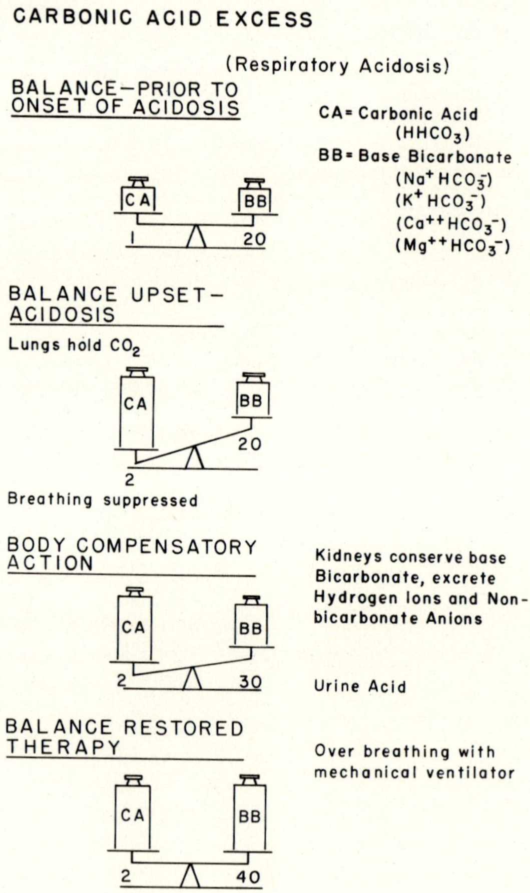

TABLE 1-8.—SUMMARY OF ETIOLOGIC FACTORS INVOLVED IN RESPIRATORY AND METABOLIC ALKALOSIS

Respiratory	Metabolic		
			Alkalosis of K^+
1. Overbreathing	Acid Reduction	Base Increase	Depletion
A. Mechanical	Loss of Acid	$NaHCO_3$, Na	
Ventilators	Gastric Juice	Lactate Administration	Deficient Intake of K^+
B. Hysterical			
2. Oxygen Lack			Excessive Loss of K^+
A. Lung Disease			A. Alimentary
B. Cardiac Failure			B. Renal
C. Blood Loss			1. Alkalosis (Artificial Ventilation)
D. Alveolar-Capillary Block			
E. Carbon-Monoxide Poisoning			2. Glucocorticoid Excess
			3. Aldosterone Excess
3. Central Neurogenic Hyperventilation			4. Diuretics
Pontine Lesions from Hemorrhage, Carcinoma, Infection			
4. Toxic Stimulation of Respiratory Center			
A. Hepatic Coma			
B. Water Intoxication			
C. Septicemia			
5. Stimulation of Respiratory Center by Drugs			
6. Prolonged Artificial Ventilation			

within the body, in which the kidneys conserve sodium and bicarbonate, excrete chloride, hydrogen ions, and non-bicarbonate anions, and the urine is acidified. The result is an increase in base bicarbonate, which helps to restore the pH to normal. The treatment involves recognition of the inadequate ventilation before severe hypoxia compounds the problem. In acute respiratory insufficiency, a patient's airway should be assured and mechanical ventilation instituted until the P_{CO_2} can be returned to normal. Fluid therapy can also be given in the form of lactate-containing solution. The lactate ions are converted into bicarbonate ions in the liver, thus increasing further the base bicarbonate in order to restore balance.

2. RESPIRATORY ALKALOSIS (CARBONIC ACID DEFICIT) (FIG. 1–8).—This is associated with a decrease in plasma P_{CO_2} + H_2CO_3 and a rise in pH due to an increase in alveolar ventilation. This may occur under a variety of conditions, such as emotional hyperventilation, encephalitis or salycylate poisoning, or the respiratory center can be directly affected. Following open-heart surgery, this may occur from the use of mechanical respirators for assisted breathing. Severe respiratory alkalosis may result in tetany plus cardiac arrhythmias from depression of ionization of calcium and in digitalis intoxication from a fall in serum potassium. In these situations, the normal balance

Fig. 1–8.—In respiratory alkalosis, the carbonic acid blood levels are depleted from overventilation. The body compensates by depleting the base bicarbonate. Full balance can be restored by giving chloride solutions or, if the patient is on a respirator, by discontinuing mechanical ventilation.

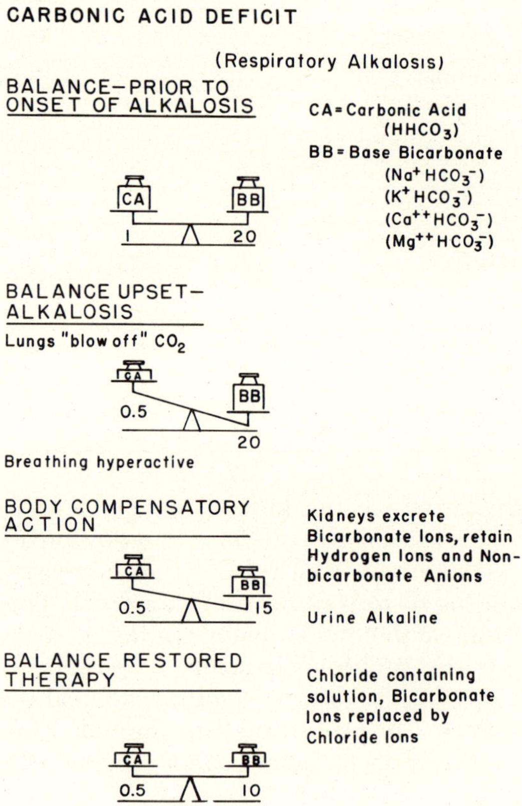

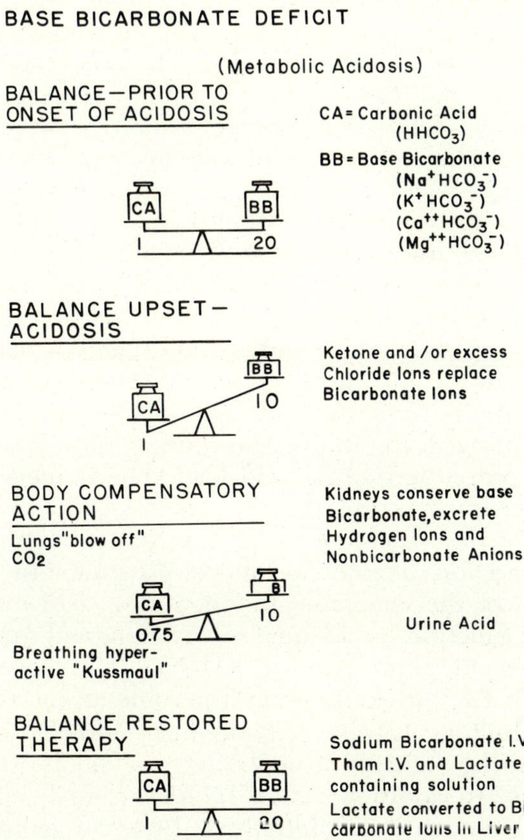

Fig. 1-9.—In patients with metabolic acidosis, the base bicarbonate is depleted. Compensation is afforded by the lungs and intravenous buffers, such as sodium bicarbonate, THAM (Tris buffer) and lactate solutions.

of 1:20 is upset, with the lungs blowing off the CO_2. Thus, the carbonic acid is lowered, upsetting the balance towards the alkalotic side. Early compensatory mechanisms which come into play are excretion of bicarbonate, Na^+ and K^+ by the kidneys, resulting in an alkaline urine. Hydrogen and non-bicarbonate anions such as Cl^- are retained. If the patient is being ventilated by a respirator, acid-base balance can be temporarily restored by discontinuing the mechanical ventilator. Since K^+ is excreted in the urine, solutions containing both K^+ and Cl^- should be given. The latter ion will replace the HCO_3^- excreted in the urine.

3. Metabolic acidosis (base bicarbonate deficit) (Fig. 1-9).—This is associated with an increase in nonvolatile acids or a

loss of bicarbonate from the extracellular fluid. It is commonly encountered in uncontrolled diabetes with the replacement of bicarbonate by ketonic acids, in azotemia in which H^+ cannot be excreted by the kidneys, and lactic acid accumulation from tissue anoxia, which can occur following trauma, hemorrhage and peritonitis. Lactacidemia may also occur from low-flow perfusion during cardiopulmonary bypass and is observed as a result of low cardiac output following open-heart surgery. In both instances, it is due to hypoxia from subliminal tissue perfusion with accumulation of lactic acid to such an extent that it cannot be metabolized by the liver. In the postoperative period, severe diarrhea and renal tubular dysfunction can precipitate loss of bicarbonate and sodium. The balance is upset from a replacement of the bicarbonate ions by ketones or excess chloride ions.

In any event, the 1:20 ratio is disturbed, with the base bicarbonate decreased in proportion to the acid load. The immediate body compensatory mechanisms entail the removal of CO_2 by the lungs and the conservation of base bicarbonate by the kidneys with the excretion of hydrogen and non-bicarbonate anions. Treatment includes remedying the cause of the excessive production of acid metabolites, improving renal function by adequate hydration, and replacing the depleted bicarbonate with Na^+ or $KHCO_3$. The fixed cation often combines with Cl^- for excretion and permits an increase in HCO_3^-. The strong buffer, THAM (*tris*-[hydroxymethyl] aminomethane) buffer can also be infused to neutralize the deleterious products of tissue hypoxia. In addition, when blood lactate levels are not elevated, a lactate-containing solution can be given as restorative fluid therapy, in which case the lactate ions are converted to bicarbonate ions in the liver.

4. METABOLIC ALKALOSIS (BASE BICARBONATE EXCESS) (FIG. 1–10).—This is associated with a loss of strong acid from the body and is most often encountered in severe persistent vomiting, with a substantial loss of HCl. As H^+ and serum Cl^- decrease, Na^+ becomes available to combine with HCO_3^-, which increases as carbonic acid diminishes. To lower the increased bicarbonate, respiratory exchange is suppressed, permitting retention of carbonic acid and increased excretion of bicarbonate with Na^+ and K^+.

A common cause of metabolic alkalosis in cardiac patients is the diuresis effected by mercurial diuretics. Excessive use of these substances is often complicated by a hypochloremic alkalosis, believed to be related to the potassium deficits that occur. Cellular K^+ depletion of any origin leads to alkalosis with an elevated bicarbonate and

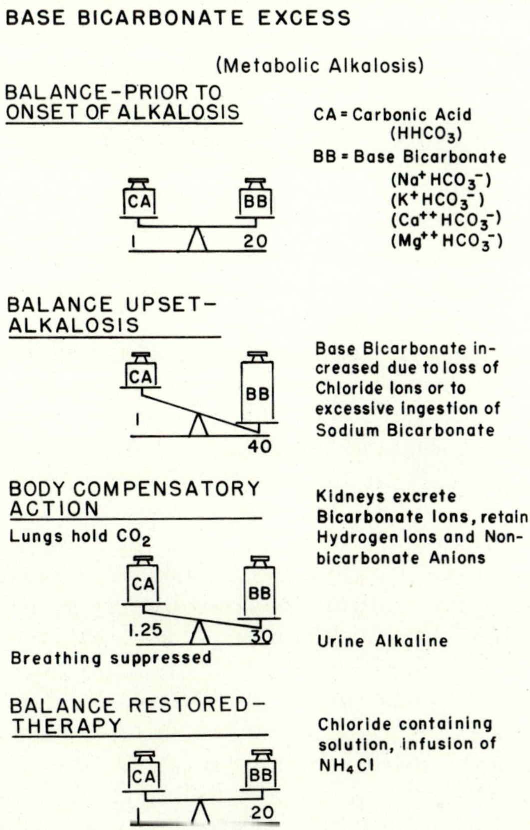

Fig. 1-10.—In metabolic alkalosis, base bicarbonate is increased. Respiration is compensatorily decreased, which increases carbonic acid blood levels. Balance is restored with chloride solution or infusion of NH_4Cl.

a lowered serum chloride, probably as a result of an intracellular fluid shift of H^+.

Administration of large doses of alkali in the form of sodium bicarbonate or sodium lactate may result in metabolic alkalosis. This is not due simply to sodium excess, since sodium is not a proton acceptor and thus does not alter the H^+ concentration. However, the increase in bicarbonate reduces H^+ concentration by forming more carbonic acid, which is excreted as CO_2 and H_2O, the binding of bicarbonate by the added cation leading to alkalosis.

Treatment of alkalosis necessitates the prevention of further acid loss, along with the replacement of anions and any potassium deficit. Both NaCl and KCl should be given in order to ameliorate the K^+

deficiency and to replace the bicarbonate ions with Cl^-. Although not recommended for therapy, NH_4Cl can be used, since the NH_4 is metabolized to urea and the Cl^- replaces bicarbonate and binds the H^+.

Electrolyte Shifts in Acidosis and Alkalosis

In metabolic acidosis the increased concentration of H^+ in the ECF causes H^+ to move into the cells and K^+ to migrate into the ECF. It has been observed experimentally that Na^+ also moves into the ECF in exchange for hydrogen when HCl is infused into nephrectomized animals. The increased amount of H^+ in the tubular cells leads to an increased excretion of H^+ in the urine in exchange for Na^+. In diabetes, deficits of sodium and potassium occur from the excretion with the ketonic anions. A deficiency of these cations is also observed in renal acidosis, since the kidney is unable to excrete adequate amounts of H^+.

Correction of the acidosis by alkaline salts such as sodium lactate will result both in an alkalosis and a profound decrease in serum K^+ until the latter ion is also replaced. Metabolic acidosis in diabetes, diarrhea or starvation is always accompanied by protein breakdown and cell fluid loss. As a result, both K^+ and Na^+ are lost in large quantities. Since Na^+ may diffuse into the cell to partially replace the lost K^+, salt depletion may occur.

Metabolic alkalosis.—When acid is lost by vomiting or through administration of excessive amounts of alkali, the decrease in H^+ concentration in the ECF produces a shift in H^+ from the cells to the ECF, resulting in both an intracellular and extracellular alkalosis. Potassium diffuses into the cell, reducing extracellular bicarbonate salt and thereby ameliorating the alkalosis. However, since renal tubular cells also have a lowered H^+ concentration, the K^+ of the tubular cell, rather than the less available H^+, is used in exchange for sodium. This results in large K^+ losses and eventually to potassium depletion.

Potassium losses.—In potassium loss, such as occurs in primary aldosteronism, sodium enters the cell to partially replace the K^+ loss. It is assumed that H^+ also moves into the cell to make up the remaining intracellular K^+ deficit. Thus, an intracellular acidosis and an extracellular fluid alkalosis are produced. In alkalosis due to causes other than potassium depletion, the increased renal tubular cell H^+ assumes the major position in the Na^+ exchange resorption, so that an aciduria is produced. Thus it is mandatory, when giving solutions to correct the alkalosis, that K^+ deficits be concurrently ameliorated, so as to halt the continued H^+ shift into the intracellular compartment.

It is important to realize that K^+ depletion alone does not produce alkalosis or even a lowering of serum K^+. ACTH, stress, or the addition of corticosteroids is also required to cause a potassium deficit. The adrenal steroids block the excretion of sodium by the kidneys in exchange for H^+, thus increasing urinary hydrogen and ammonium loss. Sodium and bicarbonate are retained, leading to alkalosis, which is actually a response of adrenocortical activity rather than potassium depletion.

The Measurement of Acid-Base Balance

Probably the easiest method of determining acid-base disturbances is by the technic of Astrup, in which, with only a small amount of blood, the pH can be obtained quickly and reliably. By use of the Siggaard-Andersen nomogram (see Fig. 1–11), the P_{CO_2}, buffer base, base excess, standard bicarbonate, actual plasma bicarbonate and total CO_2 content can be determined indirectly.

Using the Siggaard-Andersen Nomogram

The pH of the blood is first determined directly with a pH meter, the electrode of which is maintained at a constant temperature of 38°C., with the patient's Sa_{O_2} at 90% or higher. Two samples of blood are then equilibrated, one with gas of a high P_{CO_2} and the other with gas of a low P_{CO_2}, by bubbling CO_2 through each sample for 3 to 5 minutes. The pH of each sample is then plotted on the nomogram at the point where the pH value on the abscissa intercepts the horizontal lines of the predetermined P_{CO_2}.

For example, if a blood sample with a pH of 7.07 is equilibrated with a gas whose P_{CO_2} is 60 mm. Hg, a dot is placed on the nomogram at the corresponding intersection (A, Fig. 1–11). If the pH of the blood equilibrated with a gas having a P_{CO_2} of 30 mm. Hg is 7.22, another dot (B, Fig. 1–11) is inserted on the nomogram to coincide with these readings. A line drawn between dots A and B permits determination of the remaining acid-base parameters.

Point C is found by extension of the line A–B; by placing the actual pH of the blood on this line, the P_{CO_2} can be read on the ordinate. The point at which the diagonal line crosses the buffer-base portion of the nomogram indicates the buffer base in mEq. per liter. The standard bicarbonate (in mEq. per liter) can be read out at the point where this line intercepts that area of the nomogram (point E) and the base excess can be determined where the line intersects the base-excess curve. The actual plasma bicarbonate is determined by draw-

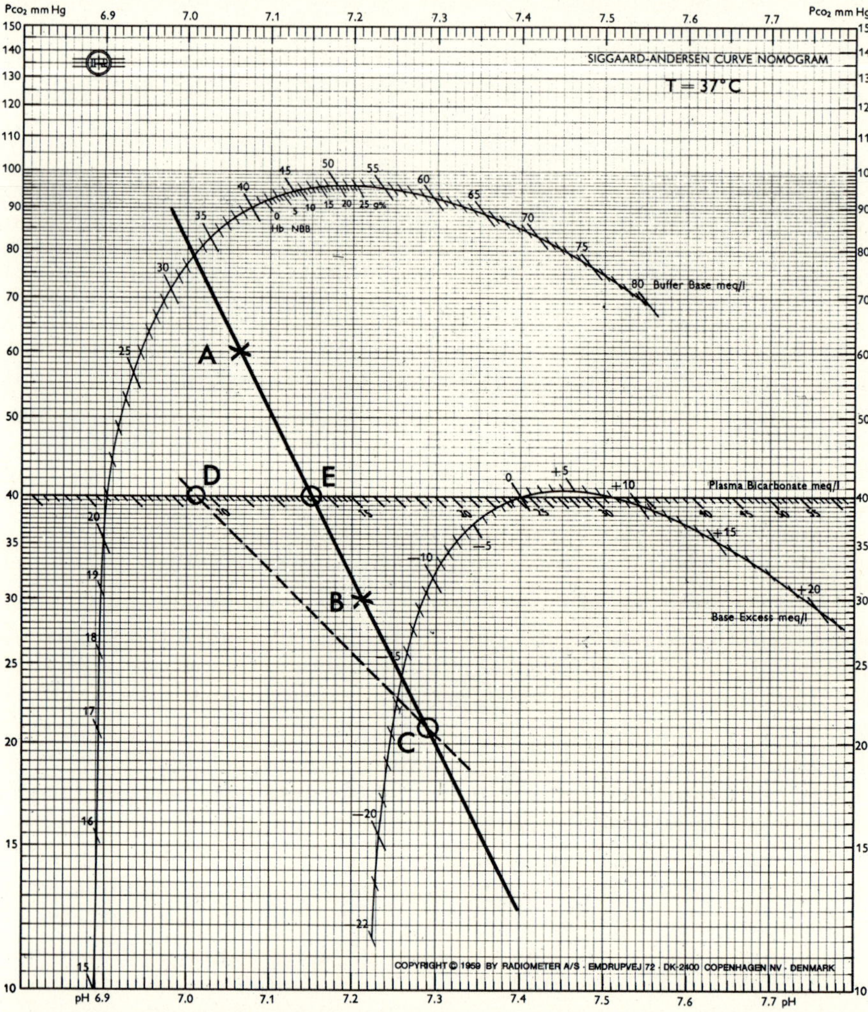

Fig. 1–11.—The Siggaard-Andersen Nomogram. (Modified from drawing courtesy of Radiometer, Copenhagen, Denmark.)

ing a line at an angle of 45° from point C until it meets the standard bicarbonate line at point D. The total CO_2 content is obtained by adding actual $P_{CO_2} \times 0.3$ to the actual HCO_3 concentration.

Two new measurements are obtained from the Siggaard-Andersen nomogram: the standard bicarbonate and concentration in base excess. These are related to the term "buffer base," introduced by Singer and Hastings in 1948 and defined as the sum of the concentrations of buffer ions, in mEq. per liter, contained in whole blood. Such buffer ions, estimated to be 45–50 mEq. per liter, include the bicarbonate and phosphates in the plasma and in the red cells, plus hemoglobin and plasma protein.

Astrup's terms, standard bicarbonate and base excess, represent metabolic changes in a slightly different way. For example, the standard bicarbonate, which has a normal value of 24 mEq. per liter, represents the bicarbonate concentration in the blood plasma equilibrated at a P_{CO_2} of 40 mm. Hg and with O_2, in order to fully saturate the hemoglobin. On the other hand, base excess represents either a deficit in base or a deficiency of acid. It is defined as 0 for blood with a pH of 7.4 at a P_{CO_2} of 40 mm. Hg. Positive values indicate an excess of base or a deficiency in fixed acids, while negative values indicate a deficit of base or an excess of fixed acid. Thus, base excess represents the amount of strong base or acid per liter of blood which has been added as a result of metabolic disturbances.

Although the exact concentration actually depends on the hemoglobin concentration of the blood sample, relatively large changes in hemoglobin cause small changes in this value. This is particularly important in patients hemodiluted during and following cardiopulmonary bypass. For this reason, the author uses this as an index of metabolic acidosis or alkalosis in preference to other values, such as buffer base. The advantages of using either the standard bicarbonate or base excess rather than buffer base is that these values can be rapidly and accurately determined by the Astrup method and, unlike buffer base, they are not influenced by the O_2 saturation of the original blood sample. In addition, the values of base excess or deficit can be used not only for diagnosis but also for the treatment of metabolic acidosis or alkalosis in patients by the Astrup formula, in which the mEq. value of base required to correct a metabolic acidosis = the body weight in kilograms $\times$ 0.3 $\times$ the base deficit. Correspondingly, to correct a metabolic alkalosis with acid, a similar formula can be used (mEq. acid = body weight in kg. $\times$ 0.3 plus base excess).

Although we rely on the base excess or deficit in treating metabolic acidosis and alkalosis, these values can be misleading when used to treat respiratory acidosis or alkalosis. With uncompensated respiratory acidosis or alkalosis, bicarbonate and base excess may be normal. Again, a patient with primary respiratory acidosis complicated by a metabolic acidosis or a primary respiratory alkalosis, who develops an independent metabolic acidosis, may also have a normal standard bicarbonate and base excess despite a serious acidosis or alkalosis.

Thus, a normal base excess cannot always be used as a guide to treatment.

In essence, the standard bicarbonate and base excess represent a balance between metabolic acidosis and alkalosis, which may exist simultaneously in a patient. For example, an individual in metabolic acidosis will usually develop a compensatory respiratory alkalosis. Similarly, if a respiratory acidosis should develop independently, there will be a tendency for a compensatory metabolic alkalosis to occur. Thus, normal standard bicarbonate or base excess values in such a patient merely indicate that a *metabolic* balance is present. Hence it can be seen that it is mandatory for the physician to use the base excess only in association with the pH and the P_{CO_2}, to obtain full knowledge of the total acid-base balance in the extracellular fluid.

BIBLIOGRAPHY

Ad Hoc Committee on Acid-Base Terminology: Conference on current concepts of acid-base measurement, Ann. New York Acad. Sc. 133:251, 1966.

Astrup, P., *et al.:* Acid-base metabolism: A new approach, Lancet 1:1035, 1960.

Best, C. H., and Taylor, N. B.: *The Physiological Basis of Medical Practice* (8th ed.; Baltimore: Williams & Wilkins Company, 1966).

Bland, J. H.: *Clinical Metabolism of Body Water and Electrolytes* (Philadelphia: W. B. Saunders Company, 1963).

Elkinton, J. R., and Danowski, T. S.: *The Body Fluids* (Baltimore: Williams & Wilkins Company, 1955).

Gamble, J. S.: *Chemical Anatomy, Physiology and Pathology of Extracellular Fluid* (Cambridge, Mass.: Harvard University Press, 1950).

Ganang, W. F.: *Review of Medical Physiology* (3d ed.; Los Altos, California: Lange Medical Publications, 1967).

Goldberger, E.: *A Primer of Water, Electrolyte and Acid-Base Syndromes* (Philadelphia: Lea & Febiger, 1965).

Irvine, W. T.: *The Scientific Basis of Surgery* (Boston: Little, Brown & Company, 1965).

Maxwell, M. H., and Kleeman, C. R.: *Clinical Disorders of Fluids and Electrolyte Metabolism* (New York: Blakiston, 1962).

Moore, F. D.: *Metabolic Care of the Surgical Patient* (Philadelphia: W. B. Saunders Company, 1959).

Parks, C. R.: Operative fluid shifts: A review of the literature, Anesth. & Analg. 45:495, 1966.

Randall, H. T.: Fluid and Electrolyte Therapy, in *Manual of Preoperative and Postoperative Care,* Committee on Pre- and Postoperative Care, American College of Surgeons (Philadelphia: W.B. Saunders Company, 1967).

Robinson, J. R.: *Fundamentals of Acid-Base Regulation* (6th ed.; Philadelphia: F. A. Davis Company, 1967).

Siggaard-Andersen, O., and Engel, K.: A new acid-base nomogram, Scandinav. J. Clin. & Lab. Invest. 12:186, 1960.

Smith, J. W.: *Manual of Medical Therapeutics* (Boston: Little, Brown & Company, 1969).

Statland, H.: *Fluid and Electrolytes in Practice* (3d ed.; Philadelphia: J. B. Lippincott Company, 1963).

Weisberg, H. F.: *Water, Electrolyte and Acid-Base Balance* (2d ed.; Baltimore: Williams & Wilkins Company, 1962).

Welt, F. G.: *Clinical Disorders of Hydration and Acid-Base Equilibrium* (2d ed.; Boston: Little, Brown & Company, 1958).
Wilkinson, A. W.: *Body Fluids in Surgery* (2d ed.; Baltimore: Williams & Wilkins Company, 1960).
Wynn, V.: Water and Electrolyte Metabolism, in *The Scientific Basis of Surgery,* W. T. Irvine (ed.) (Boston: Little, Brown & Company, 1965).

CHAPTER

2

The Adult Cardiac Patient

PART 1.

Cardiac Output

WILLIAM E. NEVILLE, M.D.,
ROBERT D. LYNCH, M.D.,
and ROBERT VANECKO, M.D.

A COMPREHENSIVE UNDERSTANDING of the physiology of cardiac output is essential for a logical approach to cardiac surgery. Though knowledge in this field is rapidly expanding, a great deal is already known about normal cardiac output, the multiple factors regulating it, and the alterations caused by disease. Surgical correction of heart disease is aimed at restoring altered cardiac output toward normal. The closer this restoration approaches normal, the more successful the surgical procedure. The better one understands cardiac output, the better one can cope with cardiac surgery and the care of the diseased and surgically altered heart.

Cardiac output is dependent upon the condition of the heart itself, its contractile force, its rate, blood supply and anatomic integrity. It is also dependent upon peripheral factors such as the resistance against which the heart works, the tone of the autonomic nervous system and the rate of venous return. The volume and viscosity of the circulating blood as well as its pH, oxygen tension (PO_2), and carbon dioxide tension (PCO_2), and electrolyte levels influence the cardiac output.

MEASUREMENT OF CARDIAC OUTPUT

The two basic methods of determining cardiac output in clinical practice are the Fick and the indicator dilution method. The Fick method is based on the general assumption that, in any fluid system in a steady state, the rate of flow can be determined if (*a*) a detectable substance can be added to the system at a known rate, and (*b*) the concentration of that substance can be determined at points proximal and distal to the portal of entry. This method has its widest use in the cardiac catheterization laboratory. The measured substance is O_2, the portal of entry is the lung. The O_2 concentration is measured on either side of the lung. The formula then becomes:

$$\text{cardiac output} = \frac{\text{oxygen consumption (ml./min.)}}{\text{arterial } O_2 - \text{venous } O_2 \text{ (ml./liter)}}$$

The O_2 consumption is measured by collecting the patient's expired air for a given length of time and analyzing its O_2 concentration. The difference between the concentration of O_2 in the inspired air and the expired sample times the total volume expired gives the O_2 consumption.

In obtaining the proximal and distal blood samples, there is one qualified condition: The sample must represent a uniformly mixed portion of blood representing the entire circulation. The arterial sample may be obtained from any artery. Blood leaving the lungs is thoroughly mixed in the left side of the heart and the O_2 concentration is uniform from the left ventricle to the arterioles. No O_2 is added or extracted until the blood reaches the nutrient vessels.

Obtaining an upstream sample is more difficult. Because of the various rates of O_2 extraction in different organs and parts of the body, a truly mixed venous sample is not obtainable until blood from various parts of the body is mixed together within the right side of the heart. Due to laminar flow from the superior vena cava, the inferior vena cava and the coronary sinus, blood in the right atrium is not really mixed. Samples must be taken from the outflow tract of the right ventricle or preferably the pulmonary artery in order to obtain a sample of uniformly mixed venous blood for O_2 concentration analysis.

Within the environments of the catheterization laboratory, facilities are adequate to make these measurements routine. Obviously, considerable equipment and technical assistance are necessary. The value of this measurement in diagnosis is established; however, it cannot be made in the recovery room or at the patient's bedside.

The essentials of the indicated dilution method consist of injecting a bolus of indicative substance into the venous side of the circulation and the continuous measurement of the concentration of this indicator as it passes a point in the arterial circulation. In order to measure cardiac output, the dye must pass through one or both chambers of the heart. Only in this way can the dye be diluted with mixed blood from the total body circulation; if it is not so mixed, it will not reflect cardiac output. The time course of appearance and disappearance of variable concentrations of indicator is related to the amount of cardiac output. Although a staggering number of indicator substances may be used, the more satisfactory ones are dyes. Thus this method is frequently called the dye-dilution method.

The study is carried out clinically by placing a plastic catheter in a peripheral artery—for example, the radial—for measurements of dye concentration. Another catheter is passed through a peripheral vein (usually in the antecubital area) into the right atrium, right ventricle or pulmonary artery for dye injection. This ensures the delivery of a bolus of dye into the central circulation where it will form a truly mixed venous sample. As the dye is injected through the centrally placed venous catheter, blood is withdrawn at a constant rate from the peripheral artery. As it is withdrawn, it passes through a densitometer, an optical electronic device for continually detecting varying concentrations of dye. The densitometer is coupled to a recording device which makes a permanent visual record of the concentration in relation to time. This record forms a dye-dilution curve. Cardiac output is calculated from mathematical analysis of this curve. Small portable computers are also available which can be coupled to the densitometer and provide almost instantaneous calculations of the cardiac output. The equipment necessary for this method can be made highly mobile and consequently very useful at the patient's bedside as well as in the catheterization laboratory. Both these methods, if carefully done, yield comparable results.

NORMAL VALUES.—The normal cardiac output at rest is usually considered to be 6 liters/minute. The resting cardiac output gradually decreases with patient age. In order to compare the cardiac output of individuals of different size, cardiac output is frequently expressed as cardiac index. This is the cardiac output in liters/minute divided by the surface area of the individual in square meters. The cardiac index is normally about 3 liters/minute/meter^2. Although this index is very useful, it would probably be more accurate if it were based on a weight ratio. This becomes particularly evident in small infants, where the ratio of weight to surface area is markedly different from that of the adult. Thus, in the infant, the cardiac output expressed as cardiac index is much lower than in the adult. However, on a weight-for-weight basis, it is much greater.

FACTORS INFLUENCING CARDIAC OUTPUT.—The regulation of cardiac output is quite complex. No one unifying concept is presently available to explain the interaction of all the known factors and feedback mechanisms which participate in its regulation. Undoubtedly there are many that are still unknown. Some of the more important determinants of cardiac output follow.

a) Resistance, or Starling's law of the heart.—The heart itself has an autonomous ability to adapt to an increased volume of blood or to increased resistance. Either of these events results in a larger volume of blood remaining in the ventricle at the end of systole. This stretches the ventricular muscle which in turn increases the force of the next contraction. Thus, within physiologic limitations, the heart automatically adjusts to the increased load and maintains a fairly steady or slightly adjusted cardiac output.

The resistive forces vary from about one-half to twice normal during most circulatory phenomena. Automatic adjustments by the heart itself within this range are as follows: With a decrease of resistance of one-half normal, the cardiac output increases about 10%. With an increase of resistance to twice normal, cardiac output decreases about 30%. Both ventricles are capable of adjusting independently. With a decrease in systemic load, the cardiac output increases only about 10% because the right ventricle is a limiting factor and is little affected by systemic resistance. With an increase in systemic load, the cardiac output decreases in the more nearly proportional manner because the left ventricle is directly influenced by the systemic resistance.

b) Autonomic nervous system.—Sympathetic stimulation increases the cardiac output. It is capable of producing outputs of up to 20–25 liters/minute when maximally stimulated. Under normal circumstances there is a normal minimal sympathetic stimulation. If this normal sympathetic tone is eliminated (as in total spinal anesthesia) or diminished, the cardiac output diminishes. Sympathetic stimulation produces its effect by increasing the strength of the myocardial contractility and the heart rate.

The parasympathetic nervous system has the opposite effect. Stimulation in parasympathetics produces a falling cardiac output. It produces its effect not by altering the contractile strength but by diminishing the heart rate.

c) Effective heart rate.—Within the limits of each individual heart, the rate will affect cardiac output. Increased rate up to a certain optimal rate, approximately 120 beats/minute, will increase the cardiac output. Beyond this point and up to a rate of about 160/minute, cardiac output will be above normal but not as great as at the optimal rate. Beyond this limit the cardiac output will fall below normal because there is insufficient time for the heart to fill with blood between beats. Slowing of the heart rate to very low rates—for example, 40 beats/minute—will also diminish the cardiac output.

d) Disease.—Any disease of the heart, such as coronary occlusion, myocardial infarction, cardiac trauma, myocarditis or valvular disease, diminishes the effectiveness of the heart as a pump. Continued activity of the compensatory mechanisms is required to maintain near-normal cardiac output even at rest. The ability of the heart to react to increased demand is seriously diminished.

e) Peripheral factors.—An explanation of all the affects of peripheral circulation on cardiac output is beyond the scope of this introduction. Nonetheless, it is important to be familiar with them. The peripheral resistance which greatly affects the cardiac output is itself affected by the volume and the velocity of the blood, the tone of the autonomic nervous system, the pressure and composition of the interstitial fluid, the affects of hormonal substances such as epinephrine and norepinephrine, the pH, O_2, CO_2, and lactate content of the blood. Also important is the ability of the venous side of the circulation to adapt by the "pooling" of blood in the various venous reservoirs, such as the portal circulation, and in the pulmonary circulation. External forces exert considerable effect on the low-pressure, highly distensible venous bed, which can be favorably or adversely affected by such factors as positive-pressure breathing, abdominal compression, gravity and body position.

CLINICAL SITUATIONS.—Certain clinical situations frequently encountered in cardiac surgery have a considerable effect on cardiac output. These include the following:

a) Open-chest and positive-pressure breathing.—Cardiac output is affected by the pressures around the heart. Under normal circumstances the negative interpleural pressure enhances the transpleural pressure of the right atrium (i.e., the intra-atrial pressure minus the intrapleural pressure). This in effect enhances the effective filling pressure of the heart. Positive pressures that result from opening the chest and from positive-pressure respiration, which occurs during endotracheal anesthesia, produce the opposite effect. This requires a greater right intra-atrial pressure to maintain the same cardiac output. In other words, compensatory mechanisms must come into play. The sympathetic nervous system is activated. This produces a vasoconstrictive effect in the peripheral circulation, which elevates the mean systemic pressure. Sympathetic stimulation also directly strengthens the heart. The positive pressure within the lungs forces into the systemic circulation a portion of the blood "stored" in the pulmonary circulation, also increasing the mean systemic pressure.

b) Transfusion.—Transfusions of blood are usually intended to restore the volume of the circulating blood to normal. At times over-transfusion may result in a greater than normal blood volume. Cardiac output is increased, right atrial pressure is elevated. The pressure increase is transmitted throughout the circulation. At the capillary level, fluid is forced into the interstitial spaces. Gradually, over a period of hours, the fluid thus lost from the circulation returns the main systemic pressure to normal levels. The venous return to the heart and the right atrial pressure return to normal, as does the cardiac output.

c) Hemorrhage.—Hemorrhage and shock produce profound effects throughout the whole organ and initiate numerous compensatory adjustments. Basically the cardiac output will drop precipitously in response to a drop in the mean systemic pressure. Within seconds to minutes, sympathetic reflexes will return the mean systemic pressure toward normal and make the heart a more effective pump. Over the next few hours, fluid is mobilized from interstitial spaces into the vascular bed, compensating for the lost volume, further enhancing the mean systemic pressure and raising the cardiac output toward normal. Continued blood loss or prolonged activity of the compensatory mechanisms may exhaust the ability to maintain cardiac output. An irreversible stage is entered. The cardiac output is depressed. Anoxia affects the responsiveness of the heart and the peripheral circulation. The cardiac output falls further, anoxia increases, death ensues. If the heart itself is diseased, it may not be able to react to the peripheral compensatory mechanisms and cardiac output will remain low. This is a form of cardiac shock.

d) Tamponade.—Pressure within the pericardial space affects the right atrial pressure adversely. The right atrial pressure increases, necessitating an increase in mean systemic pressure to maintain the venous return of blood to the heart. This is accomplished initially by sympathetic reflexes acting on the heart and the peripheral circulation. The heart becomes more effective. Blood is "squeezed" out of the heart and lungs into the systemic circulation which, together with sympathetic stimulation of the periphery, raises the mean systemic pressure. If the need for higher cardiac outputs arises, the heart responds by increasing its volume to increase its effectiveness (Starling's law). The increased volume of the ventricle transmits an increased pressure to the fluid confined within the pericardium. This sets in motion a self-defeating cycle.

General Considerations after Open-Heart Surgery

The mechanics necessary for the proper postoperative care of the adult cardiac patient begin prior to the operation and continue until the patient leaves the hospital. Although the majority of the patients have been observed in the hospital for a period of time and are presumed to be in optimum condition for surgery, the day before the operation an electrocardiogram should be made and a chest x-ray obtained. As noted earlier, the serum chloride, potassium, sodium, calcium and blood urea nitrogen are quantitated and a complete blood count is made. Since the majority of the patients have been digitalized and have been on prolonged diuretic therapy, the serum electrolytes, especially the serum potassium, may be altered.

For reasons not completely understood, postperfusion cardiac arrhythmias are prone to occur in the digitalized, hypokalemic patient. For this reason, digitalis is withheld for 48–72 hours prior to the operation, and diuretic agents are discontinued the day preceding surgery. If the serum potassium is depleted, supplementation is given orally. If facilities are available, the total circulating blood volume should be determined 24 hours before the surgical procedure and the red cell mass and plasma volume calculated.

Prior to anesthesia, the radial artery is exposed and cannulated with a plastic tube. This is attached through a three-way stopcock and a suitable length of tubing to a strain gauge through which a continuous recording of the arterial blood pressure can be obtained on an oscilloscope. The patency of the radial artery catheter is maintained following surgery by intermittent flushing with dilute heparin solution (10 mg. of heparin in 500 ml. of Ringer's lactate solution). Of all the cannulae used by the authors, that which has proven most satisfactory for long-term oscillographic monitoring of the blood pressure has been the variety used by the Renal Dialysis Unit. This consists of a short section of Teflon tubing inserted into a segment of silastic rubber. Although direct measurement of the peripheral-arterial blood pressure is not essential during perfusion, it is mandatory during induction of anesthesia, and is helpful in the early postoperative period. It is also useful in permitting frequent withdrawal of arterial blood for acid-base determinations. This obviates the necessity for multiple needling of the peripheral vessels, which may result in thrombosis. However, it is our present policy to remove the catheter as soon as acid-base determinations are no longer necessary.

The central venous blood pressure is measured in centimeters of water with a commercially available saline manometer through a small polyethylene tube passed into the right atrium from an upper arm vein. An alternative technic is the use of the external jugular or the subclavian vein just below the clavicle for passage of this catheter. Monitoring of the venous blood pressure is desirable during oxygenator reinfusion at the termination of bypass and is a guide to the adequacy of blood replacement following surgery. The left atrial pressure may be measured in a similar manner from a small catheter inserted into this area of the heart at the completion of the intracardiac procedure. Although this has not routinely been done, it is useful as an index of left ventricular function in the early postoperative period.

The endotracheal tube used for anesthesia is left in place for 24 hours following surgery and the patient ventilated with a respirator. In order to accomplish this, maximum sedation must be afforded with intravenous morphine sulfate or meperidine. The beneficial effects of oxygenation are vitiated if breathing is asynchronous with the machine. On the first postoperative day the patient's ability to oxygenate his blood without ventilatory support is ascertained before removal of the endotracheal tube. If he is unable to maintain an O_2 saturation above 85%, either the endotracheal tube is not removed at this time or a tracheostomy is performed, with insertion of a cuffed tube. This decision is dependent upon the condition of the patient and the need for long-term respiratory support. Because of the difficulty of tolerating an orotracheal tube, it is prudent to do a tracheostomy as soon as it is obvious that prolonged ventilatory assistance is required. This also facilitates the removal of the pulmonary secretions, which are more prevalent in adult cardiac patients. The disadvantages of a tracheostomy are entirely related to infection, which is introduced extrinsically by careless handling of the tube and suction equipment. This can be mitigated by meticulous attention to asepsis by personnel responsible for the tracheal toilet.

Prior to closing the chest, two intrathoracic tubes are inserted, one draining the heart anteriorly, and the other placed in the posterior aspect of the thorax just above the diaphragm if the pleural cavity has been entered. These are independently connected to underwater seal drainage and suction applied through a three-bottle system. To assess the drainage of blood from the thorax postoperatively, it is extremely important to note the position of each tube and to accurately mark the fluid level in the drainage bottles at hourly intervals. This maneuver, together with serial x-rays of the chest, permits an accurate estimate of intrathoracic bleeding. In addition, intravenous fluid bottles are marked by the nurse when the patient enters the recovery room, and an accurate measurement of the intake and output from the various indwelling tubes and catheters is recorded on the chart.

Upon arrival of the patient in the intensive care area, base-line determinations of the cardiovascular state are clinically established. These include the body temperature and the color of the skin, extremities and face. The peripheral arterial pulsations and the rate of urine production are recorded at regular intervals. The fullness of the superficial veins of the feet is observed, and the central venous pressure, arterial blood pressure and electrocardiogram are constantly monitored on an oscillograph.

If this service is available, the total circulating blood volume should be determined immediately upon entrance into the recovery room. Although the general condition of the patient prevents using laboratory data as a stringent guide to therapy, reliable blood volume studies are helpful, especially with the authors' method of totally priming the pump oxygenator with Ringer's lactate solution. However, with increasing experience and the inability to correlate the blood volume determinations with the momentary condition of the patient, we have abandoned this modality. Previously repeated studies of the circulating blood volume showed that although the total blood volume is near the control level, the plasma volume is increased and the red cell mass is decreased in the early postoperative period. From these results, the right atrial pressure reading, the subsequent drainage from the chest tubes, the need for whole blood replacement was determined. If there was no bleeding from the thorax and a deficiency in red cell mass was within 500 ml. of normal, the patient did not need to receive a transfusion. If the red cell mass was depleted in excess of half a liter and the plasma volume was concomitantly increased, a unit of packed red cells was given instead of whole blood. However, with experience gained in over 700 patients perfused with only Ringer's lactate solution, it is apparent that the venous and arterial blood pressures, the urinary output, the chest drainage, and the color and temperature of the extremities are much more reliable indices for blood replacement than a computerized machine.

In addition, blood is removed from the catheter in the radial artery for determination of O_2 saturation (with an oximeter) and the acid-base balance is assessed. The pH is measured by the Astrup method and the standard bicarbonate, buffer base, P_{CO_2}, and base excess or deficit determined from the Siggaard-Andersen nomogram (see Chapter 1). If a base deficit is recorded, this is ameliorated with infusions of sodium bicarbonate or *tris* buffer, as described in Chapter 1.

The serum sodium, chloride, potassium and calcium electrolytes are immediately measured and deviations from the normal are corrected. Ordinarily, the only serious alteration observed in the early postoperative period has been a low serum potassium. When this exists, the intravenous-therapy fluid should contain supplemental potassium chloride. As a result of the authors' method of perfusion with Ringer's lactate, there has been a slight increase in chloride and sodium in the early postoperative period, which is not detrimental.

Exclusive of blood replacement, intravenous-fluid therapy, consisting of Ringer's lactate solution, is limited to 1,000 ml. within 24 hours for the first 3–4 days. The reason for this is that the patients have an increase in serum water and are actually overhydrated following perfusion. As a result, they need only to replace the amount of fluid excreted through the lungs and the skin. This amounts to approximately 800–1,000 ml. of Ringer's lactate for the first 48–72 hours. Penicillin, staphcillin and KCl are added in the appropriate amounts, which vary from group to group.

Management of Specific Problems

SHOCK

The term shock refers to that state in which the cardiovascular system is unable to provide adequate tissue perfusion. It invariably results from failure of one or more of four separate but interrelated components of the vascular system: 1) the heart, 2) the fluid which is pumped, 3) the peripheral arterial resistance (resistance vessels), and 4) the capacity of the venous bed (capacitance vessels).

Four general types of shock can be delineated according to their primary etiologies:

1. *Hemorrhagic shock* results from blood loss and initially represents relatively pure hypovolemia.

2. *Traumatic or wound shock* is consequent to loss of blood plasma and other fluids secondary to tissue injury and may include bacterial contamination.

3. *Septic shock* is secondary to infections, primarily from gram-negative organisms. Infection may also play a role in late shock from other causes.

4. *Cardiogenic shock* is caused by the inability of the myocardium to maintain an adequate cardiac output. This primarily occurs in patients with myocardial infarction, valvular lesions, cardiac arrhythmias or pathology, such as pericardial tamponade, which obstructs the venous return to the heart.

GENERAL PATHOPHYSIOLOGY.—The progression of events following the onset of shock is similar regardless of the etiology. Thus, it is imperative to comprehend these changes and the compensatory mechanisms which occur, if proper therapy is to be instituted. These alterations are 1) *hypovolemia,* which is the primary problem in hemorrhagic and traumatic shock, 2) *decreased venous return,* 3) *diminution in cardiac output,* 4) *decline in blood pressure,* and 5) *decreased capillary blood flow.* The combatant physiologic processes include a redistribution in blood flow to the essential organs such as the heart and brain and a replenishment of the intravascular volume with fluid derived from the interstitial fluid compartment. The decline in arterial blood pressure stimulates the baroreceptors in the arch of the aorta and carotid sinus, which increases the heart rate and force of cardiac contraction. Neural stimulation causes arterial and venous vasoconstriction while endocrine activity promotes the increased secretion of ADH, ACTH, 17-hydroxycorticosteroids and catecholamines. In addition, it is believed that diminished blood flow through the kidneys incites a release of renin. This in turn combines with one of the plasma proteins to form angiotensin, which is postulated either to act directly on the blood vessels to produce vasoconstriction or induce the adrenal glands to secrete aldosterone, which permits the kidneys to retain salt and water.

The decreased central nervous system blood flow results in hyperventilation and a respiratory alkalosis. As tissue hypoxia progresses, a metabolic acidosis is observed. The decreased aerobic oxidation via the Krebs tricarboxilic acid cycle with increased aerobic glycolysis by Embden-Meyerhof pathway leads to a rise in lactic and pyruvic acids with potentiation of the metabolic acidosis. In addition, tissue ATP is decreased together with glucose utilization. Further deterioration of the physiologic state depresses the reticuloendothelial system, increases the lysozyme hydrolysate enzymes, and sludging of the formed elements of the blood with intravascular red cell agglutination is observed.

The signs and symptoms of well-established shock are classical and usually quite easy to recognize. However, the differential diagnosis of shock can be extremely difficult in the postoperative period. It is usually secondary to either hemorrhage, pericardial tamponade, cardiac failure, cardiac arrhythmias, vasodilation, acid-base imbalance, adrenal exhaustion, or pulmonary emboli. Following open-heart surgery, the most frequent cause is on a hemorrhagic basis, with cardiogenic shock assuming a second position.

Postoperative Hemorrhage (Figs. 2-1 and 2-2)

Hemorrhage is one of the major hazards of any surgical procedure. This is particularly true after cardiopulmonary bypass. Statistically, it is usually due to inadequate hemostasis; however, coagulation defects must be considered. The diagnosis of overt hemorrhage is simple and requires only recording the volume of obvious blood loss from chest and pericardial tubes. On the other hand, concealed hemorrhage into pleural, pericardial, mediastinal and abdominal cavities is more difficult to detect. Usually the patient presents a picture of reduced blood volume, with increasing restlessness and irritability. The extremities are cool, pale, and show a reduced capillary filling time. Peripheral venous constriction is easily appreciated on the dorsum of the foot, where the veins become empty. Arterial vasoconstriction also predominates and, if the arterial blood pressure is used as the main index of decreased blood volume, the diagnosis of hypovolemia will be delayed. Ordinarily, a decreasing central venous pressure is a reliable index of blood loss; however, this may be misleading if there is an element of pericardial tamponade. Under these circumstances, the venous pressure will remain elevated in the face of continued exsanguination, due to compression of the right atrium by accumulated blood. As the shock state progresses, there is a de-

Fig. 2-1.—Postoperative hemorrhage with pericardial tamponade following an aortic valve replacement. The patient was taken back to surgery and the blood was evacuated.

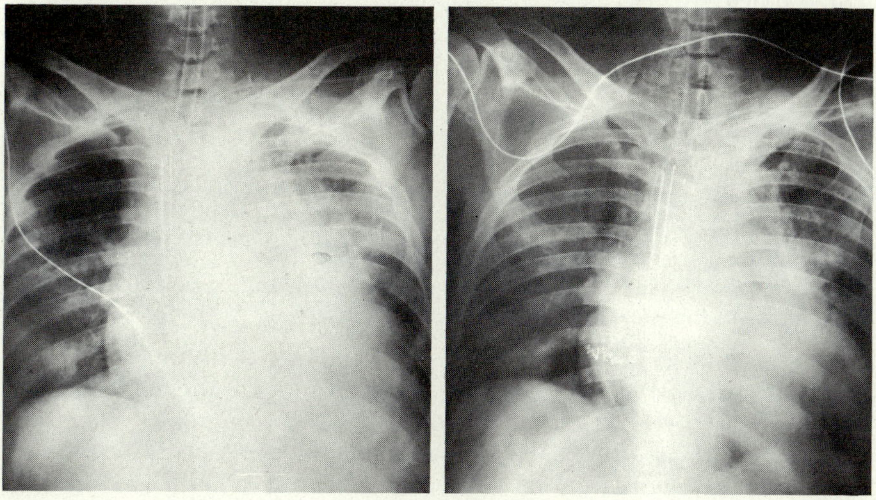

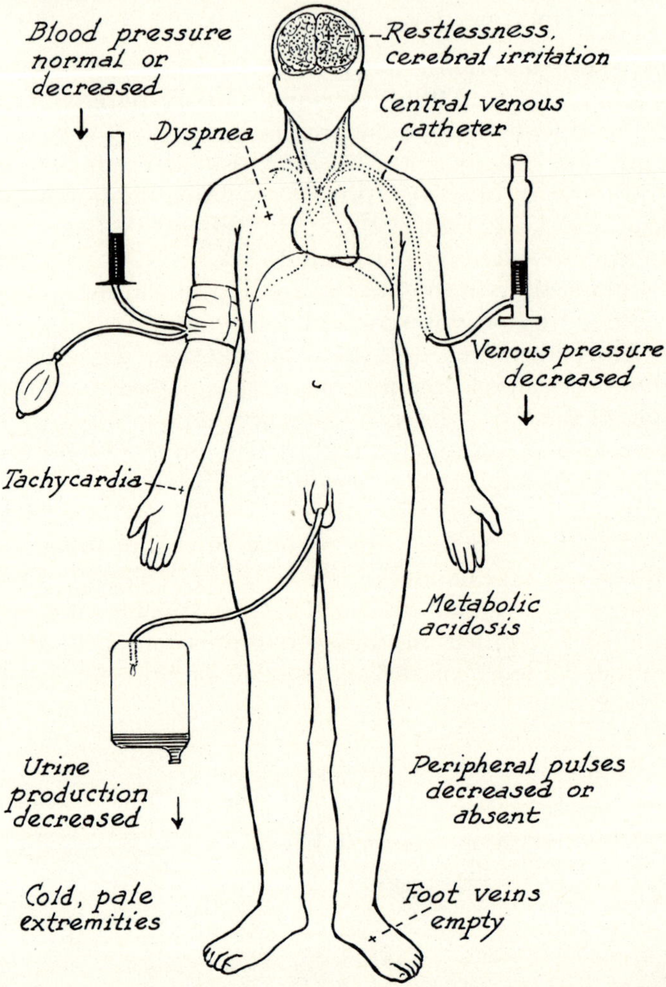

Fig. 2-2.—The pertinent features of patients in hemorrhagic shock are shown in this drawing. It should be stressed that the arterial blood pressure does not always reflect the severity of the blood loss because of the body's temporary adaptive physiologic mechanisms. Other parameters, such as the central venous pressure, the urinary output, the fullness of the peripheral veins and the color and temperature of the extremities, should be assessed.

crease in urinary output and the venous O_2 saturation falls, from tissue hypoxia prior to the development of a metabolic acidosis.

The recognition of the late stages of hypovolemic shock is not difficult, since the patient is cold and pale, with essentially complete peripheral vasoconstriction. The central venous pressure is low, the arterial blood pressure is reduced, cerebral irritation is evident and urinary output is markedly curtailed.

From the foregoing, it is obvious that the maintenance of a normal blood volume is the most important factor in the immediate postoperative period. Hypervolemia causes an over-loading of the left ventricle with an increase in the left atrial pressure, which reduces pulmonary compliance and eventually progresses to pulmonary edema. On the other hand, hypovolemia causes vasoconstriction with inadequate tissue perfusion, metabolic acidosis and shock. Thus, hemorrhage without adequate replacement therapy results in a reduction in cardiac output and a low circulating blood volume. Compensation is temporarily afforded by an increase in sympathetic nervous tone together with a rise in the secretion of adrenaline, noradrenaline, adrenal corticoids and the antidiuretic hormone from the posterior pituitary. Urine volume is diminished as well as intestinal secretion and salivation, to conserve fluids. The A.V. oxygen difference is widened from an increased extraction of O_2 by the tissues, and hypoxic acidosis may occur from the low cardiac output. Continued blood loss causes peripheral vasoconstriction in order to maintain the blood pressure and distribute the blood flow to the brain and myocardium. Under these circumstances the venous pressure will fall slightly, but a reflex tachycardia helps to maintain the blood pressure. Further decrements in the blood volume are temporarily compensated at the expense of proper tissue perfusion. After 20 to 30% of the blood volume has been depleted, the blood pressure begins to fall. At this point maximal vasoconstriction is prominent. Cold, cyanotic extremities can be perceived, and the venous pressure falls. During this period, flow through the skin and splanchnic area is drastically reduced and acute tubular necrosis may occur from the diminished renal blood flow. Coronary blood flow is diminished as a result of the low aortic pressure and the tachycardia, in spite of the reduction in coronary vascular resistance. Critical reduction in blood pressure and consequent poor coronary perfusion lead to a mechanically ineffective heart.

In addition, poor blood flow to the brain causes damage to the vasomotor and respiratory centers. Failure of the former allows venous pooling while failure of the respiratory center diminishes oxygenation of the blood, which worsens the hypoxic acidosis. Compensatory hyperventilation from the increased metabolic acidosis may lower the CO_2, thus further aggravating cerebral ischemia. Another vicious cycle is created by the diminished blood flow as a consequence of blood clots developing in the small vessels. This further reduces the available venous return, and the progressively more sluggish flow of blood through peripheral vessels causes more and more blood clotting. Endotoxins are also formed in the liver and the intestines during prolonged ischemia which, combined with electrolyte shifts, may make the situation irreversible.

Ordinarily the blood volume is maintained by replacing the blood loss in the intravascular compartment as it occurs. However, in the postoperative period, the problem is complicated by the fact that there is a delay of varying degree from the loss of blood from the circulation and its appearance in the chest drainage bottle. In addition, the vascular compartment may alter by a liter or more because of changes in arterial and venous tone. Thus a blood volume that is adequate for vital organ perfusion when the patient is vasoconstricted becomes inadequate when blood is sequestered in splanchnic vessels. For this reason, an accurate measurement and assessment of blood loss is mandatory following cardiac surgery, plus continued and critical observation of the patient.

To ensure adequate drainage of blood from the thoracic cavity and prevent accumulation in the pericardium and mediastinum, two large-caliber tubes with multiple side holes should be inserted. One is placed just above the diaphragm and the other into the apex. Their position is maintained by skin fixation with a stitch outside the chest. In our institution the thin-walled plastic argyle tubes are routinely used. These are comfortable for the patient, and clotting is lessened but not entirely prevented. Unfortunately, clots can collect along the side holes and block the tubes, with resultant accumulation of blood within the chest. For this reason, frequent x-rays are necessary to assess the condition of the intrathoracic cavity.

Adequate pericardial drainage is as important as chest drainage because of the danger of cardiac tamponade. This may result in postoperative tachycardia or occasionally cause death. The pericardium should be closed loosely, to allow for the evacuation of serous fluid and blood. Occasionally the pericardium is not closed at all, so that the blood may escape freely into the pleural cavity. Postoperative dislocation of the heart need not be feared following cardiac operations, since the lungs are intact. Following a median sternotomy, if the pleural cavity has not been entered, the tubes are placed superiorly and inferiorly. In fact, it may be wise to insert the lower tube into the pericardial cavity at the apex of the heart. If the pleural cavity has been entered, it is desirable to make an opening in the posterior pericardium to allow free access of accumulated blood into the pleural cavity. Drainage should be assisted by continuous suction applied separately to each tube. This should be instituted during closure of the chest in order to prevent clotting within the tubes. In addition, milking the tubes by hand sometimes assists in removing the clot, and moving the patient from side to side, in addition to raising the head of the bed, will facilitate evacuation of undrained areas. Despite these maneuvers, a radiograph is mandatory to exclude unsuspected accumulation of clotted blood and fluid. However, the film may be misleading, since 500 to 1,000 ml. of blood may lie posteriorly without appearing on the film, if the x-ray is taken with the patient in the dorsal recumbent position. For this reason, the roentgenogram should be made with the patient lying at an angle of 45 degrees head up. Even in this position, a considerable amount of blood can be trapped in the gutter and behind the dome of the diaphragm. For these reasons, replenishment of the intravascular volume should remain well ahead of the calculated loss through the chest tubes.

Adequacy of the peripheral circulation is assessed clinically by the urinary output, the appearance of the extremities, and the body temperature. Progressive depletion of the circulation is manifest by restlessness, sweating, tachycardia and pallor, and by dyspnea if the patient is without ventilatory support. A marked diminution in urinary output with mottling of the extremities and cyanosis of the nail beds is ominous.

Since the blood pressure is maintained for a time by adaptive physiologic means, blood should be replaced proportionate to the amount draining into the bottles and by the central venous pressure, regardless of the arterial pressure and the pulse rate. An absolute decrease in cardiac output is apparent only by the foregoing clinical manifestations and repetitive measurements of the acid-base balance. A metabolic acidosis gradually occurs from decreased tissue perfusion; this can be temporarily ameliorated by sodium bicarbonate or THAM. If blood is unavailable, buffered Ringer's lactate solution or dextran will temporarily support the circulation when the bleeding has been controlled. However, in the face of continued exsanguination, these solutions are ineffective, due to the lack of the strong buffer hemoglobin. In addition, Isuprel (isoproterenol) or epinephrine may be advantageous for relatively short periods to sustain the faltering heart. However, without the oxygen-carrying capacity inherent in blood, despite tissue perfusion, hypoxic acidosis is inevitable.

The dilemma in treating postoperative bleeding following open-heart surgery is in the timing necessary for returning the patient to the operating room. Many cardiac patients have a preoperative hematologic profile which suggests that postoperative bleeding may occur. Circulating fibrinolysins may be present in the blood, or the bleeding and clotting time may be prolonged. If abnormal bleeding occurs, fresh blood, frozen plasma, Amicar (aminocaproic acid), protamine, and vitamin K can be given. However, during this interlude, a false sense of security may be achieved, particularly when the chest-tube drainage temporarily abates. In the authors' institution, when the intrathoracic bleeding continues in excess of 100 ml. per hour over a 4-hour period despite drug therapy and continued transfusions, the patient is returned to the operating room for exploration of the chest. Although this is usually not rewarding in discerning a specific bleeding area, the blood clots can be evacuated and the inside of the chest minutely combed with the cautery. Ordinarily this is effective in repressing further hemorrhage.

PERICARDIAL TAMPONADE (FIG. 2–3).—One of the adverse sequelae of hemorrhage is a collection of blood or fluid in the closed pericardial sac, causing a rise in intrapericardial pressure. This increases right atrial pressure and interferes with diastolic ventricular filling, thus reducing the stroke volume. The pulse pressure narrows and the blood pressure falls. However, an initial rise in venous pressure, tachycardia and vasoconstriction compensate for the tamponade in early phases. As compression of the heart progresses, the cardiac output diminishes, coronary artery perfusion is progressively decreased, and cardiac failure eventually occurs.

Pericardial tamponade following open-heart operations seldom resembles the classic description of a chronic tamponade. The latter presents a picture of a low pulse pressure, a reduction in arterial blood pressure, and a paradoxic pulse with an increased jugular venous pressure which rises markedly on inspiration. Faint heart sounds and a pericardial friction rub may be heard. The heart size is usually found to be increased radiographically and by percussion. On the other hand, acute tamponade requires a high index of suspicion and a readiness to operate to exclude the diagnosis. This suspicion should be highest when active bleeding is occurring, since the degree of bleeding from the mediastinal tubes does not necessarily substantiate the diagnosis. However, when pericardial tamponade occurs, deterioration proceeds in a characteristic fashion. Tachycardia and a mild hypotension are evident although there is a wide fluctuation in both the heart rate and the arterial blood pressure. With each temporary improvement there is further physiologic degradation. A decline in blood pressure on inspiration is common

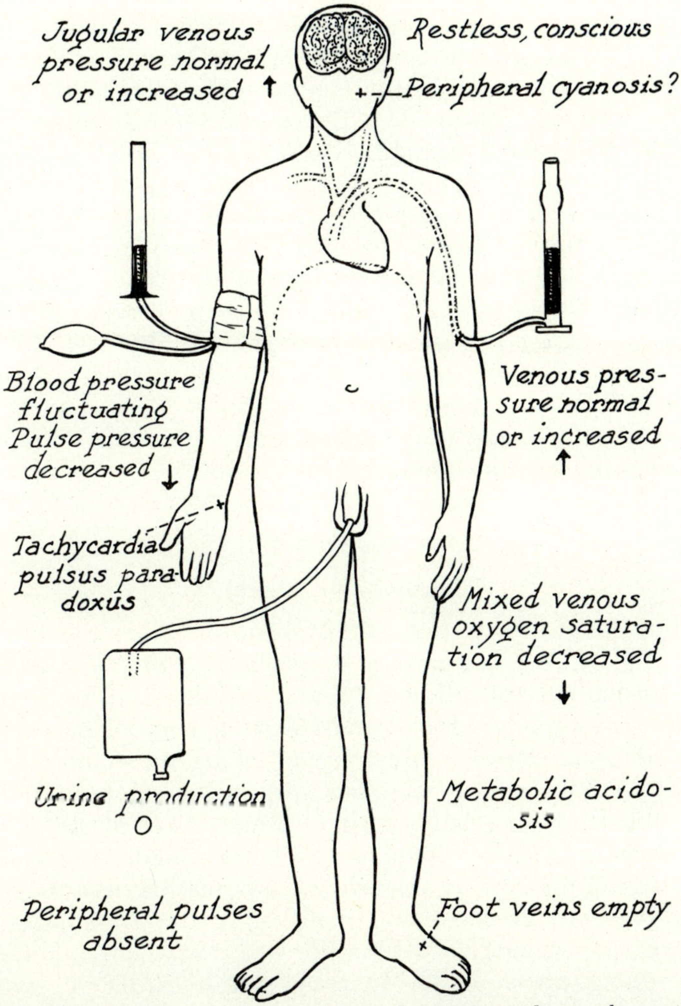

Fig. 2-3.—The changes in postoperative cardiac tamponade are shown in this diagram. Note that the jugular venous pressure and central venous pressure are not necessarily elevated. In fact, early diagnosis requires a great deal of suspicion because the patient may suddenly deteriorate before any of the textbook signs are evident.

but this should exceed 15 mm. Hg to be significant. If the patient is on positive-pressure respiration, the pulse may improve with inspiration and disappear on expiration. Inspection of the jugular venous pulsation will reveal a dominant descent of the V wave, which helps to differentiate tamponade from cardiac failure which reveals a dominant y descent. However, it must be remembered that tamponade may occur in the absence of increased central venous pressure when hypovolemia is also present. Significantly, pericardial tamponade is the only condition in which a pulseless patient may be fully conscious. The urine output is reduced but the heart sounds are essentially normal; however, a decreased cardiac thrust may be noted. Even the usual portable chest x-ray following open-heart surgery may be misleading, due to the positioning of the patient and the quality of the film. It should be remembered that even though the clinical picture of acute tamponade is fluctuant, the diagnosis can be made through steady deterioration of the patient as evidenced by tachycardia, hypotension, paradoxic pulse, a raised central venous pressure and oliguria. If the diagnosis is in doubt, 100–200 ml. of blood given rapidly will elevate the venous pressure steeply without significantly affecting the systemic pressure. The dictum should be that when tamponade is suspected, early operation is imperative without awaiting the appearance of the cardinal signs.

THE LOW CARDIAC OUTPUT SYNDROME

(Cardiogenic Shock)

A. PATHOPHYSIOLOGY (FIG. 2–4).—Cardiogenic shock implies failure of the heart as a pump. It is frequently observed as a result of a low cardiac output following massive pulmonary or myocardial infarction, arrhythmias which produce such a rapid or slow heart rate that adequate tissue perfusion cannot be maintained, and deficient myocardial reserve following intracardiac operations. The inability of the heart to sustain a blood pressure results in decreased tissue perfusion, cellular anoxia and metabolic acidosis. The peripheral manifestations are characterized by restlessness leading to agitation, cyanosis, coolness and mottling of the extremities, a decreasing urinary output, a low blood pressure with normal or slightly elevated venous pressure, and increasing tachycardia. As in hemorrhagic shock, an effort is made to maintain perfusion to the vital organs by increased sympathetic tone from stimulation of the baroreceptors. Secretion of epinephrine and norepinephrine produces vasoconstriction and increases the peripheral resistance in order to supply blood to the essential areas.

Initially, the blood volume remains unchanged and the rise in central venous pressure reflects the degree of cardiac failure. In addition, stagnation in the under-perfused areas of the viscera and the skin eventually reduces the effective circulatory blood volume, which causes further sympathetic response. Cardiac failure occurs

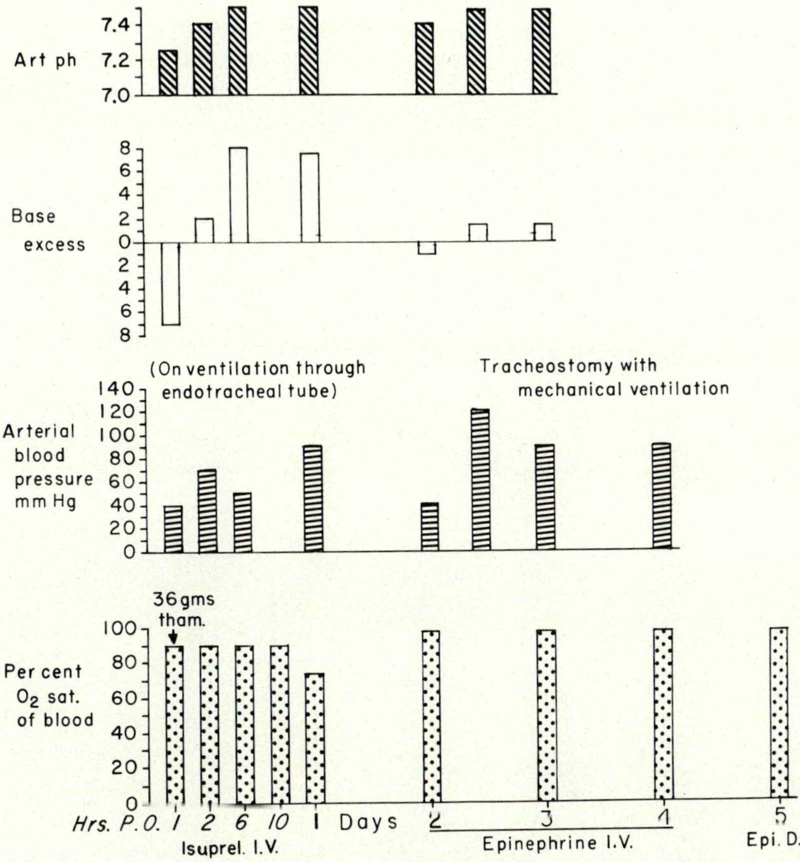

Fig. 2-4.—Graph depicting the parameters measured in a patient with a low cardiac output syndrome following a double valve procedure. Notice the low arterial pH, the low oxygen saturation, the low blood pressure and the marked base deficit immediately after surgery. THAM buffer, continuous intravenous drip of Isuprel helped to ameliorate the situation. On the second postoperative day his failure to respond to Isuprel prompted the use of epinephrine infusion (4 mg. in 250 ml. G/W). The mechanical ventilation was continued as was the epinephrine drip until the 5th day, when his physiologic response was adequate to discontinue artificial stimulation.

when the compensatory mechanisms fail and the heart becomes overdistended in diastole. The rise in diastolic pressure in the ventricle leads to an increase in the left atrial and pulmonary venous pressures. From progression of the latter, an associated rise in right atrial and peripheral venous pressure occurs, with liver distention. The cerebral and coronary circulation are maintained with priority; however, there is a progressive decrease in renal blood flow, leading to oliguria, salt and water retention, a rise in BUN and acute tubular necrosis. The hepatic blood flow is similarly reduced, with resultant physiologic aberrations. Preoperative cardiac failure is seen in patients with valvular disease, A.V. shunt, coronary insufficiency or primary myocardial disease. In the postoperative period, cardiac decompensation may be the result of hypervolemia, arrhythmias, or a reduction in coronary blood flow.

Fig. 2–5.—One of the earliest signs of left ventricular failure is a diminution in urinary output. In the more advanced form depicted here, the patient is peripherally vasoconstricted, the central venous pressure is elevated, metabolic acidosis exists and a tachycardia is present. Accumulation of fluid in the lung accounts for the dyspnea. Frank pulmonary edema occurs later unless the condition is ameliorated.

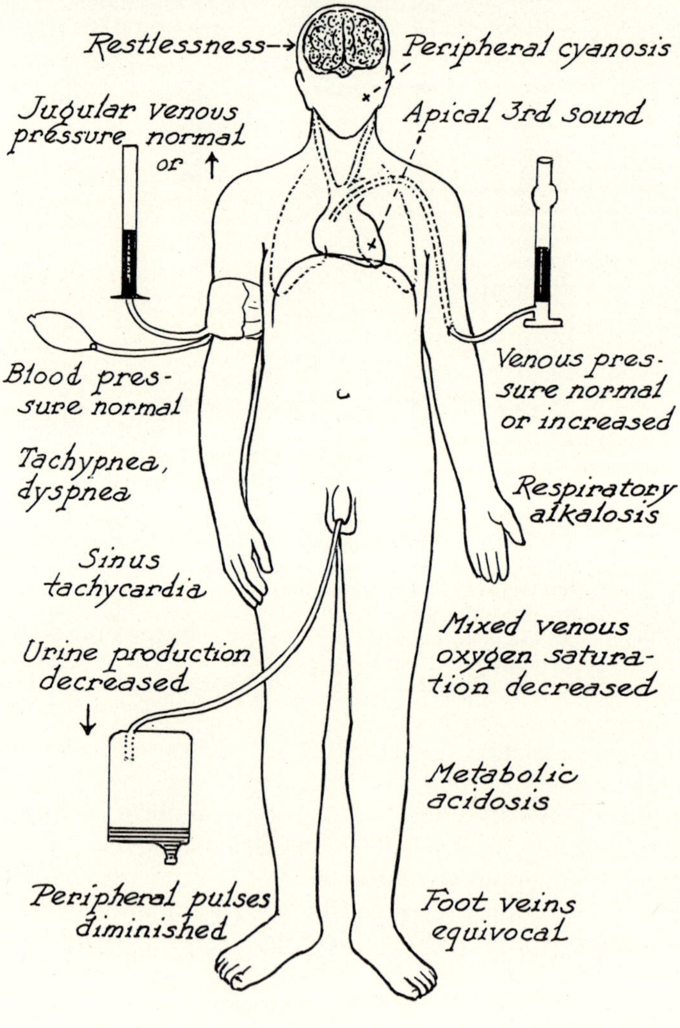

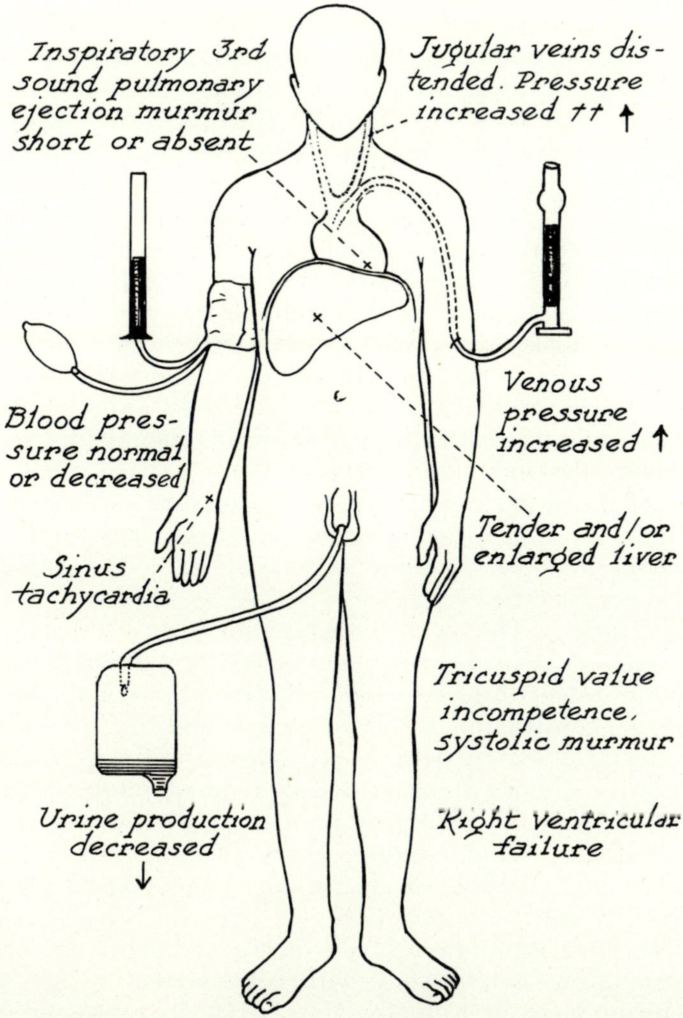

Fig. 2–6.—In right ventricular failure the findings are limited to the right side of the heart. Increased venous pressure is evident from distended jugular veins; an enlarged, tender and pulsating liver can be palpated. A murmur of tricuspid insufficiency is audible.

Clinically, it is helpful to divide heart failure according to whether the right or left ventricle is primarily involved. Left ventricular failure can be diagnosed by an elevation in left atrial pressure and increased pulmonary compliance. As the cardiac output declines, an increasing arteriovenous O_2 saturation difference occurs due to the extraction of O_2 from the blood as a result of insufficient tissue perfusion. The physical signs of left ventricular failure include tachycardia, raised jugular venous pressure, and a third heart sound. As the left ventricle weakens, cardiac output progressively falls, with evidence of cerebral ischemia ranging from irritability to stupor. Moist rales in the lungs are evident and the pulmonary compliance continues to decrease, with marked dyspnea and orthopnea. The P_{CO_2} falls, due to hyperventilation, and as the blood pressure decreases, vasoconstriction is evidenced by poor peripheral pulses, cold, cyanotic extremities and decreased capillary filling. Urine output is concomitantly reduced, with the process continuing until metabolic acidosis develops. The chest x-ray will reveal patchy consolidation and congestion and eventually frank pulmonary edema (see Fig. 2–5).

Right ventricular failure may occur separately or in combination with left ventricular failure. Auscultation may reveal a systolic murmur from tricuspid insufficiency. The right atrial pressure will be elevated and venous tracing will show a pronounced V wave with a sharp, wide descent. The arterial pressure is usually low and the presence of increased pulmonary artery pressure confirms the diagnosis. In addition, abdominal pain and tenderness due to liver engorgement may be present, with ascites, pleural effusion and peripheral edema (see Fig. 2–6).

B. TREATMENT.—The therapeutic regimen is directed at increasing the inotropic effect of the heart and reducing the peripheral resistance, thus re-establishing an equitable blood flow to all the tissues. Relief of vasoconstriction can be accomplished by 1) the reduction of the effects of sympathetic nerve stimulation (alpha-adrenergic blockade with phenoxybenzamine), 2) beta-adrenergic stimulation with isoproterenol, 3) saturation of the sympathetic nerve system with epinephrine, which reduces the vasoconstrictive response of the sympathetic stimulation, and 4) a still-undefined mechanism which occurs with massive doses of adrenal corticosteroids. In addition to drug stimulation of the heart, metabolic acidosis must be concomitantly ameliorated with alkalinizing agents such as sodium bicarbonate or tromethamine (THAM). Frequent determinations of the pH and the base deficit are mandatory to determine the metabolic state in addition to monitoring the other parameters.

The marked inotropic and chronotropic effect of isoproterenol on the heart makes it the drug of choice; 1 mg. of this drug dissolved in 500 ml. of G/W should be used initially with the aid of a microdrip. Because of the propensity of a rapid infusion or too large a dose to cause ventricular tachycardia and even fibrillation, the electrocardiogram and the arterial blood pressure should be visualized on an oscillograph screen. As a rule, by adjusting the dose to the requirements of the heart, one can usually support the circulation for long periods.

Initially, sodium bicarbonate should be infused according to the dictates of the acid-base deficit. A useful formula to correct the acidosis is $0.3 \times$ base deficit $\times$ kg. body weight equals the amount of sodium bicarbonate to be given. However, in the authors' opinion, the amount of sodium bicarbonate calculated from this formula is usually not enough to relieve the acid load. The more practical principle to follow is that proposed by Dr. Mörch in Chapter 5 on Respiratory Failure. In his opinion, when the base deficit approaches 10 mEq. per liter and the pH is low, because of the amount of sodium bicarbonate required to replenish the buffer stores, THAM is the drug of choice. At this level of metabolic acidosis, 36 gm. of THAM dissolved in 200 ml. of G/W can be rapidly infused if the patient is on a respirator. When the individual is breathing spontaneously, the buffer should be administered slowly, since apnea can occur from suddenly lowering the P_{CO_2} and creating a respiratory alkalosis. Needless to say, the base deficit should be frequently determined in order to effectively ameliorate the condition.

In the majority of patients, Isuprel will support the circulation for a considerable period of time. Others, however, fail to respond to this drug and in these individuals, epinephrine should be substituted. Four milligrams of adrenaline can be dissolved in 250 ml. of G/W and infused at a rate sufficient to elevate the blood pressure and increase the heart rate. This drug has the ability to stimulate both the alpha and beta myocardial excitatory and the peripheral depressor receptors. This results in augmentation of myocardial force and rate, a decrease in peripheral resistance, and in coronary vasodilation. In doses exceeding 1.5 μg./kg./min., peripheral vasoconstriction becomes dominant, resulting in decreased peripheral venous return and cardiac output and thus defeats the purpose. In smaller doses, epinephrine produces primarily a cardiotonic response with an increase in peripheral and splanchnic blood flow without evidence of significant vasoconstriction. Regardless of the drug used, the metabolic acidosis must be concomitantly corrected.

Considerable information has accrued as to the value of adrenergic blocking agents such as phenoxybenzamine (Dibenzyline). This drug may be worth using when the two previously mentioned cardiotonic drugs are ineffectual. However, one must be certain that volume deficits do not exist, as the marked fall in blood pressure may result in cardiac arrest.

Corticosteroids have also been found beneficial in shock, although their modus operandi is not clear. However, it is apparent that in large doses they can decrease peripheral resistance and increase tissue perfusion and venous return, thereby eradicating the stagnant pools of blood which occur in the shock state. Thus they tend to improve oxygenation of the tissue and reduce cellular anoxia and metabolic acidosis. In addition, it has been suggested that corticoids may directly diminish accumulation of lactic acid in the cell by enhancing conversion of lactate to glucose.

Added to the hemodynamic effects of corticoids may be their secondary effect on the maintenance of tissue integrity. Under normal conditions the subcellular particle, the hormone and its powerful hydrolic enzymes appear to play an essential role in intracellular digestion. Various noxious stimuli apparently cause loss of the lysosomal integrity and allow lysosomal enzymes to escape within the cell. Although much about the lysosomal response remains to be learned, it appears that lysosomal enzymes, once released, digest their host cell and then damage the neighboring cells. Studies of animals in shock demonstrate that massive doses of corticoids may stabilize cell walls and prevent lysosomal enzyme release.

The dose which we have used corresponds to that advocated by Lillehei and his group: 1) methyl prednisolone (Solu-Medrol) 30 mg./kg., 2) dexamethasone phosphate (Decadron) 6 mg./kg., and 3) hydrocortisone sodium succinate (Solu-Cortef) 150 mg./kg. body weight.

The Management of Cardiac Pacemakers

The use of permanent artificial pacemakers for the prevention of Adams-Stokes syndrome, the treatment of intractable heart failure due to persistent bradycardia, congenital and iatrogenic heart block, and heart block associated with myocardial infarctions is well established. In addition, temporary pacing is indicated in patients with acute myocardial infarction who have 1) a 2nd and 3rd degree A.V. block, 2) normal sinus rhythm with interventricular conduction disturbances such as bundle branch blocks, 3) episodes of cardiac arrest, 4) bradycardia or prolonged P-R interval causing congestive heart failure, or 5) tachyarrhythmias refractory to drugs. In some clinics, pacemaker wires are routinely inserted into the myocardium after open-heart operation.

Technic of transvenous pacemaker insertion.—Since the methodology has some bearing on the problems encountered postoperatively, the operative technic is pertinent. Under local anesthesia, a short transverse skin incision is made over the sternocleidomastoid muscle just above the right clavicle, and the latter is separated between its medial and lateral insertions. The internal jugular vein is exposed and ligated distally and a tourniquet ligature is positioned proximally. An incision is made in the vein between the ligatures and a catheter electrode is passed under fluoroscopy through the vein into the apex of the right ventricle. After satisfactory pacing has been achieved and the threshold determined, which is usually less than 1.5 milliamperes, the stylets are removed and the catheter electrode is secured firmly to the internal jugular vein by placing a heavy silk ligature around the vein and the electrode. The distally placed ligature on the internal jugular vein likewise is tied around the catheter electrode. No attempt should be made to anchor the electrode to adjacent structures.

The catheter electrode should form a gentle curve in the right atrium in order to transmit slight tension to the tip wedged in the apex of the right ventricle. The proper amount of tension can be ascertained by evidence under fluoroscopy of minimal buckling of the catheter near its tip with each cardiac systole. The patient is instructed

Fig. 2–7.—Medial position of the electrode as it courses over the head of the clavicle. This position prevents the movements of the clavicle from causing motion on the electrode.

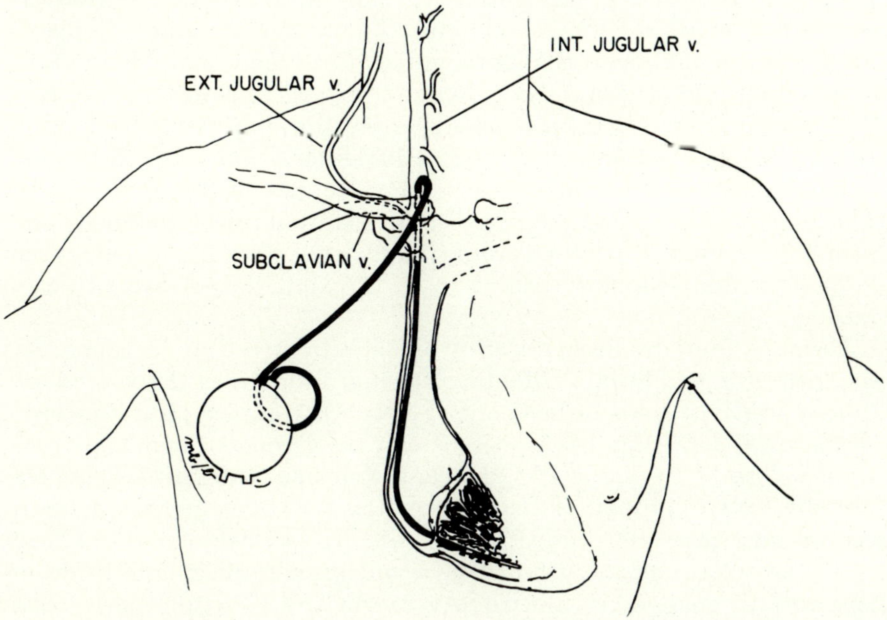

to cough and breathe deeply while the position and stability of the intercardiac electrode is observed under fluoroscopy (see Fig. 2–7).

A transverse skin incision is then made 3 to 4 cm. above the right nipple and over the lateral border of the pectoralis major muscle. A pocket is fashioned beneath this muscle by blunt and sharp dissection. This is connected with the cervical incision by creating a tunnel, with a long, curved Kelly clamp, between the layers of the pectoralis major and minor muscles. The instrument is then brought through the pectoralis major muscle and passed anteriorly over the medial end of the clavicle to the cervical incision.

The ends of the catheter electrode are placed inside a Penrose drain and fixed in place with a heavy ligature. In this manner the electrode can be brought easily through the tunnel without damage to the wires. The pulse generator is connected to the electrodes and inserted into the previously fashioned pocket after hemostasis has been obtained. A final view of the entire course of the catheter electrode is made by fluoroscopy in order to eliminate any sharp angulations before closing the incision. The lateral edge of the pectoralis major muscle is sutured to the fascia overlying the lateral chest wall. This helps to prevent the pulse generator from eroding through the skin from pressure necrosis. After the procedure, the patient is returned to the intensive care unit, where the ECG is constantly monitored for 24–48 hours. To prevent electrode displacement, complete bedrest is maintained for 1 to 2 days, with instructions to avoid lying on the right side. When temporary pacing is advisable, the transvenous electrodes are inserted through either the antecubital, cephalic, femoral or external jugular veins and positioned in the right ventricle under fluoroscopic control, if this is available. The electrodes are then attached to an external pulse generator and pacing instituted. If pacing is required for over 3 weeks, it is essential to convert the temporary pacing to an implantable permanent pacemaker.

Drugs.—Digitalis and diuretics are administered as indicated by the patient's condition. Dilantin 100 mg. four times daily is given intravenously if signs of myocardial irritability appear, and lidocaine (Xylocaine) 1 mg./kg. body weight can be given intravenously as a single dose if frequent PVC's occur. Cardiac arrhythmias are extremely rare if proper electrode position has been obtained; their occurrence may be indicative of electrode dislodgment. Chest x-rays are obtained daily for 3 days and prior to discharge in order to ascertain changes in electrode position and to detect pericardial effusion. Antibiotics are given for 5–7 days.

Complications

Infection.—Infection remains one of the most important and dangerous complications of permanent transvenous pacemaker insertion. In order to minimize bacterial contamination, the operation should ideally be performed in the operating room with a portable image intensifier. However, since this is not ordinarily possible, the procedure has to be done either in the x-ray department or the cardiopulmonary laboratory.

By using the internal jugular vein for the insertion of the electrode, manipulation of the electrode catheter has been reduced, which minimizes the chance of contamination. Also, skin necrosis, another source of infection, is avoided by placing the pulse generator pocket under the pectoralis muscle, and carefully suturing the lateral edge of the pectoralis muscle to fascia overlying the lateral chest wall.

Hemostasis is mandatory, especially in the pulse generator pocket. Although many groups have advocated the use of drains in this area, we have found them to be unnecessary and believe they may be a source of pocket contamination. However, if hemostasis is inadequate, a drain should be used to avoid a hematoma, which has a propensity to become infected.

The use of antibiotics in the postoperative period is controversial, but we believe that whenever a foreign body is placed in the vascular system, sepsis may be avoided by administration of postoperative antibiotics.

Once an infection is established, three principles must be adhered to if recovery is to be expected. 1) All foreign material must be removed before the infection can be eradicated. 2) A new permanent pacemaker should be implanted in a clean area, preferably after the infection has been eliminated. 3) Electrical pacing of the heart must be uninterrupted while the infection is treated.

These principles are at times in conflict and therefore it is essential to stage the treatment. The first step consists in the percutaneous placement of a temporary transvenous electrode via the femoral vein. This electrode is connected to an external power source. All the foreign material is then removed. This may require a thoracotomy if the previously placed electrodes are epicardial or the previously placed endocardial electrode has become firmly fibrosed to the endocardial wall. The transvenous electrodes should be removed from proximal to distal so far as possible, thus avoiding the proximal extent of infection. The pulse generator pocket should be left open so that it can close by secondary intention. After the infection has cleared and all wounds are healed completely, the third stage is undertaken. This consists of the insertion of a new permanent transvenous pacemaker in a site as far from the previous site of insertion as feasible. Following the insertion of the new pacemaker, the temporary pacemaker leads are removed from the femoral vein.

Dislodgment of electrodes.—The diagnosis of dislodgment is suspected by intermittent pacing or failure to pace and usually occurs within 48 hours after insertion. The diagnosis is confirmed by a PA chest x-ray, which will show the electrode displaced either into the right atrium or into the right ventricular outflow tract. Once this has occurred the electrode must be repositioned under fluoroscopic control.

Since we began using the right internal jugular vein for insertion of the electrode, we have not encountered electrode dislodgment, which frequently occurred when the catheter was inserted through the external jugular vein. The electrode is secured 1 cm. distal to the point of entrance into the vein and passes in front of the clavicle. If possible, a gentle curve in the electrode is established as it enters into the right ventricular apex. The catheter tip should flex very slightly with each ventricular systole if the electrode is properly positioned in the trabeculae of the right ventricle.

Myocardial perforation.—Myocardial perforation can be prevented by proper insertion of the electrode. If the curve in the electrode is too acute or the electrode catheter too stiff, excessive pressure may be exerted on the myocardial wall and perforation of the right ventricle will occur. This complication is most often encountered during positioning of the electrode, and its incidence has been markedly reduced with the advent of the more flexible transvenous catheters. However, a rising pacemaker threshold, a pericardial friction rub and diaphragmatic pacing are suggestive of a myocardial perforation. If suspected, a chest x-ray should be obtained and a fluoroscopic examination performed to confirm the diagnosis.

While pericardial tamponade has been reported, usually repositioning of the electrode is all that is necessary for the correction of this complication. It is advisable to obtain daily serial x-rays for 3 to 4 days following repositioning to guard against a fatality. If pericardial tamponade occurs, unless it is massive, it should be aspirated on two occasions, and if it recurs, open operation should be performed.

Wire fracture.—This complication is most frequently diagnosed by intermittent pacing which the patient may or may not relate to position. If bipolar electrodes are used, the patient may note pacing of pectoral muscles, which frequently can be heard with a stethoscope. The chest x-ray may demonstrate the site of fracture. When a fixed-rate pulse generator is used, the ECG will reveal pacemaker spikes that have no relationship to the cardiac action. However, if a demand pacemaker unit has been inserted, the ECG will reveal no pacing spikes. It then becomes essential to determine if the problem is one of a fractured wire or a pulse-generator failure. By using the external rate control and setting it at a rate in excess of the heart rate, the function of the pulse generator can be determined.

Correction consists of replacement of the electrode wire. If the fracture occurs prior to fibrosis of the electrode to the endocardium, the wire can be removed and a new electrode inserted. However, if fibrosis has occurred, there is danger of evulsing part of the ventricular wall with removal of the electrode. In this situation, it is more feasible to cut the first electrode and insert a new transvenous electrode through a secondary venous route. Rarely, it may even be necessary to splice an electrode but this is definitely not recommended.

Electronic failures.—Although an occasional malfunction of the pulse generator may be encountered, premature battery failure remains one of the most frequent causes of pacemaker failure. The diagnosis is suspected when the electrode position and continuity are confirmed by a chest x-ray and fluoroscopy. Once the malfunction is established by special testing devices, a new pulse generator can be inserted.

ORGANIZATION OF A PACEMAKER CLINIC.—Institutions which insert a moderate number of transvenous pacemakers might well consider the organization of a pacemaker clinic. This clinic should be located where both medical and electronic facilities are available and where follow-up procedures can be carried out in a routine manner. Due to the advanced age of the majority, the patients in whom pacemakers are inserted may suffer from purely medical disabilities or from problems associated with malfunction of the pacemaker or from a combination of these.

One to two days prior to discharge, control values are established for subsequent comparison. The apex rate is accurately measured and a prolonged recording of one ECG lead is made to detect ectopic beats. A penetrated PA and lateral chest films are taken to establish the position of the transvenous electrode. If a calibrated oscilloscope for the measurement of impulse duration, form and height of the stimulus deflection in millivolts is available, a photograph of this should be taken prior to discharge. Upon discharge, the patient is given a card stating that he is being treated with a particular type of artificial pacemaker, the date of its insertion, the rate of the pacemaker, and the name of the hospital where the operation was performed.

The patient is instructed to return to the clinic if at any time he is concerned about the integrity of the pacemaker system. He is informed that the usual indications of pacemaker failure are: 1) syncopal or near syncopal attacks, 2) pulse variation of more than 5 beats per minute from the control rate, 3) palpitation or mis-beats, 4) pain around the pacemaker site, 5) evidence of infection of the pacemaker system.

In the absence of the above signs and symptoms, the patient is asked to return to the clinic in 1 month and then at 3-month intervals. At each visit, a careful history is taken and a thorough clinical examination is carried out. The pacemaker rate is checked and a prolonged strip of the ECG tracing is printed out to confirm stable pacing. Measurement of the impulse duration, stimulus amplitude and form are taken, if equipment is available. The patient also obtains a chest x-ray to evaluate the position and continuity of the system.

PART 2.

Cardiac Arrhythmias and Cardiopulmonary Arrest

WILLIAM E. NEVILLE, M.D.

CARDIAC ARRHYTHMIAS are a frequent and troublesome complication in the course of patients after cardiopulmonary surgery. The lethal potentiality of an arrhythmia depends upon its effect on the cardiac output. Benign arrhythmias such as premature ventricular contractions (PVC's) may proceed to a grave arrhythmia such as ventricular tachycardia, if unrecognized and inadequately treated. Avoidance of well-known factors that can precipitate abnormalities in sinus rhythm is mandatory. These include correction of electrolyte imbalance, hypoxia, hypovolemia, restlessness, pain, and digitalis

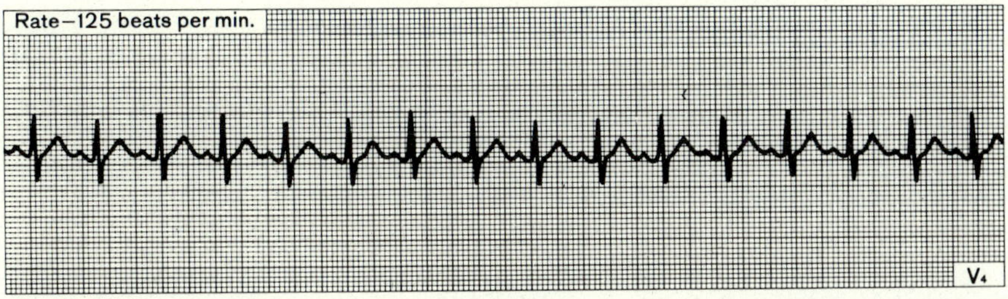

Fig. 2–8.—Sinus tachycardia. Sinus rhythm with rates above 100 beats per minute and below 160 (adult).

intoxication. Needless to say, constant monitoring of the electrocardiogram is essential.

Supraventricular tachycardia is a term used to denote an abnormality in which the ventricles receive a regular stimulus from the A.V. node in the usual manner regardless of the rhythm of the auricles. It is differentiated from some of the other atrial arrhythmias by the presence of P waves and a fast, regular rhythm, whereas in nodal tachycardia, P waves appear before, within, or after the normal QRS complex. In both instances, the heart rate is usually greater than 140 beats/min. Supraventricular tachycardia can be distinguished from ventricular tachycardia by the complete absence of any sign of an atrial contraction in the latter condition. That is extremely important because of the more ominous signs of ventricular tachycardia (see Fig. 2–8).

Atrial extrasystoles, or premature atrial beats, may arise in any part of the auricle muscle. On the electrocardiogram, the premature beats are difficult to detect but their presence is often suspected when the intervals between the QRS complexes become irregular. The abnormal P wave is often swallowed up in the preceding QRS complex or it may occur on top of the T wave. The significance of atrial premature contractions is not fully understood, since they may occur in both conscious and unconscious patients and in normal and abnormal hearts.

Atrial tachycardia (see Fig. 2–9) is a rapid, regular supraventricular rhythm commonly seen postoperatively. The rate is usually between 140 and 180 beats/min. Carotid sinus massage will occasionally cause an abrupt cessation of the tachycardia.

As a rule, atrial tachycardia will respond to sedation. Preoperative digitalization is a good preventive measure. If the administration of digitalis was interrupted 24–48 hours prior to cardiac surgery, the

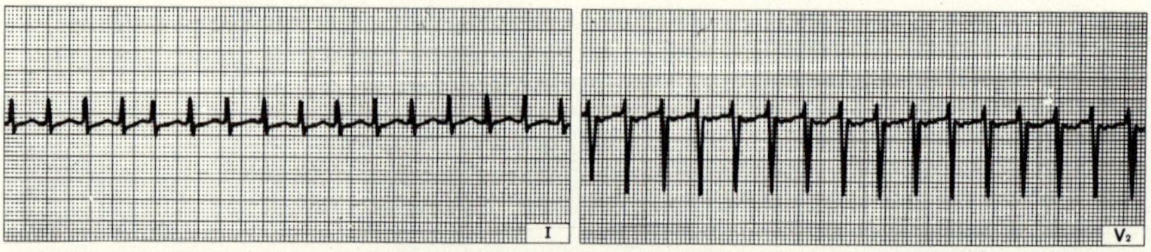

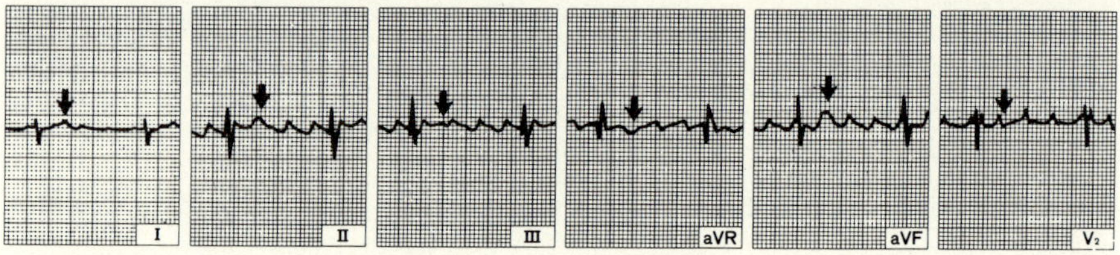

Fig. 2–9 (above).—Paroxysmal atrial tachycardia. Ectopic atrial focus; buried P waves in I, present in V_2. Rhythm regular. May show minor ST segment depressions in precordial lead.

Fig. 2–10 (below).—Atrial flutter. Sawtooth flutter waves may occur at rates of 220–350 per minute. Sawtooth flutter waves seen in II, III, aVF. Regular atrial rhythm 4:1 ventricular response. 2nd flutter wave (indicated by arrows) altered by superimposition on T wave.

administration of a regular daily dose of the digitalis preparation will control the tachycardia in most cases.

Atrial flutter (see Fig. 2–10) is generally associated with significant heart disease and is more difficult to manage than atrial fibrillation. In this condition, the rate is generally between 200–350 beats/min. and is nearly always associated with some degree of atrioventricular block, so that the ventricle beats at one-half or one-quarter of the auricle; thus there is a 2–1 or 4–1 block. The saw-toothed appearance of the ECG is due to the presence of numerous F waves, which in reality are multiple P waves of relatively high voltage. The P-R interval is absent and the ventricular rate may be regular or irregular. When there is no A.V. block, the presence of F waves with a saw-toothed appearance may be difficult to recognize. The treatment of choice is electronic cardioversion.

Atrial fibrillation (see Fig. 2–11). The essential difference between atrial fibrillation and atrial flutter is that in the latter, the atrial twitches occur at a slower rate. In both conditions, the impulse often reaches the A.V. node when it is in a refractory state, so that some degree of heart block is always present. The ventricular response is closely irregular, with short and long cycles occurring without reason. This arrhythmia is frequently encountered in patients with mitral valvular pathology, ischemic heart disease, or following pneumonectomy in elderly patients.

Although it may be innocuous, atrial fibrillation can become a problem. Ventricular rates between 130 and 160/min. require active therapy, since diastolic filling is impeded and cardiac output is decreased. Correction is usually accomplished with the administration of a digitalis preparation until the ventricular rate is controlled in the range of 60 to 80 beats/min. at rest.

Occasionally when the arrhythmia has occurred postoperatively, it may revert spontaneously to a sinus mechanism. Often, reversion of atrial fibrillation requires the administration of quinidine sulfate or the application of electric cardioversion.

Nodal rhythm (see Fig. 2–12) occurs when the pacemaker wanders to atrioventricular node or even to the bundle of His. This may occur for a few isolated contractions or the whole rhythm of the heart beat may be controlled from this site for long periods of time. The impulse passes to the ventricles in the normal manner, so that the ventricular complex is unchanged; it reaches the atria, however, in the reverse manner, so the atrial contraction occurs either immediately before or just after the ventricular complex. If the focus of origin is near the atrial A.V. node, it will reach the atrium rapidly and a short P-R interval will be seen on the electrocardioscope. On the other hand, if the focus of origin is low down in the bundle of His, the impulse may not reach the atrium until after the ventricle is contracted or it may be swallowed up in the QRS complex. Thus, nodal rhythm is exemplified by a short P-R interval and an occasional

Fig. 2–11 (above).—Atrial fibrillation. Asynchronous atrial contractions. Rapid, irregular f waves. Totally irregular ventricular response.

Fig. 2–12 (below).—A.V. nodal tachycardia. A.V. node becomes pacemaker. Rate 182. P waves which should be negative in II, III, and aVF, are obscured in all leads. P waves may be identified in special esophageal leads.

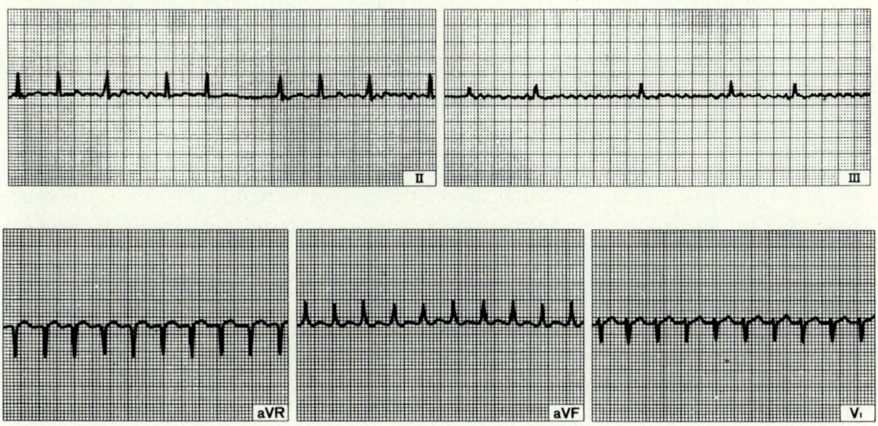

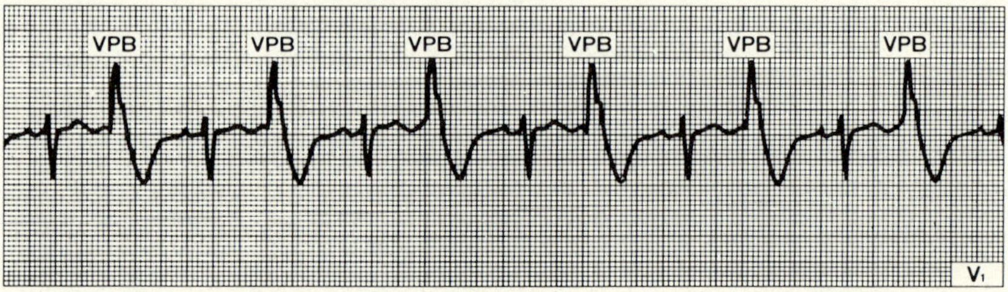

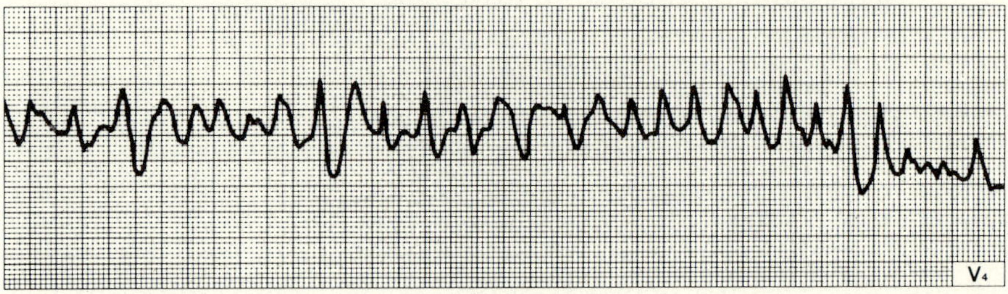

Fig. 2–13 (above).—Ventricular bigeminy. Alternating sinus beats and VPB's. Interval between sinus beat and VPB is constant, suggesting that sinus beat is related to discharge of ectopic focus in ventricle. VPB's are not triggered by the sinus P waves that immediately precede them.

Fig. 2–14 (below).—Ventricular fibrillation. Rapid rate; irregular rhythm. No discrete complexes. May terminate in asystole as terminal event.

absence of P waves, which are superimposed segments. This type of rhythm leads to a reduction in cardiac output.

Ventricular extrasystoles (premature ventricular contractions) (see Figs. 2–13 and 2–14) arise from ectopic foci in any part of the ventricular muscle. The spread of this impulse is abnormal, so that the result and potential differ from the normal. The shape and size depends upon whether the impulse arises in the left or right ventricle and whether in the basilar or apical region. Usually the complexes are large and broad but occasionally they are coarsely notched, with the T wave pointing in the direction opposite to the main deflection. After this contraction, the ventricle is refractory when the atrial impulse occurs, so that it fails to elicit a ventricular response. Therefore, the heart must await the next impulse before it can make another response. Sometimes ventricular foci occur regularly with every second beat (bigemini) or with every third beat (trigemini). Their appearance may foreshadow the onset of ventricular fibrillation (V.F.) and for this reason should be a cause for concern in the postoperative period. This type of rhythm is prone to occur in the presence of hypoxia or raised carbon dioxide tension and is seen in digitalis intoxication, hypokalemia, congestive heart failure, myocardial ischemia and infarction.

Treatment

The first step in the treatment is an attempt to correct the precipitating factors, following which drug therapy can be instituted (see Table 2-1). Lidocaine (Xylocaine) is preferable, and 1 mg./kg. of body weight may be given intravenously as an initial dose. If this does not abolish the arrhythmia, additional 1 mg./kg. doses are infused every 3 to 5 minutes until the PVC's disappear or a total dose of 5 mg./kg. is given over a period of 15 to 20 minutes.

The recurrence or persistence of frequent PVC's may warrant the administration of a continuous intravenous drip of lidocaine (2,000 mg. in 1,000 ml. of 5% D/W, to drip at a rate of 1 ml./min. and therefore deliver 2 mg. of lidocaine/min.). To avoid central nervous system side effects, the dose should not exceed 300 mg./hr.

Diphenylhydantoin (Dilantin), 100 mg. given intravenously every 8 hours, or procainamide (Pronestyl) are occasionally helpful but are not employed as frequently as lidocaine.

When PVC's are secondary to digitalis intoxication, an intravenous infusion of potassium chloride (40 mEq. in 250 ml. of 5% dextrose in water, given over a period of 2-3 hours) may be very rewarding. When the arrhythmia is refractory to the preceding drugs, 1-3 mg. of propranolol (Inderal) administered intravenously has also been used with excellent results

Ventricular tachycardia (see Fig. 2-15) is produced by a succession of ectopic beats which arise from a single focus or multiple foci. The heart rate is usually above 140 beats/min.; the QRS complex is widened, and frequently the S-T segment is masked by the next QRS complex. The P waves are absent, although, by using different leads, it is sometimes possible to pick up isolated beats. The onset of ventricular tachycardia is particularly ominous in that the increased irritability is the precursor of ventricular fibrillation and suggests myocardial ischemia. Quinidine may restore sinus rhythm but it must not be prescribed in the presence of an A.V. block, since it may cause ventricular fibrillation. Intravenous procainamide (Pronestyl) (250 mg.) or procaine (1 gm., or 10 ml. of 10% solution) may stop ventricular tachycardia. However, both these drugs may produce a severe fall in blood pressure when injected intravenously and for this reason lidocaine is probably the drug of choice. In addition, Pronestyl and procaine cause a prolongation of the P-R on the

TABLE 2-1.—TREATMENT OF ARRHYTHMIAS

Ventricular Premature Beats

Lidocaine: 50 mg. or 1 mg. per kg. body weight, given I.V. as a bolus (2–5 min.). If not effective, give 1/2 the dose in 5 min. If effective: 2,000 mg. lidocaine in 1,000 ml. 5% D/W, to drip at a rate of 1 ml. per min. (2 mc. per min.).
Dilantin: 100 to 250 mg. given within a few minutes (largely replaced by lidocaine).
Procainamide (Pronestyl): 50 mg. every 2–3 min. I.V. up to 1,000 mg. until the arrhythmia is abolished. (Constant monitoring of ECG and B.P. needed.)
Quinidine sulfate: 0.2 to 0.4 Gm. every 2 hr. for 5 doses, or every 6 hr. (Maintenance dose: 0.2 to 0.4 Gm. q. 6 hr.)

PVC's Secondary to Digitalis Intoxication

KCl: 40 mEq. in 1,000 ml. 5% D/W.
EDTA: (Ethylenediaminetetraacetic acid): 50 mg. per kg. in 200 ml. of 5% D/W infused over 30 min.

Sinus Bradycardia After Acute Myocardial Infarction

Atropine: 0.3 to 1.2 mg. I.V. or I.M. every 2 to 4 hrs.
Isuprel: 1 mg. diluted in 500 ml. 5% D/W intravenous by microdrip.

Ventricular Tachycardia

Lidocaine: 50 mg. bolus at once I.V., followed by 100 mg. if not effective. If not successful:
Synchronized electrocardioversion: 10 to 200 watt-seconds.

Ventricular Fibrillation

Artificial respiration (endotracheal tube and Ambu bag) and closed-chest cardiac massage.
Electrocardioversion: 200 to 400 watt-seconds.
Sodium bicarbonate: I.V. 40 mEq. every 5–8 min. to combat acidosis, if resuscitation must be continued for any length of time.
Once defibrillation is accomplished, continue prophylaxis as described for PVC's.

Atrial Flutter

Digitalis or quinidine sulfate may be tried, but the treatment of choice is cardioversion.

Complete A.V. Block (After Acute M.I.)

Atropine: 0.3 to 1.2 mg. I.V. (repeat q. 4 hrs. if necessary). If effective give:
Isuprel: 5–15 mg. sublingually q. 1 to 6 hrs. or 0.2 mg. I.V. (slowly). Better: 2 mg. in 1,000 ml. 5% D/W and titrate. About 2 ml. per min. or 20 to 30 drops per min.
Epinephrine: 4 ml. of 1:1,000 (4 mg.) in 1,000 ml. of 5% D/W. (Run about 1 ml. per min.) Watch for ventricular irritability!
Steroids: Solu-Cortef: 100 mg. I.V.) Repeat 2–6 hrs.
Solu-Cortef: 40 mg. I.V.)
Transvenous catheter pacemakers.

Atrial Tachycardia

Sometimes can be terminated by carotid sinus pressure or induced vomiting. Morphine S.C. or I.V. if patient is on a respirator may cause conversion. Digoxin may relieve; in hypotensive patients, phenylephrine HCl (Neo-Synephrine) may be beneficial. This is given as a dose of 0.3 ml. of 1% solution diluted to 1 ml.

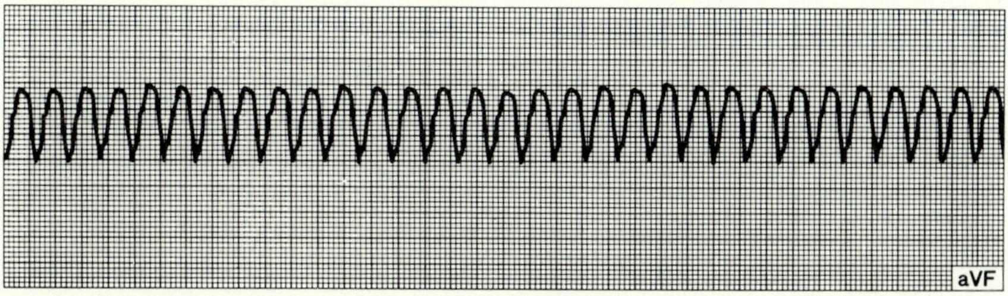

Fig. 2-15.—Ventricular tachycardia. Rate variable from 140 to 250 beats per minute. Slightly irregular rhythm. Wide, slurred QRS complexes of ventricular premature beats. S-T segment and T waves indistinguishable. There is an independent slower P rate, but the P waves are often obscured.

Q-T interval, with widening of the QRS complex, and may precipitate ventricular ectopic beats.

If lidocaine, given intravenously at up to 300 mg./hr., does not elicit a response, Inderal can be infused. The latter drug should be used cautiously and in low doses, since abolition of the sympathetic drive to the heart may precipitate cardiac arrest. In all probability, when synchronized cardioversion technics are available, electric shock should be instituted prior to treatment with beta-adrenergic blocking agents. An initial shock of 100–300 watt-seconds may convert the tachycardia to sinus rhythm.

If conversion cannot be established by the foregoing methods, it may be feasible to insert an intravenous electrode through a peripheral vein into the right ventricle. An external pacemaker can then be applied and, with repetitive stimuli, the ventricular rate may be slowed. The disadvantage of this technic is that it should be done under fluoroscopic control, which is not available in the intensive care unit.

Heart block (see Fig. 2–16) designates some form of delay in the

Fig. 2-16.—Complete A.V. block (third degree block). Independent regular atrial and ventricular rhythms. Atrial rate 72/min. Ventricular rate 54. S.A. impulses do not depolarize the ventricles.

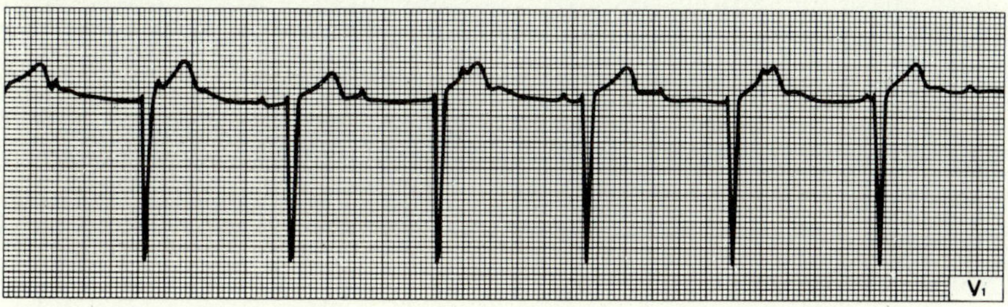

passage of impulses through the main conducting pathway of the A.V. node or the bundle of His. In a mild case, the length of the time (the P-R interval) taken for an impulse to traverse its junctional tissue is lengthened. As the defect increases, the electrical impulses from auricles find it increasingly difficult to reach the ventricles, until one impulse finally is blocked. In this manner, there may be two or three atrial beats for every ventricular contraction; thus a two-to-one or three-to-one heart block occurs. In severe cases, the defect may be such as to block all conduction and a complete heart block occurs. In these instances the atria, dictated by the S.A. node, continue to contract at their own rate, while the ventricular rhythm is controlled by a pacemaker, which arises immediately below the block in the A.V. node or the bundle of His. Since the inherent rhythmicity of the ventricles is slow, the rate is regular but is only 30 beats or so a minute.

Differential diagnosis between complete and partial heart block is made by following the P waves. In partial heart block, two or more P waves occur to each ventricular beat. However, a ventricular contraction occurs regularly following a P wave and there is an increase in the P-R interval. In complete heart block, there are regular P waves in the QRS complexes, each of which is totally unrelated to the other. There is a widely varying P-R interval and a slow ventricular rhythm of about 30 beats/min.

A bundle branch block is caused by disease in one or other of the conducting bundles below the bundle of His. The principal features of a bundle branch block are (1) a normal rhythm, (2) widening and sometimes notching of the QRS complex, and (3) a T wave which moves in the direction opposite to the main deflection. The direction of the main deflection in leads I and III signifies whether the left or the right bundle is defective.

Treatment

Several drugs are useful in the management of complete heart block. Atropine sulfate (0.3 to 1.2 mg.) given intravenously is efficacious and may be repeated every 4 to 6 hours. However, Isuprel is the most effective drug at present. It may be given sublingually in doses of 5–15 mg. every 1 to 6 hours or intravenously as a drip. In our institution, 1 mg. of Isuprel dissolved in 500 ml. of 5% dextrose in water is infused at the rate of 20 to 30 drops/min. Epinephrine may also be used in a dilution of 4 ml. of a 1:1,000 solution (4 mg.) in 1 liter of 5% dextrose in water, infused at a rate of 1 ml./min. Both epinephrine and Isuprel may produce ventricular irritability, so careful monitoring of the electrocardiogram is required.

Individuals with frequent syncopal attacks should have a temporary bipolar-electrode pacemaker catheter inserted into the right ventricle as soon as possible. The frequency should be set high enough to overcome the idioventricular focus. Preparations can then be made for the insertion of a permanent pacemaker.

Cardiopulmonary arrest is defined as the sudden cessation of cardiac output which can occur from (1) ventricular fibrillation, (2) cardiac asystole, and (3) profound cardiovascular collapse. Since the effective circulation of oxygenated blood suddenly ceases, irreversible death of the brain occurs within 4 to 6 minutes.

Causes of cardiac arrest.—Hypoxia, secondary to inadequate pulmonary ventilation, is the etiologic factor in the majority of cases of cardiac arrest. Cardiac standstill may also occur during intubation, from a vagovagal reflex, and certain anesthetic agents are known to produce ventricular irritability which, in the absence of hypoxia, may result in ventricular fibrillation. Prolonged preoperative administration of digitalis and diuretics may cause electrolyte imbalance which, combined with hypoxia or anesthetic agents, may result in cardiac arrest.

Cardiovascular collapse may develop during a prolonged operation during which blood-volume replacement has been inadequate. For this reason, blood loss should be carefully monitored and adequately replaced.

Coronary-artery patients undergoing operation require monitoring of the blood pressure, inasmuch as a fall in arterial pressure may initiate a coronary occlusion from thrombosis. This may precipitate ventricular fibrillation or profound cardiovascular collapse.

Cardiopulmonary resuscitation.—Constant monitoring of the patient during the operation and in the postoperative period is fundamental in the diagnosis of cardiopulmonary arrest, since the outcome will depend upon early recognition. Once the diagnosis of cardiac arrest is made, regardless of the cause, immediate action should be taken.

1. Artificial circulation must be maintained either by external or direct cardiac massage.
2. The lungs must be effectively ventilated.
3. Metabolic acidosis must be corrected.
4. The type of cardiac arrest must be determined from an electrocardiogram.
5. Coexisting hypovolemia must be ameliorated.

Although closed-chest massage is the treatment of choice in cardiac arrest, direct massage of the heart is indicated when the chest is already open or when cardiac tamponade is present.

External cardiac massage is best accomplished by the compression of the heart between the sternum and the spine by rhythmically depressing the lower third of the sternum 3–4 cm. from 60 to 80 times per minute. The compression is maintained for one-half second with rapid release. To accomplish this, the patient must be placed on a firm surface which will support the spine and thus allow the heart to be compressed between it and the sternum. In nonintubated patients, an endotracheal tube should be inserted as soon as possible.

When direct cardiac massage is indicated, an incision is made in the left fifth intercostal space. The heart is grasped with the hand and compressed 60 to 80 times per minute through the pericardium or against the sternum. If this is unsatisfactory, the pericardium should be opened so that both hands can be used, one placed anteriorly and the other posteriorly to the heart, to achieve better compression. As soon as possible, a rib spreader must be inserted to ease the pressure on the wrists of the operator.

Adequate oxygenation is paramount. Outside the operating room this is best accomplished by mouth-to-mouth or mouth-to-nose resuscitation by one person while another initiates cardiac massage. In the operation room, the anesthesiologist should ventilate the patient's lungs with 100% O_2 and the anesthetic discontinued.

The type of cardiac arrest should be determined as soon as possible by an electrocardiogram if the chest has not been opened. Ventricular fibrillation requires electrical defibrillation, accomplished by applying the electrode paddles directly to the heart or by placing the electrodes on the chest wall, one over the apex and the other over the base of the heart. A direct-current (D.C.) type of defibrillator delivering a shock of 20 to 60 watt-seconds is used when the paddles are in contact with the heart; if alternating current (A.C.) is employed, an electrical impulse of 110 to 180 volts for 0.1 to 0.2 seconds is delivered. For external defibrillation, the D.C. shock is 100 to 400 watt-seconds and the A.C. shock is 400 to 800 volts for a duration of 0.25 seconds.

An injection of epinephrine (5 to 10 ml., 1:10,000) solution will increase the cardiac muscular tone and facilitate defibrillation in many instances. When the heart has arrested in asystole and does not resume effective contraction, drug therapy to stimulate contraction must be initiated. As mentioned previously, both epinephrine and isoproterenol (Isuprel) increase the rate and force of myocardial contraction and can be used individually or alternatively. Calcium chloride also has a direct effect on myocardial contractility, increasing the strength as well as the duration of the contractions (5 to 10 ml. of diluted 1% solution). These three drugs, in a poorly oxygenated heart, may produce ventricular fibrillation, which should be treated as previously discussed.

Metabolic acidosis inevitably accompanies prolonged attempts at resuscitation. This must be corrected, since it is detrimental to spontaneous cardiac action and may result in a low cardiac output. Sodium bicarbonate in doses of 44.6 mEq. (50 ml. containing 3.75Gm.) can be given intravenously every 20 to 30 minutes as long as resuscitation attempts are continued. Measurements of arterial pH and base deficit, as described elsewhere, are the ideal guides to a more precise management. In severe degrees of metabolic acidosis, THAM (trometamol; Talatrol) is administered intravenously (0.3 M solution at a rate of 5 mg./kg. body weight per hour). As soon as the base deficit is normal, the drug should be discontinued. Since the administration of THAM may result in respiratory paralysis, a respirator should be available.

As soon as respiration and circulation have been restored, a route for intravenous therapy should be provided. A peripheral venous cutdown with the insertion of a long catheter is probably the most expeditious way. If this can be advanced into the right atrium, it may be used to determine central venous pressure. Immediate blood replacement is mandatory when the hypoxia leading to cardiac arrest is due to hypovolemia from blood loss. Often, blood replacement by itself will renew effective cardiac action in patients with profound cardiovascular collapse.

When resuscitation has been successfully achieved, the patient should be continuously monitored in an intensive care unit. Recurrent PVC's or ventricular tachycardia are controlled with an intravenous drip of lidocaine, the blood volume is replenished and, if necessary, an intravenous drip of isoproterenol or epinephrine may be used to support the blood pressure. Frequent determination of the arterial or mixed venous blood gases is mandatory. Controlled ventilation with adequate sedation may be desirable for a period of time.

To prevent permanent brain damage after cerebral hypoxia, the use of external hypothermia has been advocated and the administration of a massive dose of glucocorticosteroids (methylprednisolone sodium succinate [Solu-Medrol] 30 mg./kg.) may be beneficial.

PART 3.

The Coronary Patient for Myocardial Revascularization

WILLIAM E. NEVILLE, M.D., *and*
ROBERT D. LYNCH, M.D.

IMPLANTATION OF ONE OR TWO mammary arteries and aorta-coronary autogenous vein bypass grafts are accepted surgical procedures for myocardial revascularization. Since psychologic factors play such an important role in the development of angina pectoris, it is of the utmost importance that the surgeon establish rapport with the patient. It is imperative to explain that angina may persist for 2 to 3 months after an internal mammary myocardial implant, since anastomotic communications between the internal mammary artery and the branches of the coronary artery cannot immediately be established. The patient should be told that he may expect maximum improvement in 6 to 12 months, when the anastomotic channels have reached the peak of their development. However, when a vein bypass graft is possible, the relief of angina should be immediate.

Although the management of these patients is continuous from the time the decision for operation is made, for the sake of clarity the discussion is divided into three parts.

A. PREOPERATIVE MANAGEMENT.—The patient should be admitted to the hospital several days prior to operation in order to have him in optimum condition for surgery. Individuals with chronic bronchitis and emphysema will benefit from intermittent positive-pressure breathing. Two daily treatments of one-half hour duration are helpful in lessening cough and mucus formation, which in turn enhances ventilatory function. Positive pressure with acetylcysteine (Mucomyst) and bronchodilators may be indicated, and abstinence from smoking is mandatory.

The majority of patients are taking nitroglycerin and isosorbide-dinitrate (Isordil); these should be continued until surgery is performed. Since there is arteriographic evidence of the ability of Isordil to dilate the coronary arteries, 5 mg. of this drug is administered sublingually prior to induction of anesthesia. Its action is almost as powerful as that of nitroglycerin and its duration is much longer.

The use of digitalis in these patients is controversial, especially without overt signs of cardiac failure. However, we are of the opinion that digoxin can benefit cardiac patients who have a decreased myocardial reserve even though there is no evidence of cardiac decompensation. Our experience and that of others suggests that it is safer to digitalize a patient 4 or 5 days prior to surgery than to do so as an emergency procedure following the operation. Digoxin is preferred, since these short-acting glycosides allow adjustment of the dosage so that digitalis intoxication or underdigitalization can be avoided.

In the absence of heart failure, diuretics are not administered. In doubtful cases, a trial dose of meralluride injection (Mercuhydrin) or sodium mercaptomerin (Thiomerin), 2 ml. I.M., is given. A loss of 3 or 4 pounds of body weight indicates evidence of fluid retention, while in the absence of failure there is no weight loss. Diuretics should be discontinued 3 to 4 days before surgery; but it is still essential to give potassium supplements until operation, to minimize postoperative hypokalemia.

Anticoagulants are discontinued when the patient is admitted. The routine use of lactated Ringer's solution, as the only fluid administered in the operating room, makes the use of blood rarely necessary for single implants. However, it should be stressed that coronary patients do not tolerate a low hematocrit and bank blood should be available. A persistent tachycardia during surgery may respond to a transfusion of blood that brings the hematocrit to the normal level. Even though aorto-coronary bypass vein grafts are performed with cardiopulmonary bypass, again no blood is required during the procedure, since the pump oxygenator is primed with Ringer's lactate solution. Following surgery, blood is infused according to the dictates of the various physiologic parameters which are routinely monitored after open-heart operations.

It is important to have the patient's blood pressure recorded several times a day for 2 to 3 days prior to surgery, to establish a guide for the anesthesiologist. During the operation, it is mandatory that the arterial blood pressure be maintained at or above the average preoperative value, since hypotension may cause arrhythmias and a myocardial infarction.

The patient is informed that he will remain in the Intensive Care Unit for 2 or 3 days, and that the endotracheal tube will be kept in for 24 hours or longer.

B. Intraoperative management.—*Premedication.*—Unless the

patient arrives in the operating room well sedated, he may have an attack of angina. We prefer morphine sulfate (10–15 mg.) and promethazine hydrochloride (Phenergan) (0.5 mg. per kg. of body weight) given I.M. 1 hour preoperatively. With this premedication, dryness of the mouth, tachycardia, hypotension, nausea and restlessness are minimized or prevented. Atropine is not used because it may cause tachycardia and initiate arrhythmias.

Prior to the induction of anesthesia, isosorbide dinitrate 5 mg. is administered sublingually. Anesthesia is induced with intravenous sodium thiopental (Pentothal sodium), followed by *d*-tubocurarine and endotracheal intubation. Succinylcholine chloride (Anectine) is not used because of its vagotonic action. The anesthesia is then continued with methoxyflurane (Penthrane), with ventilation controlled mechanically throughout the procedure. A fairly deep and constant level of anesthesia will help to prevent ventricular arrhythmias during the operative manipulation of the heart. The arterial and central venous blood pressures and electrocardiogram are continually monitored. At the end of the operation, the patient is transferred to the Intensive Care Unit with the endotracheal tube in place, and controlled ventilation is instituted for 24 to 48 hours.

The midline sternal splitting incision is used for all myocardial revascularization procedures. With the use of the Favaloro retractor, one or both internal mammary arteries are easily dissected. The advantage of this operative approach is that the patient remains flat on his back and the lungs are not compressed during surgery. When an aorto-coronary bypass vein graft is combined with an internal mammary artery implantation, the left internal mammary artery is dissected prior to the onset of cardiopulmonary bypass. Once the pedicle is free, it is left attached distally and implanted after completion of the vein graft.

It is imperative that the arterial blood pressure be maintained at the preoperative level in order to avoid undesirable sequelae. If hypotension develops, an intravenous drip of isoproterenol is begun; the operation is terminated if the drug does not sustain the arterial blood pressure, since an acute myocardial infarction may occur. If the hypotension is only transient without evidence of infarction, the operation can proceed.

Premature ventricular contractions and runs of ventricular tachycardia are not uncommon during manipulation of the heart for tunneling and internal mammary implantation. As mentioned earlier, good premedication and the use of *d*-tubocurarine and methoxyflurane will virtually eliminate ventricular arrhythmias. However, if they occur, treatment should be instituted immediately. An intravenous bolus of lidocaine (1 to 2 mg. per kg. of body weight) is usually effective in controlling the arrhythmia. Recurrent premature beats may be prevented or reduced by a continuous intravenous infusion of lidocaine (2,000 mg. in 1,000 ml. 5% D/W, to drip at a rate of 1 ml. per minute). The toxic effects (convulsions, hypotension and depression of the central venous system) can be avoided by using less than 250 mg. per hour. A good prophylactic measure is to administer a bolus of lidocaine (100 mg.) intravenously, and a tablet of nitroglycerin (0.4 mg.) sublingually, prior to manipulation of the heart for implantation. The heart-lung machine with a disposable oxygenator is in the operating room as a standby unit. If progressive hypotension or an uncontrolled ventricular arrhythmia should develop, temporary support with the pump oxygenator may be lifesaving.

Blood loss is recorded and blood replaced accordingly during the operation. With the use of Ringer's lactate solution in the routine case, blood is unnecessary. However, in patients with severe coronary artery disease and diminished cardiac reserve, the maintenance of ventricular filling pressure by sustaining the blood volume is very important. A blood loss of even 500 ml. should be replaced in these individuals. In addition, frequent determinations of blood gases are essential in order to detect metabolic derangements before they become detrimental.

C. POSTOPERATIVE MANAGEMENT.—*Controlled ventilation.*—At the end of the operation, the patient is transferred to the Intensive Care Unit with the endotracheal tube in place. Controlled ventilation with a volume respirator is maintained for 24 to 48 hours. During this period, the cuff on the endotracheal tube should be deflated periodically and the branched secretions aspirated. If further ventilatory support is required, a tracheostomy is performed. During the period of mechanical ventilation, the patient is sedated with morphine sulfate (5–10 mg. every 1–4 hours). We have found that 5 mg. every 1–2 hours intravenously produced less hypotension than 10 mg. every 3–4 hours and maintains a more uniform sedation.

Controlled ventilation not only relieves the patient of the work of spontaneous breathing but prevents hypoxemia and acidosis, which often lead to ventricular arrhythmias. According to our experimental studies, ventilation should be maintained with a humidified gas mixture containing from 30 to 40% oxygen. Higher concentrations of O_2 administered for long periods of time may lead to "oxygen-lung toxicity." An arterial Po_2 of around 150 mm. Hg is the ideal level to prevent ventricular fibrillation. Since this method was adopted, premature ventricular contractions are seldom seen in the postoperative period.

Blood-gases are analyzed regularly while the patient is on the respirator, and base deficits are treated with sodium bicarbonate. In addition, frequent radiographs of the chest and serial electrocardiograms are obtained during the first 24 hours together with serum enzymes and electrolytes.

Fluid and Electrolyte Administration

The serum electrolytes are measured immediately after the operation. Although there is no clear explanation, the K^+ is consistently low even in patients who have not received diuretics preoperatively. This hypokalemia following myocardial revascularization may be related to the myocardial injury that follows the production of the myocardial tunnel and implantation of the internal mammary artery. In any event, 40 mEq. of KCl dissolved in 100 ml. of D/W is given empirically by I.V. drip during the first 2 hours after surgery, and in subsequent hours 60 mEq. of KCl are added to each 1,000 ml. of fluid administered. An effort is made to maintain a serum potassium level above 4.5 mEq. per liter. To achieve this level, it has been necessary in certain instances to administer up to 200 mEq. of KCl within 24 hours.

The patient receives 1,500 ml. of 5% dextrose in lactated Ringer's solution. Urinary output and specific gravity are measured hourly during this time as a guide to the adequacy of fluid replacement and cardiac output.

Temperature control.—Some elevation of the temperature (up to 39.2°C. or 102.6°F. rectal) is common in patients kept on controlled ventilation. When temperature increases above this level, alcohol sponges are applied to the exposed skin area. The increased heat loss results in a lowering of the temperature.

Cardiac drugs.—Although every patient undergoing myocardial revascularization is digitalized preoperatively, the majority have a rapid ventricular rate in the postoperative period. For this and for previously mentioned reasons, digoxin is continued postoperatively.

Nitroglycerin (0.4 mg.) is administered sublingually every hour for the first 48 hours and thereafter as needed for angina. In addition, 5 mg. of Isordil is given sublingually every 6 hours. Diuretics are not used routinely, except in patients who have had preoperative heart failure.

In order to immediately ascertain disturbances in cardiac rhythm, the electrocardiogram should continuously be monitored for 2–3 days after surgery. Frequent PVC's can cause a reduction in cardiac output and may be a precursor of ventricular tachycardia and fibrillation. Lidocaine is the drug of choice in these circumstances; an intravenous dose of 50–100 mg. will ordinarily stop premature ventricular contractions. However, if they become frequent and recur after several injections, a slow I.V. drip should be started. Diphenylhydantoin sodium (Dilantin) 100 mg. I.V. every 8 hours may be helpful in some cases.

The etiology of the ventricular arrhythmias should be ascertained as soon as possible. Hypoxemia, metabolic acidosis and even digitalis intoxication may be responsible. Since a frequent cause is hypokalemia, an intravenous infusion of KCl may stop a ventricular arrhythmia that is refractory to lidocaine and other drugs.

Arterial blood gases.—During the first 48 hours, frequent determinations of the Sa_{O_2}, Pa_{O_2}, Pa_{CO_2}, pH, standard bicarbonate, buffer base and base excess are made. The Pa_{O_2} should be maintained between 100 and 150 mm. Hg; higher levels for prolonged periods may result in oxygen-lung toxicity. Optimally, the Pa_{CO_2} should remain between 34 and 46 mm. Hg. However, it is lower with controlled ventilation because of the respiratory alkalosis incumbent on the use of mechanical respirators.

Metabolic acidosis is corrected with appropriate amounts of sodium bicarbonate (2 mg./kg. body weight per hour) until the base deficit is normal. The administration of THAM may result in respiratory paralysis, so a respirator should be available.

Thoracotomy tubes.—If both pleural spaces have been opened, one thoracotomy tube is left in each pleural cavity. If only one pleural space has been entered, one tube is left in the mediastinum and the other is placed in the open thorax. These tubes are attached to separate water-seal bottles and the drainage from each tube is checked every hour during the first 24 hours. Ordinarily, the amount of drainage is less than 500 ml. during 24 hours. Any sudden increase in drainage accompanied by hypotension and tachycardia should arouse suspicion of possible active bleeding which may require immediate reoperation. The chest tubes are removed when the drainage is less than 100 ml. in 24 hours. This is usually possible on the second or third postoperative day.

Discharge from the hospital.—After an uneventful recovery from myocardial revascularization, the patient may be discharged from the hospital in 12 to 15 days. A long-acting coronary vasodilator (Isordil) is prescribed for at least 3 months and nitroglycerin is used as needed. Digitalis and diuretics are continued only in those patients who have been in cardiac failure. In addition, a low-fat diet is strongly recommended and the patient is made aware of the necessity to quit smoking; there should be no compromise in this respect if the patient is to have complete relief from his angina. Gradual exercise short of experiencing angina is advised, since this may be the best stimulus for the development of myocardial collateral circulation.

Where an aorto-coronary bypass graft has been possible, myocardial revascularization is accomplished immediately, with relief of the patient's symptoms. However, after indirect myocardial revascularization, it is imperative to inform the patient that it may take from 3 to 6 months to obtain complete relief from angina. He should understand that during the first 6 to 8 weeks his myocardial blood supply is no different than before the operation. Reassurance that the collateral circulation increases week by week, up to a year, is very helpful.

PART 4.

Action of and Indications for Adrenergic Drugs

RAYMOND A. DIETER, JR., M.D., *and*
WILLIAM E. NEVILLE, M.D.

THE FAILING CIRCULATION can be assisted by several classes of drugs. These are divided into the *inotropes,* which increase myocardial contractility, the *chronotropes,* which affect the heart rate and rhythm, and the *vasoconstrictor* and *vasodilator* drugs, which influence the tone in the capacitance and resistance blood vessels. Since a close relationship exists between the dose of the drug and the receptor sites and effector mechanisms in the heart and vessels, knowledge of their mode of action and precise indications for their judicious employment is mandatory.

One of the most important factors in determining the effects of a sympathomimetic drug is to realize that there are two types of receptor sites with which it can elicit a response in sympathetic effector cells. These have been classified as alpha (α) and beta (β), on the basis of their responses to a variety of sympathomimetic amines and to adrenergic blocking agents. In general the effect on α-receptors is excitatory and on β-receptors is inhibitory. The adrenergic blocking action of many compounds such as phenoxybenzamine (Dibenzyline) is selective for α-receptors, whereas other blocking agents, for example, pronetalol, act only on β-receptors.

Sympathomimetic Drugs

As mentioned, certain drugs activate adrenergic receptors or increase the free norepinephrine at the receptor site (see Table 2–2). Ahlquist, in 1948, suggested that the varied effects of sympathetic activity were due to different receptor types. Thus it is believed that the alpha- and beta-adrenergic receptor stimulators directly activate the receptor site, whereas the indirectly-acting sympathomimetic

TABLE 2-2.—Sympathomimetic Drugs

I. *Direct: Adrenergic Receptor Stimulators*
- A. Alpha
  1. Epinephrine (Adrenalin)
  2. Norepinephrine (Levarterenol)
  3. Phenylephrine (Neo-Synephrine)
  4. Methoxamine (Vasoxyl)
  5. Metaraminol (Aramine)
  6. Dopamine
- B. Beta
  1. Isoproterenol (Isuprel)
- C. Alpha and Beta
  1. Ephedrine
  2. Mephentermine (Wyamine)

II. *Indirect: Increase Free Norepinephrine*
- A. Norepinephrine Release from Nerve Ending
  1. Tyramine (Uteramine)
  2. Ephedrine
  3. Amphetamine
  4. Reserpine—acute effect
  5. Guanethidine—acute effect
- B. Decreased Norepinephrine Inactivation
  1. Prevention rebinding
     - a. Cocaine
  2. Prevention metabolism

drugs increase the free norepinephrine either by an increased release of this drug from the nerve ending or by decreased inactivation of norepinephrine by rebinding or metabolism. There is no direct effect of α-adrenergic stimulation on the heart. However, there are β-adrenergic receptors mediated by norepinephrine within the heart. These receptors lead to increased cardiac rate by stimulation of the S.A. node and subsidiary ectopic sites, to increased contractility and metabolism of the heart. Alpha-adrenergic receptor stimulation by norepinephrine results in vascular constriction in most tissues, but β-adrenergic receptor stimulation, probably due to norepinephrine, leads to arterial dilatation in skeletal muscle. Lastly, acetylcholine, through a cholinergic receptor site, causes a sympathetic cholinergic vasodilatory effect on the arteries. Within the veins, norepinephrine-mediated alpha- and beta-adrenergic receptors lead to venous constriction; however, the β-receptors may also lead to dilatation in some veins. It should be noted that most vasodilatation is passive and that there is no definite proof of active nerve-mediated adrenergic vasodilatation.

Sympathetic Antagonists

The sympathetic antagonists (see Table 2–3) prevent normal norepinephrine stimulation of the receptor site. These drugs produce receptor blockade by occupying the adrenergic receptor site. With this type of blockade, the nerve terminals and effector (receptor) cells remain functional. Another group of antagonists function by inactivation of the nerve terminal, thus decreasing the free norepinephrine. They may do so by prevention or release, by inhibition of synthesis, or by depletion of norepinephrine from the nerve ending. However, the nerve axon and effector cell receptors remain functional.

The β-adrenergic blocking agents selectively antagonize the increased discharge of the cardiac pacemakers, the increased myocardial contractility and the increased metabolic glycogenolysis. They may also counteract the effects of catecholamines and exercise on the heart rate and cardiac work in the human. In addition, β-adrenergic blocking drugs exert antiarrhythmic actions by receptor blockade and by nonspecific cardiac depression. On the other hand, α-adrenergic blocking agents may suppress ventricular arrhythmias by antagonizing vasopressor catecholamine, blood pressure elevation and cardiac stimulation. Systemic arterial and arteriolar vasoconstriction and venous vasoconstriction are prevented by α-adrenergic blocking drugs but not by β-blocking agents.

TABLE 2-3.—SYMPATHETIC ANTAGONISTS

I. Adrenergic Receptor Blockers

- A. Alpha
  1. Phenoxybenzamine hydrochloride (Dibenzyline)
  2. Phentolamine hydrochloride (Regitine)
  3. Ergot derivatives (Hydergine)
  4. Azapetine (Ilidar)
  5. Tolazoline hydrochloride (Priscoline)
  6. Piperoxan hydrochloride (Benodaine)
  7. Chlorpromazine hydrochloride (Thorazine)
- B. Beta
  1. Dichloroisoproterenol (DCI)
  2. Pronethalol (Alderlin)
  3. Propranolol hydrochloride (Inderal)
  4. Sotalol hydrochloride (MJ 1999)

II. Blockade Nerve Terminal

- A. Prevention Norepinephrine Release
  1. Bretylium tosylate (Bretylan)
- B. Synthesis Inhibition
  1. Methyltyrosine
  2. Methyldopa (Aldomet)
- C. Depletion Neural Norepinephrine
  1. Reserpine—chronic effect
  2. Guanethidine sulfate (Ismelin)—chronic effect

Clinically, α-adrenergic blockade is used to antagonize sympathetic arterial and venous constriction, thus producing a reduction in peripheral resistance, an increase in venous return and a compensatory tachycardia.

ALPHA-ADRENERGIC RECEPTOR STIMULATORS (TABLE 2–4)

Epinephrine.—Epinephrine is a very potent peripheral vasoconstrictor and myocardial stimulator capable of causing an increase in the cardiac rate. Splanchnic and renal arterioles are strongly constricted by epinephrine, as are the arterioles in the skin and mucous membranes, but the muscular arterioles are dilated. Epinephrine stimulates the effector cells of the cardiac accelerator nerves and reflexly stimulates the vagus nerve. The resultant cardiac rate may be slow but the beats are forceful. This vagal effect of epinephrine is abolished by atropine. Systole is shorter and more powerful and the cardiac output is enhanced by the inotropic action on the myocardium but the overall peripheral resistance is diminished. Coronary flow is increased by virtue of a rise in aortic pressure and an increase

TABLE 2-4.—ALPHA-ADRENERGIC RECEPTOR STIMULATORS

DRUG	DOSE
1. Epinephrine	0.22 ml. 1:1,000 solution I.V. 0.5 to 1 ml. 1:10,000 I.V. 4–6 mg./250 ml. 5% D/W
2. Norepinephrine	1 ml. (4 mcg.) of base/250 ml. 5% D/W as a drip
3. Isoproterenol	0.4 mg./250 ml. 5% D/W as a drip
4. Phenylephrine	0.8 mg. I.V. 5 mg. S.C. 250 mg. oral
5. Methoxamine	10–20 mg. I.M. 5–10 mg. I.V.
6. Metaraminol	5–10 mg. I.M. 1–2 mg. I.V.
7. Phenoxybenzamine	1 mg./kg. I.V. (slowly)
8. Phentolamine	5 mg. I.V. 20 mg. in 1,000 ml. 5% D/W as a drip
9. Guanethidine	25–50 mg. orally per day initial 10 mg. per day
10. Propranolol	Oral 10–30 mg. T.I.D. for arrhythmias 1–3 mg. I.V. (ECG monitoring)
11. Chlorpromazine	2.5–5 mg. I.V. 0.5–10 minutes

in diastolic time. However, premature ventricular systoles may occur, which may herald serious ventricular arrhythmias. Large concentrations of the drug may produce cardiac dilatation and ventricular fibrillation (see Table 2–5).

Epinephrine also increases the arterial and venous pulmonary pressures, and a direct pulmonary vasoconstriction can be shown under suitable conditions. In man, however, the increase in pulmonary pressure is predominantly secondary to an increase in the left atrial pressure. Redistribution of blood from the systemic to the pulmonary circulation plays an important role in the increase in pulmonary pressure. Thus an overdose of epinephrine may produce pulmonary edema and death by precipitating an elevated pulmonary capillary filtration pressure.

For therapy of hypotension secondary to a low cardiac output, 4 to 6 mg. of epinephrine is dissolved in 250 ml. of glucose and water. This is given at a rate sufficient to maintain an adequate blood pressure while not appreciably increasing the cardiac rate. Since ventricular tachycardia and fibrillation must be avoided, the heart rate and blood pressure should be continuously monitored. For the treatment of cardiac arrest in the average adult patient or to stimulate myocardial activity following open-heart surgery, 0.2 ml. of 1:1,000 solution is effective either intravenously or by intracardiac injection. If a larger volume is desired, 0.5 to 1 ml. of a 1:10,000 solution may be used.

Norepinephrine.—This drug is the chemical mediator liberated by postganglionic adrenergic nerves. It differs from epinephrine by lacking the methyl substitution in the amino group. It acts predominantly on the alpha or vasoconstrictor receptors and has little action on beta receptors except in the heart. Peripheral resistance increases in most vascular beds, and the blood flow is reduced through the kidney, brain, liver and skeletal muscle. However, glomerular filtration rate is maintained unless the renal blood flow is markedly diminished. Splanchnic and hepatic blood flow are reduced.

Norepinephrine is the most potent peripheral vasoconstrictor drug available but has only a weak inotropic effect on the heart. In actuality, there is no increase in cardiac output, due to the intense peripheral vasoconstriction and the reflex bradycardia mediated through the vagus nerve. Local tissue gangrene has followed intravenous administration, and long-term therapy has resulted in hepatic and renal failure. Thus, its use in oligemia is extremely dangerous. Norepinephrine is a primary coronary vasoconstrictor and produces an increase in O_2 extraction and a decrease in coronary venous O_2 saturation. Because of these adverse manifestations, its use following open-heart surgery is limited and may even be contraindicated.

Phenylephrine.—Phenylephrine (Neo-Synephrine) differs from epinephrine only in lacking an OH group in position 4 on the benzene ring. It is a powerful α-receptor stimulant, with little effect on the β-receptors of the heart. Intravenous, subcutaneous, and depot administration produce a rise in systolic and diastolic pressures which are sustained for approximately 20 to 50 minutes. A reflex bradycardia may occur through vagal stimulation; this can be blocked by atropine. Circulation time is slightly prolonged, the venous pressure is slightly increased, pulmonary vessels are constricted and the pulmonary artery pressure is elevated. Phenylephrine is a powerful vasoconstrictor but lacks almost completely any chronotropic and inotropic action on the heart. It is used by the anesthesiologist but has no inherent value following open-heart surgery.

Methoxamine and metaraminol.—Methoxamine is a β-hydroxyisopropyl amine which produces a rise in blood pressure by peripheral vasoconstriction. It has no stimulatory action on the heart and lacks β-receptor action on smooth muscle. Its action lasts for 60 to 90 minutes. Metaraminol, 3-hydroxyphenylisopropanolamine, produces a sustained rise in systolic and diastolic pressure accompanied by marked reflex bradycardia. Peripheral resistance is increased and the renal and cerebral blood flows are diminished.

Isoproterenol (Isuprel).—Isuprel is the most potent of the sympathomimetic amines and acts almost exclusively on the β-receptors in the myocardium. Its main effects are on the heart, the smooth muscle of the bronchi, skeletal muscle vasculature and alimentary tract. In man, an intravenous infusion of Isuprel lowers the peripheral vascular resistance in the skeletal muscle and the renal and mesenteric vascular beds, with a concomitant drop in the diastolic pressure. The coronary venous O_2 saturation is increased and the cardiac output is elevated by its inotropic and chronotropic action, combined with the increased venous return to the heart.

With the usual doses of Isuprel, the increased cardiac output is generally enough to maintain a rise in systolic pressure although the mean pressure is reduced. Because of its dual action of producing peripheral vasodilation and a positive inotropic effect on the heart, it is extremely useful in cardiac patients to maintain adequate heart action in the postoperative period. It should be given with extreme caution because of its propensity for increasing the cardiac rate and thereby precipitating ventricular tachycardia with resultant fibrillation. A microdrip solution (0.4 mg. in 250 ml. dextrose and water) will allow one to observe the effect on the heart and the pulse rate. In many patients, when this drug is ineffective, an epinephrine drip may be more beneficial. In our institution, isoproterenol is begun first, and if this does not stimulate cardiac activity or ventricular tachycardia ensues, epinephrine is then used. On occasions even alternating an infusion of these drugs has been efficacious.

Ephedrine.—Ephedrine stimulates both α and β receptors. The cardiovascular effects are in many ways similar to those of epinephrine but they persist much longer. The drug elevates the systolic and usually also the diastolic pressure, with an increase in pulse pressure. The pressor responses are predominantly due to cardiac stimulation, provided venous return is adequate. The force of myocardial contraction and cardiac output is augmented. Coronary cerebral and muscle blood flows are increased but the renal and splanchnic blood flows are decreased. In spite of its cardiovascular effects and more prolonged action, ephedrine is not as efficacious as epinephrine for postoperative hypotension.

Adrenergic Blocking Agents

Phenoxybenzamine (Dibenzyline).—This drug effectively prevents responses to adrenergic stimuli mediated by α receptors. Responses to circulating catecholamines are inhibited more effectively than those mediated or released locally at nerve endings. Effects mediated by β-adrenergic receptors, including the chronotropic and inotropic responses of the heart and vasodilation in certain vascular beds, are essentially unaltered. These blocking agents may be considered to act by reducing the total population of α receptors. Consequently, the actions of various sympathomimetics are inhibited to nearly the same extent. However, the net effects of different sympathomimetics on a complex parameter such as blood pressure may be antagonized to very different degrees. For example, a dose of phenoxybenzamine that completely eliminates the pressure response to epinephrine or converts it to a depressor response may produce only a 50% inhibition of the pressor response to norepinephrine. Epinephrine produces both vasoconstriction and vasodilation. Moderate inhibition of the former may allow the latter to predominate. On the other hand, norepinephrine has very little vasodilator action and all of the residual constriction is manifest in the pressor response.

The most important recent application of the α-adrenergic blocking agents has been in the field of shock. In the past, largely because of the concern for hypotension in shock, vasopressor agents have been extensively employed. However, vasoconstriction is a prominent feature of shock and there is little evidence that its accentuation by drugs is beneficial. Indeed, hyperactivity of the sympathetic nerve system or infusion of vasoconstrictors such as norepinephrine can accentuate the development of shock initiated by hemorrhage, trauma, infection. If sufficiently severe and prolonged, it can induce lethal shock in both laboratory animals and man.

Experimentally, it has been shown that these agents induce vasodilation by inhibiting sympathetic vasoconstriction. Survival rate of experimental animals subjected to various shock-inducing procedures is improved by directly relaxing vascular smooth muscle. It is apparent that these compounds produce: (1) an increase in total blood flow, particularly in the abdominal viscera; (2) local redistribution of blood flow so that a greater percentage of blood passes through channels that readily exchange metabolites with tissue cells; and (3) a reversal of the vasoconstriction-induced shift of fluid from the vascular to the interstitial compartment.

The use of phenoxybenzamine clinically in shock has been encouraging. In addition to its specific antishock effects, seen clearly in patients who have not responded to adequate replacement of intravascular volume, two other effects have been observed. The fall in blood pressure induced after its administration in the presence of hypovolemia provides a quick and reliable indication of the adequacy of intravascular fluid volume replacement. In addition, a shift of blood from the pulmonary to the systemic vascular bed associated with blockade of sympathetic vasomotor tone allows administration of large volumes of fluid more rapidly than would otherwise be possible in patients with myocardial inadequacy.

It should be emphasized that, in shock, administration of any drug is secondary to fully adequate replacement of intravascular fluid volume with blood or other appropriate fluids. This is particularly important before the administration of a blocking agent such as phenoxybenzamine, because the inhibition of vasoconstriction reflexes makes the circulation highly vulnerable to hypovolemia. The blocking agent must be administered slowly, and suitable fluids must be immediately available if a sharp drop in blood pressure indicates that replacement has been inadequate.

DCI and pronethalol.—A β-adrenergic blocking agent, dichloroisoproterenol (DCI), was reported in 1958 and discarded because of undesirable sympathomimetic activity. It produces α-adrenergic blockade and, in addition, effectively antagonizes β-adrenergic stimuli. The effects of epinephrine are inhibited and a precipitous fall in blood pressure, with a prolonged blockade of vasodepressor responses, is produced. It transiently increases the heart rate and the strength of contraction both in vivo and in vitro. However, larger repeated doses cause myocardial depression.

Pronethalol (Alderlin), another β-adrenergic blocking agent, tends to decrease the heart rate. It slows the ventricular rate in atrial fibrillation which summates with digitalis. It is more effective than digitalis in preventing the increase in heart rate associated with exercise. Pronethalol quite effectively antagonizes cardiac arrhythmias due to digitalis intoxication. It reduces the rate of discharge of ectopic pacemakers in various arrhythmias and in some cases it restores a sinus rhythm. However, it has been abandoned because of tumorigenic activity in mice.

Propranolol (Inderal).—Continued research led to the development of propranolol hydrochloride, which has profound β-adrenergic blocking properties and lacks the strong sympathomimetic activity and oncogenic propensities of pronethalol. This drug has demonstrated blockade of the chronotropic and of the inotropic action of isoproterenol, epinephrine, norepinephrine and stellate ganglion stimulation. It produces a decrease in the heart rate, a reduction in the cardiac output, a diminution in resting stroke volume and O_2 consumption, and an increase in left-ventricular end-diastolic pressure. It is indicated in the management of cardiac arrhythmias such as proxysmal atrial tachycardia, sinus tachycardia and extrasystoles of atrial and ventricular origin. In the majority of cases of flutter or fibrillation, a beneficial effect is attained by reduction of the ventricular rate to the atrial tacharrhythmia through a partial A.V. block. Digitalis-induced arrhythmias are usually reversible in minutes by intravenous Inderal. Once normal rhythm has been restored, maintenance with oral therapy is indicated. In ventricular tachycardia, when cardioversion technics are not available, Inderal may be given intravenously, slowly and in low dosage. Great care should be instituted in the administration of Inderal in this situation and constant monitoring with an electrocardiograph is essential, as the failing heart requires some sympathetic drive to maintain myocardial tone.

It is important to emphasize that, since sympathetic stimulation is a significant component in supporting circulatory function in congestive heart failure, inhibition with β-blocking agents always carries the potential hazard of further depressing myocardial contractility and precipitating cardiac failure. Thus, in frank or incipient congestive failure, treatment with Inderal should be carried out cautiously and under the protective cover of concurrent digitalization, since the drug does not abolish the inotropic action of digitalis on the heart muscle. Even in patients without a history of cardiac failure, myocardial depression over a period of time may lead to cardiac failure. Therefore, at the first sign or symptom of impending failure, patients should be fully digitalized and the response closely observed. If cardiac failute progresses, the drug must be discontinued. However, if the tachyarrhythmia is controlled, the patients should be maintained on combined therapy until the threat of cardiac failure is over.

Indications for Adrenergic Receptor Stimulators (Tables 2-5 and 2-6)

Shock.—Both the alpha- and the beta-adrenergic receptor stimulators have been used for shock therapy. The pros and cons of systemic pressure elevation through increased peripheral resistance have been extensively discussed in the recent literature. Therapy may be lifesaving by an increase in the perfusion pressure to vital organs. However, one must remember that the important factor is the total blood flow to an organ, which is determined by the ratio of pressure to resistance. Thus, an increase in peripheral arteriolar resistance may actually decrease the flow of blood to an organ despite an increase in arterial pressure. Since sympathomimetic amines increase

TABLE 2-5.—EFFECTS OF SEVERAL SYMPATHOMIMETIC AMINES ON CARDIAC CONTRACTILE FORCE AND BLOOD PRESSURE

COMPOUND	EFFECT* ON CARDIAC CONTRACTILE FORCE	EFFECT ON BLOOD PRESSURE
Norepinephrine	↑	↑
Epinephrine—Large doses	↑	↑
Epinephrine—Small doses	↑	↓
Metaraminol	↑	↑
Mephentermine	↑	↑
Ephedrine	↑	↑
Methamphetamine hydrochloride	↑	↑
Isoproterenol hydrochloride	↑	↓
Methoxamine hydrochloride	0	↑
Phenylephrine hydrochloride	±	↑

*↑ = increase
↓ = decrease
Isoproterenol is the only listed amine with no constricting effect.

arteriolar resistance, their employment should be reserved for the patient who is under strict surveillance. Furthermore, the choice of sympathomimetic amine depends upon the condition for which it is to be used. In general, the amines with cardiac-stimulating capabilities in addition to vasoconstricting properties are more effective. This is especially true in shock from myocardial infarction.

On the other hand, the β-adrenergic receptor stimulators decrease the peripheral resistance and concomitantly increase myocardial contractility. Consequently, peripheral perfusion may be enhanced and thus they may be more beneficial than alpha stimulators in shock.

Heart block.—The sympathomimetic amines with cardiac-stimulating properties are frequently used to increase the heart rate in patients with nodal or ventricular pacemakers in whom an inadequate cardiac output exists. If the condition is temporary, intravenous administration of isoproterenol on a short-term basis may be adequate. When this is protracted, a combination of either Isuprel, epinephrine or ephedrine, along with electrical pacing, should be utilized. In

TABLE 2-6.—INDICATIONS FOR ADRENERGIC RECEPTOR STIMULATORS

1. Shock
2. Heart Block
   a. Adams-Stokes Syndrome
3. Paroxysmal Atrial Tachycardia
4. Congestive Heart Failure—Low Cardiac Output Syndrome

Stokes-Adams syndrome, long-term therapy with Isuprel has been beneficial.

Paroxysmal atrial tachycardia.—Patients with paroxysmal atrial tachycardia may develop hypotension. Under these circumstances, sympathomimetic amines which do not have cardiac-stimulating effects are sometimes beneficial. Phenylephrine and methoxamine may increase the blood pressure and thereby stimulate vagal inhibitory reflexes with consequent slowing of the cardiac rate.

Congestive heart failure.—Sympathomimetic amines have been beneficial in the treatment of the low cardiac output in acute congestive heart failure. Isoproterenol has been most helpful in the treatment of bradycardia or hypotension associated with congestive heart failure and in the postoperative low cardiac output state.

Mercurial diuresis may be potentiated by these drugs. Dopamine, a naturally occurring catecholamine, has been demonstrated to increase sodium excretion in patients with congestive heart failure. Consequently, chronic congestive heart failure may eventually be amenable to amine therapy.

Indications for Alpha-Adrenergic Blocking Agents (Table 2-7)

Shock therapy.—Vasopressor and vasoconstrictor drugs have been criticized as a therapeutic modality for the treatment of shock. Simultaneously, the α-adrenergic blocking agents were proposed to produce peripheral vasodilation and decreased peripheral resistance. The systemic arterial pressure may then fall due to catecholamine blockade at the alpha receptors of the pre- and post-capillary arterioles and venules, thus diminishing the cardiac workload. Since capillary filtration is enhanced by adrenergic stimuli, alpha blockade of this mechanism prevents capillary filtration by reducing vasoconstriction, decreases the intravascular volume loss, increases the plasma volume and reduces the venous hematocrit. These effects are certainly beneficial in the therapy of shock. However, in the presence of hypovolemia, the vasodilatory effect of α-adrenergic blockade is

TABLE 2-7.—Indications for Alpha-Adrenergic Blocking Agents

1. Shock
2. Hypertension
3. Diagnosis—Pheochromocytoma

profound and may precipitate a cardiac arrest. On the other hand, in cardiogenic shock it has been reasoned that stimulation of the beta receptors and blockade of the alpha receptors could dilate the peripheral coronary bed and increase the coronary flow.

In general, the authors advocate that for patients in shock, the cardiac output should be increased through fluid administration and positive inotropic sympathomimetic amines such as Isuprel, epinephrine, or metaraminol. The central venous pressure must be monitored, and acidosis, septicemia and inadequate ventilation should be corrected. If anuria and peripheral vasoconstriction persist despite these measures, then alpha blockade is also indicated.

Hypertension.—The alpha blockers are potent antihypertensive agents. However, side effects usually occur before a therapeutic fall in blood pressure is obtained. Phentolamine hydrochloride (Regitine) has been used extensively in the diagnosis of pheochromocytoma with intermittent hypertensive episodes.

Indications for Beta-Adrenergic Blocking Agents (Table 2-8)

Angina pectoris.—In 1962, pronethalol was demonstrated to significantly increase the intensity of exercise that could be performed before angina occurred. In addition, fewer electrocardiographic abnormalities were noted during the exercise period while the patient was on pronethalol. However, as noted above, because of the

TABLE 2-8.—Indications for Beta-Adrenergic Blocking Agents

1. Angina pectoris
2. Arrhythmias
   a. Paroxysmal supraventricular tachycardia
      1. Wolff-Parkinson-White syndrome
   b. Paroxysmal atrial tachycardia with block
      1. Digitalis-induced
   c. Atrial fibrillation
   d. Atrial flutter
   e. Ventricular premature beats
   f. Ventricular tachycardia
      1. Digitalis-induced
      2. Paroxysmal
   g. Arrhythmias associated with Pheochromocytoma
3. Hypertrophic subaortic muscular stenosis
4. Hyperdynamic cardiovascular states
   a. Normal
   b. Abnormal

sarcomatous changes found in mice, pronethalol was not used for further clinical study.

Subsequently, propranolol (Inderal) has been preferred in the therapy of angina. This drug produces a decrease in cardiac contractile force and in arterial pressure. Concomitantly, an increase in coronary vascular resistance is noted and a decrease in coronary blood flow occurs. The latter two effects are thought to be largely a result of diminished myocardial O_2 requirements. Propranolol seems to provide symptomatic improvement for the patient with coronary artery disease who is limited by angina pectoris. The frequency of attacks are reduced and the duration and intensity of exercise may be increased. Dwyer concluded that the improvement was based primarily upon suppression of the positive chronotropic and inotropic responses by propranolol, these being major determinants of the myocardial O_2 consumption. However, patients treated with less than 120 mg. per day of propranolol have shown no statistically significant improvement. Furthermore, in a controlled study where propranolol and isosorbide dinitrate (Isordil) were compared with a placebo, there was no significant difference in the response of the entire group to exercise-induced angina. He cautioned that propranolol and isosorbide dinitrate may actually be harmful to patients with angina pectoris.

Arrhythmias.—The antiarrhythmic effect of the β-adrenergic blocking agents arise from both their blocking capabilities and their direct effect on the cell membrane. For example, they decrease the rate of spontaneous diastolic depolarization in pacemaker cells and decrease the rate of the action potential. Alterations in the conduction of the His-Purkinje system are a direct effect of the drug, and this effect is not mediated through the catecholamine antagonism of β-adrenergic receptor blockade. Further, arrhythmias resulting from exogenous catecholamines or from enhanced sympathetic stimulation may be suppressed. Certain anesthetic agents such as halothane and cyclopropane sensitize the heart to the arrhythmic effects of catecholamines; β-adrenergic blockade will prevent such responses and may also prevent cellular depletion of potassium.

Propranolol appears to be effective in decreasing both the frequency and severity of the paroxysms of paroxysmal supraventricular tachycardia. In addition, the Wolff-Parkinson-White syndrome with paroxysmal supraventricular tachycardia responds favorably to the drug.

Paroxysmal atrial tachycardia with block usually occurs as a result of digitalis toxicity. In these patients the arrhythmia responds quite well to propranolol, provided hypokalemia does not exist. However, when the arrhythmia is not due to digitalis therapy, the response is less favorable.

Whereas β-adrenergic blockage produces a sinus rhythm in only a small percentage of the individuals with chronic atrial fibrillation, in acute atrial fibrillation sinus rhythm may be re-established in a large percentage of patients. A uniform slowing in the ventricular rate and a delay in the A.V. conduction is noted. Patients with paroxysmal atrial fibrillation may be benefited by this modality when other therapeutic measures fail. Also, individuals with congestive failure, atrial fibrillation, and rapid ventricular rate have occasionally been improved by propranolol therapy when digitalis was ineffective. However, in one study, patients with atrial fibrillation not only failed to show improvement in their exercise tolerance, despite a slowing of their cardiac rate, but even showed some deterioration of exercise tolerance. Patients with atrial fibrillation due to mitral stenosis may be adversely affected by β-adrenergic blockade.

The therapeutic method of choice for atrial flutter is usually cardioversion. Propranolol may be effective either orally or intravenously in patients in whom it is necessary to slow the ventricular rate before cardioversion. However, ventricular slowing with an increase in A.V. block is noted in a large percentage of these patients.

The response to β-adrenergic blockade for ventricular premature contractions depends on the etiology. In general, exercise-induced premature contractions and those from digitalis and inhalant anesthetic agents (halothane and cyclopropane) respond quite favorably to propranolol.

Again, digitalis-precipitated ventricular tachycardia can be effectively treated with Inderal, while ventricular tachycardia, unrelated to digitalis responds less favorably to beta blockade. In addition, paroxysmal ventricular tachycardia, whether related to digitalis or to exercise, responds quite well to propranolol.

The arrhythmias resulting from the liberation of excessive catecholamines by pheochromocytomas are successfully treated with beta-adrenergic blocking agents. The hypertension associated with such tumors may be further controlled by the use of alpha-adrenergic blocking agents, such as phentolamine. On the other hand, the arrhythmias of myocardial infarction are not benefited by propranolol. Indeed, there is a potential hazard of precipitating congestive heart failure in these damaged hearts.

Hypertrophic subaortic muscular stenosis.—Propranolol is reported to decrease the ventricular gradient induced by exogenous catecholamine through relief of the outflow obstruction. Angina, syncope, vertigo and palpitations in these patients apparently are relieved to a considerable degree. Myocardial O_2 requirements are reduced and there is a reduction in the wall tension, velocity of contraction and heart rate.

Contraindications to Beta-Adrenergic Blockade

1. Bronchial asthma
2. Allergic rhinitis during the pollen season
3. Sinus bradycardia and heart block greater than second degree
4. Cardiogenic shock
5. Right ventricular failure secondary to pulmonary hypertension
6. Congestive heart failure—unless the failure is secondary to tachyarrhythmia
7. Patients receiving myocardial-depressing anesthetics such as chloroform and ether
8. Patients on adrenergic-augmenting psychotropic drugs, including MAO inhibitors, and during the 2-week withdrawal period from such drugs
9. Precautionary states:
   a. Patients with a history of congestive heart failure
   b. Patients prone to hypoglycemia, such as diabetics on insulin or oral hypoglycemic agents
   c. Pregnancy

BIBLIOGRAPHY

Parts 1 and 2

Alexander, J. K.: Postoperative differential diagnosis of cardiac versus respiratory problems, Am. J. Cardiol. 12:441, 1962.

Andersen, M. N., Border, J. R., and Mauritzen, C. V.: Acidosis catecholamines and cardiovascular dynamics: When does acidosis require correction? Ann. Surg. 166:344, 1967.

Ankeney, J. L., Coffin, L. H., Jr., and Littell, A. S.: Experimental evidence that vasoconstriction in hemorrhagic shock does not result in anaerobic metabolism, Ann. Surg. 166:365, 1967.

Barrow, M.: Use of central venous pressure as an accurate guide for body fluid replacement, Surg. Gynec. & Obst. 120:545, 1965.

Bendixen, H. H., Egbert, L. D., Hedley-Whyte, J., Laver, M. B., and Pontoppidan, H.: *Respiratory Care* (St. Louis: C. V. Mosby Company, 1965.)

Bjork, V. O., and Engstrom, C. G.: The treatment of ventilatory insufficiency by tracheotomy artificial ventilation, J. Thoracic Surg. 34:228, 1957.

Bloch, J. H., Pierce, C. H., Mannax, W. G., and Lillehei, R. C.: Treatment of experimental cardiogenic shock, Surgery 58:197, 1965.

Braimbridge, M. V., and Ghadiali, P. E.: *Post-Operative Cardiac Care* (Philadelphia: F. A. Davis Company, 1965).

Bresiman, R., Parks, L. C., and Benson, D. W.: Pitfalls in the clinical use of central venous pressure, Arch. Surg. 95:902, 1967.

Clowes, G. H. A., Sabga, G. A., Kontaxis, A., Tomin, R., Hughes, M., and Simeone, F. A.: Effects of acidosis on cardiovascular function in surgical patients, Ann. Surg. 154:524, 1961.

Coffin, L. H., Jr., Ankeney, J. L., and Beheler, E. M.: Experimental study and clinical use of epinephrine for treatment of low cardiac output syndrome, Circulation 33 and 34 (Suppl.) 78, 1966.

Dieter, R. A., Neville, W. E., and Pifarré, R.: Alterations in serum electrolytes following perfusion with Ringer's lactate, J. Thoracic & Cardiovas. Surg. 59:168, 1970.

Dieter, R. A., Neville, W. E., and Pifarré, R.: Hypokalemia following hemodilution cardiopulmonary bypass, Ann. Surg. 171:17, 1970.

Dieter, R. A., Neville, W. E., and Pifarré, R.: Serum enzyme alterations after open-heart surgery, Surgery 66:328, 1969.

Geha, A. S., Sessler, A. D., and Kirklin, J. W.: Alveolar arterial oxygen gradients after open intracardiac surgery, J. Thoracic & Cardiovas. Surg. 51:609, 1966.

Hardaway, R. M.: *Clinical Management of Shock—Surgical and Medical* (Springfield, Ill.: Charles C Thomas, Publisher, 1968).

Harrison, D. C., Sprouse, J. H., and Morrow, A. G.: The antiarrhythmic properties of lidocaine and procaine amide, Circulation 28:486, 1963.

Jude, J. R., and Elan, J. O.: *Fundamentals of Cardiopulmonary Resuscitation* (Philadelphia: F. A. Davis Company, 1966).

Kirklin, J. W.: Pulmonary dysfunction after open-heart surgery, Med. Clin. N. Amer. 48:1063, 1964.

MacLean, L. D., Duff, J. H., Scott, H. M., and Peretz, D. I.: Treatment of shock in man based on hemodynamic diagnosis, Surg. Gynec. & Obst. 120:1, 1965.

Mueller, H., Gianelli, S., Jr., Gregory, J. J., Ayres, S., and Conklin, E. F.: Effects of isoproterenol on ventricular work and myocardial metabolism in the postoperative heart, Circulation 36(4):11, 1967.

Neville, W. E., Kontaxis, A., Gavin, T., and Clowes, G. H. A., Jr.: Postperfusion pulmonary vasculitis: Its relationship to blood trauma, Arch. Surg. 86:126, 1963.

Neville, W. E., Thomason, R. O., and Hirsch, D. M.: Postperfusion hypervolemia after hemodilution cardiopulmonary bypass, Arch. Surg. 93:715, 1966.

Neville, W. E., Colby, C., Peacock, H., and Kronkowski, T. C.: Superiority of buffered Ringer's lactate to heparinized blood as total prime of the large volume disc oxygenator, Ann. Surg. 165:206, 1967.

Neville, W. E.: Extracorporeal Circulation, in *Current Problems in Surgery* (Chicago: Year Book Medical Publishers, Inc., July, 1967).

Neville, W. E., Faber, L. P., and Peacock, H.: Total prime of the disc oxygenator with Ringer's and Ringer's lactate solution for cardiopulmonary bypass, Dis. Chest 45:320, 1964.

Neville, W. E., and Talso, P. J.: Postperfusion compartmental fluid alterations, Surgery 63:220, 1968.

Neville, W. E.: Cardiopulmonary bypass with large volume non-blood perfusate: Experimental and clinical observation, Circulation Suppl. 31:130, 1965.

Pitts, R. F.: *Physiology of the Kidney and Body Fluids* (4th ed.; Chicago: Year Book Medical Publishers, Inc., 1966).

Raison, J. C. A.: Acid-base changes and tissue respiration in extracorporeal circulation, Ann. Roy. Coll. Surgeons England 37:93, 1965.

Shires, T., Williams, J., and Brown, F.: Acute changes in extracellular fluids associated with major surgical procedures, Ann. Surg. 154:803, 1961.

Shires, T., and Carrico, C. J.: Current Status of the Shock Problem, in *Current Problems in Surgery* (Chicago: Year Book Medical Publishers, Inc., March, 1966).

Stack, J. P. P., and Dale, N.: Beta-adrenergic receptor blockade in cardiac arrhythmias, Brit. M. J. 2:1230, 1963.

Stanzler, R. M.: Management of cardiac arrhythmias, New England J. Med. 274:1307, 1966.

Stephenson, H. E., Jr.: *Cardiac Arrest and Resuscitation* (St. Louis: C. V. Mosby Company, 1964).

Thung, N., Dammann, J. F., Jr., Diaz-Perez, R., Thompson, W. M., Jr., Sanmarco, M., and Mehegan, C.: Hypoxia as the cause of hemorrhage into the cardiac conduction system, arrhythmia and sudden death, J. Thoracic Surg. 44:687, 1962.

"The Role of the Extracellular Fluid in Shock." *Shock* (International Anesthesiology Clinics No. 2) (Boston: Little, Brown & Co., 1964).

BIBLIOGRAPHY
PART 3

Burman, S. O.: Digitalis and thoracic surgery, J. Thoracic & Cardiovas. Surg. 50:873, 1965.

Dieter, R. A., Neville, W. E., and Pifarré, R.: Hypokalemia following hemodilution cardiopulmonary bypass, Ann. Surg. 171:17, 1970.

Effler, D. B.: Anesthesia in revascularization surgery. A new advance, J. Thoracic & Cardiovas. Surg. 56:163, 1968.

Favaloro, R. G.: Unilateral self-retaining retractor for use in internal mammary artery dissection, J. Thoracic & Cardiovas. Surg. 53:864, 1967.

Gianelly, R., Von der Groeben, J. O., Spivack, A. P., and Harrison, J. C.: Effect of lidocaine on ventricular arrhythmias in patients with coronary heart disease, New England J. Med. 277:1215, 1967.

Kahler, R. L., Thombson, R. H., and Busuirk, E. R.: Studies on digitalis: VI: Reduction of oxygen debt after exercise with digoxin in cardiac patients without heart failure, Circulation 27:397, 1963.

Sewell, W. H.: *Surgery for Coronary Artery Disease* (Springfield, Ill.: Charles C Thomas, Publisher, 1967).

BIBLIOGRAPHY
PART 4

Abboud, F. M.: The sympathetic nervous system and alpha-adrenergic blocking agents in shock, Med. Clin. N. Amer. 52:1049, 1968.

Ahlquist, R. P.: Study of the adrenotropic receptors, Am. J. Physiol. 153:586, 1948.

Baue, A. E., Jones, E. F., and Parkins, W. M.: The effects of beta-adrenergic receptor stimulation on blood flow, oxidative metabolism, and survival in hemorrhagic shock, Ann. Surg. 1967:403, 1968.

Berne, R. M.: Effect of epinephrine and norepinephrine on the coronary circulation, Circulation Res. 6:644, 1958.

Braunwald, E., *et al.*: Symposium on beta-adrenergic receptor blockade, Am. J. Cardiol. 18:303, 1966.

Clauss, R. H., and Ray, J. F., III: Pharmacologic assistance to the failing circulation, Surg. Gynec. & Obst. 126:611, 1968.

Cohen, L. S., Buccino, R. A., Morrow, A. G., and Braunwald, E.: Recurrent ventricular tachycardia and fibrillation treated with a combination of beta-adrenergic blockage and electrical pacing, Ann. Int. Med. 66:945, 1967.

Corday, E., Gold, H., Boszormenyi, E., Enescu, V., and Bernstein, H.: Physiological rationale for the combined use of alpha-adrenergic blockers with beta-stimulators in the treatment of cardiogenic shock, Circulation 34 and 35, Suppl. III:III–79, 1968.

Cronin, R. F. P.: Effect of isoproterenol and norepinephrine on myocardial function in experimental cardiogenic shock, Am. Heart J. 74:387, 1967.

Dietzman, R. H., and Lillehei, R. C.: The treatment of cardiogenic shock: Part IV. The use of phenoxybenzamine and chlorpromazine, Am. Heart J. 75:136, 1968.

Dwyer, E. M., Jr., Weiner, L., and Cox, J. W.: Effects of beta-adrenergic blockade (Propanolol) on left ventricular hemodynamics and the electrocardiogram during exercise-induced angina pectoris, Circulation 38:250, 1968.

Elliott, W. C., and Gorlin, R.: Isoproterenol in treatment of heart disease, J.A.M.A. 197:315, 1966.

Epstein, S. E., and Braunwald, E.: Inhibition of the adrenergic nervous system in the treatment of angina pectoris, Med. Clin. N. Amer. 52:1031, 1968.

Gettes, L. S., and Surawicz, B.: Propanolol: Its use in the long-term management of life-threatening arrhythmias and its effect on the electrocardiogram, Circulation, Suppl. III to Vol. 33 and 34: III–109, 1966.

Gianelly, R., Griffin, J. R., and Harrison, D. C.: Propanolol in the treatment and prevention of cardiac arrhythmias, Ann. Int. Med. 66:667, 1967.

Hermreck, A. S., and Thal, A. P.: The Adrenergic Drugs and Their Use in Shock Therapy, in *Current Problems in Surgery* (Chicago: Year Book Medical Publishers, Inc., July, 1968).

Krasnow, N., Rolett, E. L., Yurchak, P. M., Hood, W. B., Jr., and Gorlin, R.: Isoproterenol and cardiovascular performance, Am. J. Med. 37:514, 1964.

Moran, N. C.: Adrenergic receptors, drugs, and the cardiovascular system (I), Mod. Concepts Cardiovas. Dis. 35:93, 1966.

Moran, N. C.: Adrenergic receptors, drugs, and the cardiovascular system (II), Mod. Concepts Cardiovas. Dis. 35:99, 1966.

Schwartz, W.: Sustained-action isoproterenol in the treatment of Adams-Stokes syndrome, Current Therap. Res. 11:64, 1969.

Theilen, E. O., and Wilson, W. R.: Beta-adrenergic receptor blocking drugs in the treatment of cardiac arrhythmias, Med. Clin. N. Amer. 52:1017, 1968.

CHAPTER

3

The Pediatric Cardiac Surgical Patient

MILTON WEINBERG, JR., M.D.

IT IS NOT NECESSARY to discuss here all the details of organizing, staffing, and equipping a surgical intensive care unit (ICU) for the management of pediatric cardiac surgery patients. The basic goals, facilities, and even drug and equipment categories are identical to those used in the care of adults. Certain general observations are pertinent, however.

Despite the fact that children can be taken care of in an adult unit, it is our opinion that if major pediatric surgery is to be undertaken in a general hospital, a pediatric surgical ICU should be established, separate from the adult unit, and located in a pediatric area with pediatric nurses and staff in attendance. In most general hospitals this pediatric location will probably have the undesirable effect of removing the child from the immediate area of the operating room. The advantages, however, more than compensate for this disadvantage. There can be no doubt that a pediatric area is a more desirable environment for the child. Of greater importance, of course, is the fact that the special requirements of pediatric care are learned most quickly and thoroughly when experience is concentrated. These include the simplest problems of dietary and the most complex problems of respiratory care. The proximity of the pediatric attending and house staff is invaluable. Although responsibility and authority for immediate postoperative care properly lie with the surgical staff, intimate involvement of the pediatric staff in that care is highly desirable and should be encouraged. An intangible but unmistakable and certain advantage of the pediatric location of the ICU is in the personal involvement and the dedication of the pediatric nursing staff to the care of children whom they have come to know in the preoperative period and, in most instances, during previous hospital admissions for cardiac catheterization or for medical management of cardiac problems.

The problems of size and maturity dominate the special considerations of a pediatric ICU. Attention should be directed to a careful selection of cribs, beds, and isolettes which will allow adequate access to the child. In particular, the isolettes should be as large as possible, with openings which retract widely to allow management of the ventilatory equipment that will be used for many of the infants.

No consideration is more critical than that of selection of equipment for respiratory care. Endotracheal equipment must include a full range of laryngoscopes, orotracheal and nasotracheal tubes, suction catheters, and adaptors for children, from the smallest premature infant to the largest adolescent. Metal and plastic tracheostomy tubes in all sizes should be available. The ventilators chosen should be those designed specifically for infants and children. Ventilators should be of the type whose driving mechanism is a piston providing a gradually increasing force and injection of air and a stroke volume that is not altered by airway resistance. Thorough education of all personnel in the use of this equipment is essential. The medical and surgical staff must make the effort to learn that a 7- or 8-pound infant will usually accept a #14 French orotracheal tube and that this size tube will admit passage of a #10 French suction catheter if the catheter is properly lubricated with a water-soluble lubricant. These are the critical details which will frequently determine the survival of a desperately ill infant, and similarly proper sizes for all age groups must be learned.

Preoperative Considerations

Certain aspects of preoperative management deserve special attention.

A surprising degree of effective use of intermittent positive-pressure breathing (IPPB) equipment can be achieved in the postoperative course if preoperative education is carried out in children as young as 2 or 3 years of age. The equipment should be used only with a mouthpiece held by the child himself, never with a strapped-on mask, since the forcing of the technic upon an uncooperative and frightened child is of no value and is potentially dangerous. The young child can also be taught effective deep-breathing exercises. Children thoroughly enjoy blowing up surgical gloves, which serve as balloons. It is probably as important that the child become acquainted with the technician or nurse administering the exercises as that he learn the technics, for a child will surely perform best for someone with whom he is familiar and with whom he has worked previously.

Small children should not be subjected to involved explanations of forthcoming procedures. Most children trust the medical and nursing staff about them and will accept necessary procedures when they must be performed, although not necessarily without opposition. It serves no purpose, however, to "prepare" a child by having him anticipate pain and discomfort. Questions should be answered honestly but always with accompanying reassurances. Children under 10 or 11 years of age usually are compliant and adaptable. Teenagers are at times equally manageable, but far more often than younger children may be excessively apprehensive, withdrawn, or even uncooperative and belligerent. These children deserve and should receive the sensitive attention of the surgeon, for it is he alone who must establish in these older youngsters that confidence that a proper decision has been made in subjecting them to operation and that a successful outcome may be anticipated.

Immediate preoperative studies should include coagulation surveys in addition to the more usual routine investigations. This is particularly important in cyanotic children with high hematocrits, in whom coagulation deficiencies are frequently present. Vitamin K is administered to most infants routinely at birth, but its administration should be confirmed when operation is planned in the neonatal period. Prothrombin times are occasionally altered in children with congestive heart failure and liver enlargement. Children receiving blood at a previous operation may have residual liver injury from serum hepatitis.

Most ongoing preoperative medications, including digitalis preparations and diuretics, are continued through the day prior to operation. Excessive potassium loss from dietary restriction and vigorous preoperative diuresis is seldom seen in the child to the degree that it commonly is in the adult, and the consequent arrhythmias of digitalis intoxication are rare. Potassium losses should be replaced, however, and in the child in heart failure who has lost 5 or 10 % of his body weight through diuresis, as in the adult, digitalis and diuretics should be discontinued 24 to 48 hours before operation whenever possible.

Antibiotics administered for a specific indication are usually continued into the day of operation. Nose and throat and anal cultures are taken on admission to the hospital. If a beta-hemolytic streptococcus is cultured from the nose or throat, the child is given a single injection of long-acting benzathine penicillin G. The presence of other organisms on culture usually has not been considered an indication for prophylactic antibiotic therapy, unless a staphylococcus is present in a child in whom prosthetic valve replacement is planned. In this instance, sodium methicillin or other appropriate antibiotic is begun the day prior to operation. In all patients undergoing prosthetic valve replacement, methicillin or sodium cephalothin is added to the pump-oxygenator prime and is continued in a prescribed regimen postoperatively. In all adults, this prophylactic regimen is begun the day prior to operation, but in children, unless the staphylococcus is demonstrably present, the disturbance of the child with the intravenous medication does not seem justified. The furuncles of acne should receive attention before admission to the hospital. The wound of a recent cardiac catheterization should be carefully evaluated, and if infection is present, operation should be postponed.

Preanesthetic medication for children 1 year of age or older should include a narcotic and an anticholinergic agent in dosages appropriate to the child's age and weight, and should be administered 1 hour prior to the call to the operating room. Children under 1 year of age are usually given no sedative or narcotic, and children under 3 months of age are given no premedication.

Restriction of oral intake for 6 to 8 hours before operation is permissible in most children over age 2, but the NPO order should include instructions to give the child oral fluids just prior to the restricted period. Younger children should receive fluids 6 hours before the time of operation, and infants, 4 hours prior to operation. The offered fluid in each instance should be water or other clear liquid rather than milk for this last feeding. Adequate hydration should be a particular concern in cyanotic children with high hematocrits, and if necessary intravenous fluids should be started to avoid dehydration.

Parents should be allowed to remain with their child until he is called to the operating room, and they should be allowed to see the child as soon as possible after his return from the operating room; the child is reassured by their presence on the morning of operation, despite the occasional scene in the hallway or at the elevator. Postoperatively, the child should see his parents as often as conditions in the ICU reasonably can permit visiting. Although there are sound reasons for restricting visits in the ICU, we should not forget that children belong with their parents, and the restrictions should be based upon practical considerations rather than the exercise of authority.

The Operating Room

The stable child may be transported to the operating room in his bed or by cart. It hardly seems necessary to state that a child in oxygen on the pediatric floor should have oxygen continued, but the preoperative orders should include instructions directing its maintenance. Infants in isolettes should be transported in the isolette, and the unit's heating system should be re-established as soon as possible after arrival in the operating room. The children should wait in a quiet area, attended but not entertained or engaged in play. Ideally, the premedication should allow the child to sleep when undisturbed during this waiting period.

The induction of anesthesia should proceed before the child is disturbed in any way whatsoever, so that apprehension and agitation are avoided or minimized. All manipulations, including the placement of electrocardiographic leads and intravenous cannulas, should be postponed until the child is asleep. The induction of anesthesia in a child without an I.V. cannula entails a negligible risk compared to the risk of inducing a frantic, screaming youngster.

The selection of endotracheal tubes should come within the concern of the surgeon. The use of a nasotracheal tube in a child in whom controlled ventilation is planned postoperatively must be discussed with the anesthesiologist prior to induction of anesthesia. Whereas adults will usually tolerate an orotracheal tube for 2 or 3 days, children can be relied upon to bite the tube and to displace it with the tongue. The nasotracheal tube usually can be left in place several days if necessary. Careful fixation of the tube and control of the child's hands are essential, since replacement of any endotracheal tube several times, especially under adverse conditions, is almost a guarantee of laryngeal edema and airway obstruction in a small child. Beyond this obvious interest of the surgeon in the endotracheal tubes, he should ascertain from the anesthesiologist, and make his entire staff aware of, the size of the properly fitting endotracheal tube for the involved child. This information should be in the possession of every member of the team in the ICU, and a tube of the proper size should be attached to the child's bed. The team should also know the size of the suction catheter which best fits the endotracheal tube.

The placement of intravenous cannulas is of critical importance in the management of the children. Infants under 2 years of age will usually require a venesection for cannula placement. Unless cardiopulmonary bypass is planned, one cannula is adequate; we have usually placed this cannula in the saphenous vein at the ankle. In older children undergoing "closed" procedures, two cannulas can usually be placed by percutaneous puncture. In all children who are to undergo cardiopulmonary bypass an additional cannula is placed by venesection into the basilic vein just above either antecubital fossa and passed centrally to monitor right atrial pressure. All I.V. sets should contain a chamber for measuring administered fluids in 10 ml. increments, and the sets for infants should contain droppers which deliver 1/60 ml. per drop. The sets should also have an injection site near the vein so that medications can be injected with a minimal flushing volume. Blood in larger children may be given by drip or with pressure units in measured amounts as necessary. Blood is usually administered to infants in controlled amounts by syringe injection. All blood administered in the operating room and in the ICU is warmed to approximately 37 C. by passage through a warming coil placed in a thermostatically controlled water bath. It should be emphasized that all intravenous catheters utilized for central venous pressure monitoring should be radiopaque or contain a radiopaque line for identification on x-rays.

Arterial cannulation for pressure and blood gas monitoring can be done percutaneously or by cutdown in the radial artery, but we have found this necessary only in rare instances. Arterial pressures are monitored from the arterial line of the pump-oxygenator in the children undergoing open-heart procedures, and with the chest open, blood-gas samples are obtained from the aorta or a cardiac chamber.

We have limited the deliberate planning for control of ventilation postoperatively to relatively few patients. This group commonly includes patients undergoing complete repair of transposition of the great vessels, severe tetralogy of Fallot, and ventricular septal defects with near systemic levels of pulmonary arteriolar resistance as well as a number of less common complex defects. In each of these instances temporary prolongation of the anesthesia into the immediate postoperative period has the advantage of allowing time to return the child to the ICU while still quiet and somnolent and instituting controlled ventilation under ideal circumstances. We have preferred that all other children be extubated in the operating room, a situation requiring that they be awake and capable of maintaining an adequate respiratory rate and tidal volume, and that they be free of significant tracheobronchial secretions. If these children, including severely ill infants, are to be extubated safely, it is essential that the experienced members of the surgical team be present at the end of operation, and that the children be observed critically at this time. This period in the operating room is all too frequently a time when only the least-experienced surgeons remain, a time which should be devoted to a mature evaluation of all physiologic parameters.

All children should receive oxygen en route to the ICU, the infants in the isolette, the older children by nasal catheter. High concentrations of oxygen have been delivered to the patient up to this time by the anesthesiologist, and concentrations as high as reasonably possible should be administered during this vulnerable period. An endotracheal tube of the proper size, laryngoscopic equipment, and a hand ventilator with a proper adaptor should accompany the child to the ICU. With few exceptions, children in whom an endotracheal tube has been left in place should be ventilated continuously. The relatively small endotracheal tubes that must be utilized in children introduce a highly significant degree of airway resistance that may increase the work of breathing and can reduce total air flow. Chest drainage tubes can usually be clamped during transport from the operating room to the ICU, but if blood loss is significant or if an air leak from the lung is recognized, the chest tubes should be kept open, with the bottles secured below the level of the child's thorax. Pneumothorax occasionally occurs in any patient on positive-pressure ventilation and not infrequently occurs unrecognized with a sternal splitting incision. A significant degree of pneumothorax should be determined by auscultation and palpation of the trachea before moving the patient, and if strongly suspected, can be managed by aspiration.

The Intensive Care Unit

The ICU should anticipate the needs of cardiac surgical patients in general, with monitoring equipment, oxygen and suction apparatus, I.V. equipment, and drugs appropriate to the emergency and routine requirements of this category of patient. The Unit should also anticipate the particular needs of the specific patient, which requires that the ICU staff be aware of the child's age, size, and problem so that special needs can be met. In general, one nurse should be assigned exclusively to the returning child until his immediate needs are satisfied and his stability allows her attention to be divided among other occupants of the unit.

The arrival of the child at the ICU should be met with an immediate establishment of systems to evaluate the status of the child, to initiate the regimens of therapy designed to support him during the recovery period, and to deal rapidly and efficiently with specific problems to which these children are subject. Two areas should receive the initial attention of every member of the staff—cardiac adequacy as indicated by the heart sounds over the precordium and the volume of peripheral pulses; and ventilatory adequacy as indicated by an unobstructed and adequate exchange of air. If the patient is to be ventilated mechanically, the establishment of this system demands the first priority. In prompt sequence, the electrocardiogram should be connected for display on the oscilloscope; blood pressure and pulse should be ascertained and recorded on the chart; rectal temperature is taken; I.V.'s are positioned—usually first untangled—for management of flow rates and for easy access to injection sites; the flow status of special drugs such as isoproterenol, potassium chloride, and other medications is determined; the central venous pressure monitoring system is established; arterial or left atrial monitoring may be established: blood is drawn for indicated studies; urinary drainage is connected when a catheter is in place.

CARDIAC RATE AND RHYTHM AND THE ELECTROCARDIOGRAM.— In the child as in the adult, continuous monitoring of the electrocardiogram on an easily visible oscilloscope is established for all patients immediately upon return to the ICU. Additionally, a recording of the electrocardiogram with all leads is obtained as soon as reasonably possible, and a copy of the tracing should be placed in the ICU chart for immediate reference when needed.

Significant differences can be predicted in the cardiac performance of children in contrast to the patterns encountered in adults. In great part this is due to the fact that the majority of surgical lesions in children are congenital and the myocardium is usually normal, capable of maintaining satisfactory output in the presence of rapid rates and arrhythmias that would be intolerable in an adult. Cardiac rates of 120 to 140 per minute are commonly present in children under 8 or 10 years of age following operation, and, with temperature elevation, rates of 160 per minute or higher may be seen. These rates are well tolerated and usually require no specific treatment directed to the tachycardia.

In general, pathologic tachycardias are relatively uncommon in children and are most frequently supraventricular in origin. Ventricular tachycardias are encountered in infants with pulmonary artery origin of the left coronary artery and left ventricular ischemia or infarct. We have also encountered episodes of ventricular tachycardia in a child with an isolated congenital aneurysm of the left ventricle and in an occasional child following operation upon the left ventricle for muscular subaortic stenosis. Isolated or multiple premature ventricular contractions and ventricular tachycardia may occur postoperatively in children with rheumatic heart disease or myocarditis, digitalis excess or potassium deficiency, acidosis, hypoxia and anemia. This arrhythmia, as in the adult, may be treated selectively with intravenous lidocaine, Dilantin, quinidine, procainamide, or when indicated by electric-shock cardioversion. Far more important is the avoidance and correction of those physiologic aberrations described above, to obviate the occurrence of ventricular tachycardia.

Supraventricular tachycardias are encountered in patients with atrial septal defects, particularly those of the endocardial cushion variety. They are also seen frequently in patients with Ebstein's anomaly, corrected transposition, and following complete correction of transposition of the great vessels. When these tachycardias occur in the absence of correctable physiologic disturbances and when they are persistent, they usually respond well to digitalization. Rarely, they may require electrical cardioversion and may be recurrent. Propanolol may be useful in controlling the episodes.

Nodal rhythms with rates of 70 to 90 per minute are not uncommonly seen following repair of atrial septal defects of the primum or secundum varieties. Cardiac output is not recognizably affected and no treatment is necessary. The rhythm usually reverts to a normal sinus pattern within 3 to 6 weeks, although rarely the nodal rhythm persists. Nodal rhythms are encountered frequently after total correction of transposition of the great vessels, occasionally following repair of ventricular septal defect, tetralogy of Fallot, and mitral or tricuspid valve replacement. In these patients requiring optimal cardiac performance in the immediate postoperative period, temporary pacing wires should be implanted at the time of operation when nodal rhythms or other arrhythmias are encountered.

One electrode is usually implanted in the right ventricular myocardium and a second indifferent electrode is implanted subcutaneously. The heart rate is maintained at 100 to 110 per minute. If the rhythm does not convert to a normal sinus origin, the slower rate of the nodal rhythm is usually well tolerated within 5 to 7 days after operation and pacing can be discontinued. We have implanted temporary pacing wires with increasing frequency over the past several years and now implant them in all children undergoing transposition repair or prosthetic valve replacement, and in many children undergoing right or left ventriculotomy. We have never regretted the implantation of the wires but have lamented their absence on numerous occasions.

Complete heart block due to suture injury of the bundle of His is rare now but still may occur. Complete heart block has also been encountered with the surgical production of a right bundle branch block in a child with a pre-existing congenital left bundle branch block. Without exception, electrical pacing of the heart should be maintained in the immediate postoperative period. Not only are the demands for maximal cardiac output greatest at this time, but, just as importantly, the relatively slow ventricular rate invites ventricular arrhythmias initiated from intrinsic or extrinsic foci.

Permanent cardiac pacing is no small matter in a child but should probably be undertaken if the complete block persists with a ventricular rate less than 70 per minute. Later conversion to a normal sinus rhythm may occur, the latest in our experience being 6 months after operation, although reported as long as 2 years postoperatively. The selection of a transvenous or epicardial electrodes placed by thoracotomy must depend upon the experience of the surgical and medical team. No degree of excellence in the management of complete heart block by pacing can substitute for the avoidance of this mishap, and all surgeons who would approach the area of the bundle of His are urged to acquaint themselves thoroughly with the anatomy of the conduction system of the heart.

Bradycardia in infants that are cyanotic or in heart failure is far more ominous than tachycardia and frequently signals the presence of acute distress. Typically, the electrocardiographic pattern of acute cardiac distress in these infants is one of initial slowing of the rate to below 70 or 80 per minute, followed in sequence by prolongation of the P–R interval, atrioventricular dissociation, disappearance of the P waves, an idioventricular origin of the QRS complex, and finally cardiac standstill or, less commonly, ventricular fibrillation. In the operating room the major causes of this chain of events are anesthetic depression of the myocardium and displacement of the heart and great vessels by the surgeon. Postoperatively, the cardiac deterioration is almost always due to hypoxia, and immediate therapy should begin with controlled ventilation of the child. Metabolic acidosis frequently precedes and always follows the episode, and sodium bicarbonate, in increments of 4–5 mEq. should be administered in infants. Circulation is maintained by manual external cardiac compression and the appropriate drugs for cardiac resuscitation—calcium chloride, isoproterenol, and epinephrine—are given by intravenous or intracardiac injection, as indicated.

RESPIRATORY CARE.—The overwhelming majority of children subjected to cardiac surgical procedures should have the endotracheal tube removed in the operating room and should be returned to the ICU awake and capable of maintaining adequate respirations. Infants up to 12 to 14 pounds in weight, if not limited by length, are maintained in an isolette, with high humidity supplied by an ultrasonic nebulizer and with oxygen concentrations approximating 40%. The head end of the tray upon which the infant rests is elevated 15 to 20 degrees. The infant is turned to the sides, face, and back at intervals not exceeding 2 hours. Tapping of the back or elevated side by the nurse with each turning appears to be useful. The chest should be tapped several times daily for dependent drainage of tracheobronchial secretions by a nurse or technician trained in this technic. The occasional introduction of a catheter into the oropharynx may stimulate a productive cough in some infants, but frequent use of a catheter through the nose or mouth is likely to cause nosebleed or an increase in the pharyngeal secretions by trauma, and occasionally may cause epiglottic or pharyngeal edema sufficient to obstruct the airway. Accumulated tracheobronchial secretions are best aspirated in an infant by introduction of a small suction catheter into the trachea under direct vision with a laryngoscope. Suction should be limited to no more than −20 cm. of water, to avoid excessive trauma to the tracheal mucosa, particularly at the level of the glottic structures. To alternately aspirate and hyperventilate an infant over several minutes, an endotracheal tube may be inserted for a few minutes. These procedures must be carried out expertly if laryngeal edema is to be avoided. A strong, vigorous baby with a lusty cry will seldom have postoperative respiratory problems. The weak, debilitated infant will require the utmost in the persistent, gentle and patient application of the art of respiratory care.

Older children can usually be induced to hyperventilate and cough by persuasion and occasionally by threat. As in the infant, the trachea cannot be entered easily by the nasal or oral route by blind intubation in small children, and repeated use of the catheter is futile and may be detrimental. In a child of 10 years of age or over, nasotracheal intubation is more often successful and may be used as indicated. A Coudé catheter with a curved tip is more easily introduced into the trachea than a straight catheter. Most reasonably bright youngsters will require nasotracheal introduction of a catheter to evacuate tracheobronchial secretions just once, and thereafter cough enthusiastically at the mere mention of its repetition. It should be emphasized that such vigorous assaults are seldom necessary in children. High humidity in a tent with oxygen, frequent turning, and sympathetic assistance in coughing and deep breathing will suffice to adequately ventilate and eliminate tracheobronchial secretions in all but an occasional child.

Chest tubes are painful and should be removed as soon as drainage ceases. After the first 48 to 72 hours, a high-humidity tent may become a detriment to respiratory care by restricting movement and inhibiting the conversation and interest in surroundings that stimulate normal excursion of the thoracic wall. Bronchoscopy is rarely necessary for removal of tracheobronchial secretions, and atelectasis of even substantial segments of the lung can be managed by the technics described above. Tracheostomy has been necessary for controlled ventilation but not for the management of tracheobronchial secretions in children.

The desirability or necessity for ventilatory control in cardiac surgical patients should in most cases be anticipated and imposed electively rather than as an urgent measure. That unpredictable situations will arise occasionally, however, is unfortunately but inevitably true. Unconsciousness and uncertainty regarding the adequacy of ventilation may follow cerebral embolism of air or a thrombus or a convulsion of any etiology. In cardiac arrest, ventilatory control is essential to resuscitation and for an indefinite period thereafter. The persistence or progression of metabolic acidosis is most effectively combatted when respirations are controlled, as is the acute onset of pulmonary edema in the immediate postoperative period. With the onset of an acute emergency requiring respiratory control, positive-pressure ventilation should initially be delivered with a face mask for at least a few breaths before endotracheal intubation is attempted.

Immediate oxygenation can be achieved in virtually all children with the mask and a hand ventilator, whereas even in the most expert hands the child remains hypoxic for the seconds required to introduce the endotracheal tube, and in less than expert hands the time consumed for intubation may be fatal. With the child oxygenated by mask, an endotracheal tube of the proper size, the laryngoscope, suction apparatus, and connectors can be made ready and intubation then carried out under far more favorable conditions. Because of relative ease of insertion, an orotracheal tube is usually inserted during the emergency. A bite block may be taped in place if necessary. As soon as the emergency situation is controlled and expert assistance is available, the orotracheal may be replaced with a nasotracheal tube.

When the cardiac surgical procedure to be performed can be expected to produce a temporary but serious compromise of cardiac performance, controlled ventilation should be planned from the induction of anesthesia. A nasotracheal tube is inserted and firmly secured in place by the anesthesiologist, and a proper ventilator, connectors, catheters, and an appropriate bed for control of the child are made ready. These preparations and the imposition of ventilatory control are carried out in all children subjected to complete repair of transposition of the great vessels where cardiac output is subject to variation because of the unpredictable influence of the intra-atrial baffle upon systemic and pulmonary venous return to the heart; in severe tetralogy of Fallot requiring extensive resection or a patch in the outflow tract of the right ventricle and similarly in muscular subaortic stenosis where resection of left ventricular myocardium is performed; in closure of ventricular septal defect in the presence of near systemic levels of pulmonary vascular resistance; in prosthetic valve replacement; and in a variety of other procedures now being undertaken for the correction of complex congenital anomalies of the heart. Mechanical ventilation in these children assures an unfailing adequate O_2:CO_2 exchange; with proper rate and inspiration:expiration ratio, ventricular filling is enhanced by the positive intrathoracic pressure; the caloric expenditure and O_2 consumption of the work of breathing is virtually eliminated; and a controlled respiratory alkalosis may effectively compensate metabolic acidosis. In our opinion there is no place for assisted ventilation in these children, and complete control of respiration should be accomplished by the delivering of adequate oxygenation and the reduction of the partial pressure of carbon dioxide in arterial blood (Pa_{CO_2}) to levels which eliminate the child's stimulus to spontaneous respiration. In general, the partial pressure of oxygen in arterial blood (Pa_{O_2}) should range from 80 to 100 mm. Hg and not over 150 mm. Hg; Pa_{CO_2} levels of 35 mm. Hg or less generally suppress spontaneous respirations if O_2 saturation is adequate. The respiratory rate and stroke volume of the ventilator should be at the lowest levels that will keep the child under control. Adequate sedation is indispensable to the management of a child on a respirator; we have used most effectively intravenous morphine sulfate, 0.1 mg. per kilogram of body weight, or chlorpromazine, 0.1 mg. per kilogram of body weight. In the occasional child with pulmonary insufficiency, oxygenation can be achieved only by hyperventilation with a rapid rate and high stroke volume that excessively lowers the Pa_{CO_2} and imposes undesirable levels of respiratory alkalosis. The ability of hemoglobin to release O_2 at tissue levels is inhibited by extreme alkalosis, and severe urinary potassium losses accompany the compensatory excretion of bicarbonate. It is useful under these circumstances to add CO_2 to the air–O_2 gas mixture being delivered through the ventilator, a 1 to 2 percent concentration usually being adequate to elevate the arterial P_{CO_2} to acceptable levels. Additional details regarding the management of ventilators are discussed elsewhere in this volume.

Discontinuing controlled ventilation in a child requires careful attention to blood gases and the signs of changes in cardiac output as well as signs of fatigue. If possible, before discontinuing the ventilator, the O_2 concentration being delivered should be reduced to that of room air, and rate and stroke volume should be reduced to a minimum. The inside diameter of the lumen of the connector which delivers O_2 and high humidity to the open endotracheal tube should be the same as that of the lumen of the tube. Under careful observation, the child is left off the ventilator initially for 30 minutes and blood-gas determinations are made. If these are satisfactory, the child is placed on a schedule of off–ventilator for 2 hours, then on–ventilator for 1 hour. The off interval is gradually extended, again with careful attention to the factor of fatigue as well as other physiologic considerations.

Although nasotracheal tubes are being left in place for increasing periods of time, in some institutions for 2 weeks or more, we have usually performed a tracheostomy if it is obvious that ventilation will be required for more than 4 or 5 days. Other indications for tracheostomy, including laryngeal edema, are well recognized. Tracheostomy should, however, never be performed in a struggling, hypoxic child. In all cases, an endotracheal tube should be inserted if one is not already in place, and the operation should take place with the child under complete ventilatory control, anesthetized or well sedated. While recognizing that the facilities of the operating room afford the optimal circumstances for performance of the tracheostomy, it is also true that the movement of a child with cardiac problems in the postoperative period is not always desirable, and facilities in the ICU should be adequate for the safe and efficient performance of a tracheostomy. The tracheal incision should be at a relatively high level, between the first and second tracheal rings, so that the tube rests well on the neck and not on the clavicular head. The rings should be accurately identified, since subglottic stenosis can almost be assured if the cricoid cartilage is injured in the small trachea of a child. The ring below the incision should be divided rather than a segment removed. Before final removal of the tracheostomy tube, progressively smaller tubes should be inserted, and in small children it is frequently advisable to perform laryngoscopy and bronchoscopy to see that granulation tissue does not obstruct the trachea above or below the tracheostomy site. Careful performance of the tracheostomy, proper tube selection, adequate humidification, and attention to sterile technic in suctioning and in changing of tubes are essential if the distressing complication of tracheal stenosis is to be avoided.

Management of Cardiac Output

Arterial and Venous Pressure Monitoring

There is no need to enumerate here all the principles of management of cardiac output, the treatment of shock and the "low output syndrome." In general, these do not differ as between children and adults and are adequately discussed elsewhere in this publication. There are, however, a few special considerations in children that warrant further comment.

With attention to adequate blood replacement and hemostasis in the operating room, few children will be returned to the ICU with evidences of significantly depressed cardiac output. In small infants, loss of body heat due to exposure, with rectal temperatures falling as low as 33 C., will result in cerebral depression, loss of muscular tone and a corresponding fall in cardiac output, with a slow heart rate, distant heart sounds, and feeble peripheral pulses. These signs of depression will disappear as the child is warmed in the isolette, unless the child is also hypovolemic, acidotic or has an intolerable cardiac or pulmonary disability.

Blood replacement in the operating room is judged by accurate weighing of sponges and measurement of suction with attention to volumes of pericardial and pleural fluid and irrigating solutions. Postoperatively, chest tube drainage is measured in bottles which allow estimation of 10 ml. increments. Losses should be considered as percentages of the child's blood volume. For example, a child weighing 5 kg. has an estimated blood volume of $7\frac{1}{2}\%$ of body weight, or 375 ml.; therefore, a 35 ml. blood loss, negligible in an older child or an adult, represents 10% of the infant's blood volume and if lost rapidly should be replaced. Additional guides to blood replacement are the fontanelle and neck veins and particularly the liver, which is capable of distending or receding rapidly with gain or reduction of blood volume. We do not often use arterial or central venous pressure catheters in infants but rely on clinical signs to judge the adequacy of blood volume.

Frequent blood-gas determinations are essential in these ill infants, and metabolic acidosis should be corrected with sodium bicarbonate in amounts calculated on the basis of the determined base deficit (weight in kilograms $\times$ base deficit $\times$ 0.3 = mEq. base). We have seldom used tris buffer (THAM) in the treatment of acidosis in children. Blood samples for these determinations are obtained by arterial puncture or by heel stick after warming the foot with warm, moist packs. Comparative studies have well established the validity of specimens obtained by the heel stick if the foot is well prepared and the puncture affords a free flow of blood to the capillary tube. Digitalization when indicated is carried out with digoxin in accepted dosages calculated on the basis of weight. It should be noted here that we have digitalized most infants in whom aorta-pulmonary artery shunts have been performed. In the presence of persistently low or declining cardiac output, isoproterenol by continuous drip may improve cardiac performance. The isoproterenol is administered in a solution containing 0.2 to 1 mg. per 100 ml. of 5% dextrose in water, the drug concentrated as necessary to avoid fluid overload. Cardiac tamponade should remain a consideration in the evaluation of any infant, or older child for that matter, with a declining cardiac output.

Problems of cardiac output following operation in the older child should be and are rare except in the complex procedures previously listed as frequently requiring respiratory control. In children subjected to "closed-heart" procedures, operative blood loss and gain are usually modest and pulmonary and systemic arteriolar resistances are not profoundly changed. Complications, therefore, are for the most part those of any thoracotomy—namely, blood loss from the operative site and chest wall with failure of complete hemostasis, and pulmonary atelectasis associated with retained secretions and with splinting of the chest wall and diaphragm.

Repair of coarctation of the aorta follows a somewhat exceptional pattern. Most patients exhibit systemic hypertension, occasionally striking, following coarctation repair. The hypertension is usually associated with tachycardia, both gradually declining to near normal levels in 3 to 5 days, occasionally longer. Reduction of the blood pressure to completely normal levels frequently requires 6 weeks to 3 months. We have not considered it necessary to treat such hypertension, even when initially severe, and have not recognized ill effects from not having done so. The abdominal pain and tenderness, occasional nausea and vomiting, and very rare bowel necrosis seen following coarctation repair may be related to the hypertension, but the level of the hypertension and treatment or lack thereof does not affect the course of the abdominal problems. These are treated by withholding oral intake or by passage of a nasogastric tube for gastric aspiration, or by operation if the signs of peritoneal irritation suggest the necessity.

In older children, as in infants, congestive heart failure may follow the construction of an aortic-pulmonary artery shunt, and digitalization may be necessary. Persistence of the signs of congestive heart failure may dictate the addition of diuretics to the therapeutic regimen, usually Diuril (chlorothiazide) or Lasix (furosemide). Ethacrynic acid (Edecrin) is given only to those patients refractory to the other diuretics, since its use appears to be associated occasionally with impairment of hearing.

Neither arterial nor central venous pressure catheters are utilized in these closed-heart procedures. Blood pressure is taken by cuff with auscultation. It should be noted here that the selection of a blood pressure cuff of proper size—the width approximately two-thirds the length of the upper arm—is essential to accurate recording of the blood pressure. A narrower blood pressure cuff will give a falsely high blood pressure, a wider cuff a falsely low one. Urinary bladder catheters are not used. Blood-gas and electrolyte determinations are obtained only when indicted by clinical manifestations.

The open-heart procedures entailing limited alterations of cardiac dynamics—again, exclusive of those listed in the section on controlled ventilation—are monitored by the electrocardiogram and by measurement of the systemic pressure by cuff and the central venous pressures. Urinary drainage catheters are placed to prevent bladder distention during and following cardiopulmonary bypass but are rarely needed as an aid in evaluating cardiac output in these patients. If the urinary output is adequate, the catheter is removed the night of surgery or the following morning. In the rare instance of suppression of urinary output, the presence of the catheter directs attention at the earliest possible moment to the renal problem so that mannitol, Lasix, or ethacrynic acid in trial doses may be administered, adequate consultation may be obtained, and other therapy may be instituted as indicated. As a testimony to the rarity of renal failure in children, we had not encountered a single such instance until this year, when renal shutdown occurred in a 5-year-old following operative treatment of fixed subaortic stenosis associated with corrected transposition. The reason for renal failure in this child is not known.

Digoxin is administered routinely for ventriculotomy, since the majority of these children will exhibit signs of congestive heart failure after operation. The accepted total intravenous digitalizing dose of digoxin for children is as follows:

Age	*Dosage/lb. Body Weight*
Under 2 weeks	0.01 – 0.02 mg.
2 weeks to 2 years	0.02 – 0.03 mg.
2 to 10 years	0.01 – 0.02 mg.
10 years and over	1.0 – 1.5 mg.

The intravenous dose is two-thirds the oral dose.

Half of the calculated digitalizing dose is given in the operating room after cardiopulmonary bypass is completed and major blood loss has subsided. A fourth of the total dose is given intravenously 4 to 6 hours later. The remaining fourth of the calculated dose is given 6 to 12 hours later, after review of the electrocardiogram and electrolyte determinations. Maintenance of digitalization is by parenteral or oral routes appropriate for the status of the child. In most children with a right ventriculotomy, digoxin can be discontinued within 3 months after operation, but of course is maintained as long as indicated by the child's clinical course.

Exceptionally severe congestive heart failure may follow incomplete closure of a ventricular septal defect, particularly in tetralogy of Fallot, and early reoperation should be carried out if failure is not easily controlled with digitalization and an aggressive regimen of diuretics and fluid and sodium restriction. As indicated elsewhere, fluid and sodium restrictions are seldom necessary in a child.

Despite their relative stability and the evident reserve of cardiac output, most of these children return to the ICU with some degree of increased systemic arteriolar resistance, as evidenced by less than full peripheral pulses, mildly narrowed pulse pressure, rather cool hands and feet with empty veins and perhaps slight cyanosis of nailbeds. The blood pressure is frequently high and central venous pressure may be normal or mildly elevated. The maintenance of modest elevations of central venous pressure to 10 to 12 cm. of water by blood transfusion can be expected to be accompanied by progressive warming of the extremities, with filling of the peripheral veins and disappearance of cyanosis of the nailbeds, improvement of peripheral pulses and expansion of the arterial pulse pressure. Systolic blood pressure usually declines to a level consistent with the age of the child. The persistence of these evidences of a satisfactory cardiac output and the evident return of arteriolar resistance to normal for several hours, without significant blood loss from the chest drainage tubes, allows blood administration to be stopped and the venous pressure to gradually return to normal. Failure to achieve the response described above is usually due to excessive blood loss, although cardiac tamponade should again receive strong consideration. If blood loss is persistently at a level of 5 to 10 percent of estimated blood volume per hour, and certainly if greater, reoperation for control of bleeding should not be delayed unless a clotting defect amenable to specific therapy can be identified. It is pertinent to add that we have never regretted returning a child to the operating room for the control of bleeding, but have regretted the delay many times. In the absence of obvious bleeding to explain persistent constriction and limitation of cardiac output, chest x-rays may demonstrate widening of the mediastinum or the cardiac silhouette or accumulation of blood in a pleural cavity to dictate reoperation. The absence of the findings on x-ray should not deter the surgeon from exploring the child to evacuate a possible pericardial hematoma. If no hematoma is found, inotropic agents, principally isoproterenol, may be given in an attempt to increase the effectiveness of the myocardial contraction. These patients must then be managed with a regimen designed to achieve maximum levels of cardiac output.

In the management of a patient whose cardiac output is expected to be critically reduced by an extensive operative procedure, attention to detail in the operating room and thereafter is essential. As indicated above, nasotracheal intubation is carried out by the anesthesiologist for control of ventilation as long as necessary. Meticulous attention to hemostasis is mandatory to avoid significant postoperative blood loss. Consultation with an authority in coagulation problems is obtained prior to operation, and a coagulation profile is obtained immediately after the child's return to the ICU. At the termination of cardiopulmonary bypass, but prior to removal of the arterial line from the patient, a careful estimation of right and left atrial pressures in relation to cardiac performance is made while transfusing the patient with small increments of blood from the pump oxygenator. It is at this time that the most desirable level of central venous pressure for optimal cardiac performance can be determined and maintained in the postoperative period.

The effects of inotropic agents upon the myocardium can also be determined at the operating table. Blood-gas determinations at 2-4-hour intervals should begin prior to cardiopulmonary bypass, and should continue throughout operation and the first 24 hours following operation. Base deficits are corrected with sodium bicarbonate. Persistent or progressive metabolic acidosis should initiate the consideration of administering an inotropic agent. Vasoconstriction will usually respond to the enhancement of cardiac output by maintenance of central venous pressure at optimal predetermined levels by infusion of blood or albumin. The hematocrit should be determined at frequent intervals. Peripheral resistance is increased by an increase in viscosity, and hematocrit levels greater than 45 percent should be avoided. The choice of blood or albumin to replace blood loss or to expand blood volume should be determined by the hematocrit level. A low hematocrit in the presence of an adequate blood volume will dictate the use of packed red blood cells to restore adequate oxygen-carrying capacity. Reduction of peripheral resistance due to vasoconstriction, if not accomplished by volume enhancement of stroke volume, has most often been accomplished in our experience by the administration of a titered drip of isoproterenol, 0.2–1 mg. in 100 ml. of 5% dextrose in water. The inotropic effect of isoproterenol is accompanied by its action as a peripheral dilator. We have used but have not been impressed by the reduction in peripheral resistance produced by large doses of corticosteroids. As advised, we have administered 30 mg. of Solu-Medrol (methylprednisolone sodium succinate) per kilogram of body weight intravenously in a single injection and have repeated the dose within several hours. Chlorpromazine, in intravenous doses of 0.1 mg. per kilogram of body weight, has appeared to effectively reduce peripheral resistance in some children, and has a further beneficial sedative effect. Control of restlessness and agitation by sedation with intravenous chlorpromazine and morphine sulfate also effectively reduces muscular activity, metabolic rate and oxygen consumption without a significant detrimental effect on the myocardium.

Elevations of temperature are common immediately after cardiopulmonary bypass, probably due for the most part to the patient's inability to lose heat through the skin in the presence of vasoconstriction. Fever should be combatted with rectal aspirin, morphine or chlorpromazine to reduce metabolic rate and shivering, and if necessary for temperature elevations above 40 C., sponging or the use of a cooling mattress.

We have abandoned the use of plasma as a volume expander in favor of normal serum albumin, which appears to be completely free of the danger of viral hepatitis. Fresh frozen plasma is used when indicated for the correction of coagulation defects.

Epsilon aminocaproic acid is administered intravenously, 5 Gm. in the first hour and 1 Gm. per hour thereafter for 6 to 8 hours, when excessive fibrinolytic activity can be demonstrated. We have abandoned its routine use in open–heart patients for lack of evidence that it favorably affects postoperative blood loss.

Postoperative Care

ANTIBIOTICS.—We administer intravenous sodium methicillin to all open-heart patients postoperatively, 25 mg. per kilogram of body weight every 6 hours. In patients with prosthetic valves, methicillin is replaced with oral sodium oxacillin when I.V.'s are discontinued; this drug is continued to the tenth postoperative day. In all other patients, antibiotic therapy is stopped at 5 days, or before if I.V.'s are discontinued sooner. Antibiotics are usually not administered to patients subjected to closed-heart operations. If the child has a history of mild or indistinct sensitivity to penicillin, sodium cephalothin in comparable doses is substituted for methicillin, although a 15% incidence of cross-reaction is recognized. With a clear history of a significant penicillin reaction, all penicillin-related antibiotics should be avoided and appropriate substitutes administered. Except in the patient with prosthetic valves, we have usually simply given no antibiotics with a clear history of sensitivity, and I suspect that the incidence of infection is little if at all greater.

The persistence or recurrence of fever should initiate all of the usual searches for etiology. It is often advisable to stop antibiotics, which have obviously not been effective if the fever is due to infection, to obtain additional urine, sputum, and blood cultures. It is by no means uncommon to have the fever disappear with the discontinuance of the antibiotics. It should be noted that fever frequently accompanies anemia in the postoperative period, and the hemoglobin should not be allowed to fall below 10 Gm. per 100 ml. In the presence of daily temperature elevation, hemoglobin should be maintained at 12 Gm. per 100 ml.

FLUID REQUIREMENTS AND DIET.—All children are kept on NPO until the morning following operation. Although gastric dilatation has received considerable attention in the past as a reason for interference with respirations and cardiac output, this has not been apparent to us and we do not employ nasogastric suction in the children. On the day following operation, most children will eagerly accept 30 ml. of clear liquids, which can usually be advanced to a clear liquid diet within several hours. Full liquids are usually given the following day and diet for age thereafter. Sodium and fluid restrictions are not imposed upon the children unless signs of congestive heart failure are present and persistent.

Intravenous fluids are administered in amounts of one-half the normal daily requirements for weight the first 24 hours after operation, and three-fourths the normal daily requirement minus the oral intake the second 24 hours after operation. Five per cent dextrose in water is given the first day, 5% dextrose in 0.2N saline solution the second day. Standard pediatric requirements for age and weight are given thereafter, subject to the restrictions of the cardiac status, if intravenous fluids are needed for a longer period. In the presence of fever and obvious dehydration demonstrated by a high urinary specific gravity and diminution of urine excretion, the foregoing volumes are increased as required. The following table lists the normal daily fluid requirements in children:

Weight	*Amount Per 24 Hours*
0–10 kg.	100 ml./kg.
11–20 kg.	1000 ml. + 50 ml. for each kg. > 10
21 kg. and over	1500 ml. + 20 ml. for each kg. > 20

Volumes of fluid riders for antibiotics, isoproterenol, and other medications should be included in the calculation of the daily fluid orders. At no time should more than a volume equal to one-fourth the normal daily requirement be hanging and connected to I.V.'s in a child. If this amount should accidentally be infused rapidly because of a loose clamp or regulator, it should be easily tolerated by the child.

SEDATION.—The use of morphine sulfate and chlorpromazine, as described earlier, is an important adjunct to therapy in the critically ill child. Otherwise, children under 10 years of age will require little if any sedation, and routine narcotic orders are never written. A child who is unusually restless or in distress should be seen by a physician, and, if indicated, a narcotic or sedative can be ordered as a statim dose. Older children are given PRN orders for morphine or Demerol (meperidine) according to standard age and weight tables and reasonable judgment. All narcotics are given intravenously until cardiac output appears adequate and signs of peripheral constriction have disappeared.

ELECTROLYTES.—The goals and application of electrolyte studies in adults and children are identical and need not be repeated here. It should be noted, however, that the increasing use of large dilution volumes and mannitol in the perfusate of the pump-oxygenators has introduced potassium losses that were not encountered earlier. These renal losses may be further extended by respiratory alkalosis when the child is on a mechanical ventilator. Urinary potassium should be measured as well as serum potassium, and in the presence of a good urine output, potassium is most accurately replaced by estimating the urinary loss. The kidneys are incapable of excreting urine containing less than 10 to 12 mEq. of potassium per liter, and with concentration of urine may excrete 100 or more mEq. per liter. If urinary potassium levels are determined at intervals, losses can be replaced on a current basis. Commonly used concentrated solutions of KCl —20 to 40 mEq. per 100 ml. injected as a rider—are highly irritating to peripheral veins and should be injected through the central venous catheter. If peripheral veins are used for KCl infusion, the solution should contain no more than 40 mEq. per 250 ml. of solute.

With diminution of urine output, greater reliance must be placed upon serum potassium determinations. Sodium and chloride serum levels are rarely altered postoperatively, and we have not recognized a magnesium deficiency in a child.

CHEST X-RAYS.—Portable chest x-rays are obtained immediately after the child's return to the ICU and daily while he is in the ICU. Obvious areas of concern include the presence of pneumothorax or hemothorax; expansion of the mediastinum or cardiac silhouette suggesting blood accumulation or dilatation of the heart; atelectasis and pulmonary consolidation. In children with large and hypertensive pulmonary arteries, atelectasis or air trapping may occur due to bronchial compression by the main pulmonary artery branches, usually the left. If atelectasis is extensive and persistent, pulmonary artery banding may be necessary to relieve the bronchial compression. Atelectasis of this etiology may be a preoperative indication for pulmonary artery banding or closure of an atrial or ventricular septal defect when pulmonary artery enlargement is due to increased flow.

Air trapping with disruption of lung parenchyma is likely to occur with mechanical ventilation of small infants. This is best avoided or managed by careful adjustment of the rate and stroke volume of the ventilator and by sedation of the child when necessary to prevent precipitous elevations of intrabronchial pressures with struggling or fighting the ventilator.

Particular attention should be given to the position of the central venous catheter and to the position of an endotracheal or tracheostomy tube.

A chest x-ray should be obtained whenever a child exhibits unexplained distress. It is usually wise to repeat the chest x-ray frequently if drainage of blood from the chest tubes is excessive and, when excessive bleeding stops, to be assured that the cessation is not due to impeded drainage and intrathoracic accumulation.

Finally, if in addition to expert care the surgeon will display sympathy, tenderness, patience, and perhaps love to his young patient, he will often be rewarded with a satisfaction that is matched in no other area of medicine—in the gratitude of the parents and in the joy of following the growth and development of a child whose life he has influenced profoundly.

CHAPTER

4

The Adult Thoracic Surgical Patient

HIRAM T. LANGSTON, M.D., *and*
WALTER S. BARKER, M.D.

PREOPERATIVE EVALUATION and postoperative care of thoracic surgical patients vary somewhat from other surgical disciplines. In the main, however, the principles of management follow well-recognized patterns and differ primarily in regard to the specific intrathoracic diseases encountered.

Preoperative Assessment

The preoperative asessment of pulmonary problems devolves about bacteriologic evaluation, anatomic delineation, and physiologic assessment.

Bacteriologic evaluation.—Since many intrathoracic problems can mimic infectious diseases, precise bacteriologic assessment is mandatory. Certainly routine bacteriology for pyogenic organisms and search for tuberculous and fungus diseases are required to prevent premature and unwarranted surgical treatment for these entities. Once a specific bacteriologic problem is ruled out, then resectional surgery, if indicated, can be accomplished with a greater degree of safety. If a specific microorganism is indicted, however, appropriate antimicrobial and chemotherapeutic measures can be carried out to control the infection. If residual surgical targets then remain, they can be removed more safely.

Anatomic delineation.—Once a pulmonary process is observed on the plain chest x-ray and bacteriologic evaluation has been carried out, precise anatomic localization of the process should be undertaken in order to assess whether the disease resides predominantly in a lobe or is multilobal in distribution, or perhaps would require total pneumonectomy for extirpation. In general, anatomic localization can be accomplished by appropriate use of serial x-rays, both in posteroanterior and lateral projection, by appropriate laminagrams in anteroposterior and lateral projection, and by the judicious use of bronchographic mapping. When this information is available, it is often possible to gauge precisely the amount of lung involved and hence the extent of surgical resection required.

Physiologic assessment.—Once anatomic localization is ascertained, precise physiologic evaluation is undertaken to determine how much lung-tissue loss the patient can sustain. Clinical impressions in terms of the patient's resting respiratory rate, heart rate, and blood pressure are not always the best guides of his ability to undergo extirpative surgery. More precise pulmonary functional assessment is generally deemed necessary, especially when a pneumonectomy is contemplated. In general, simple pulmonary function studies, in which the vital capacity, timed vital capacity and maximum voluntary ventilation are recorded, will provide information on the patient's ability to survive any significant removal of lung tissue. If more precise evaluation is required, determination of residual volumes, diffusion studies, arterial blood gases, differential bronchospirometry, and cardiac catheterization can all be carried out.

In some instances, the patient's preoperative status is further evaluated by differential bronchospirometry with a Carlen double-lumen catheter in association with data obtained from cardiac catheterization with balloon occlusion of the appropriate pulmonary artery. In conjunction with this, studies of arterial P_{CO_2}, P_{O_2}, and pH, both at rest and with exercise, will help determine cardiorespiratory reserve.

Cardiac evaluation.—A baseline electrocardiogram is mandatory in patients who are to undergo intrathoracic surgical procedures. The physical examination alerts the clinician to any abnormality of heart size and sound. The chest x-ray can assist in ascertaining whether cardiac enlargement exists. Cardiac abnormality seen during these simple screening tests calls for more specific cardiac evaluation.

Preoperative digitalization.—Preoperative digitalization for patients scheduled for thoracic surgical procedures is questionable. Some thoracic surgeons feel that preoperative treatment with digitalis can decrease the postoperative complications of congestive failure and particularly of arrhythmias. It is true that post-thoracotomy supraventricular arrhythmias (sinus tachycardia, atrial fibrillation, and atrial flutter) have been estimated to occur in 20–25 per cent of patients undergoing pulmonary resections, and it is generally believed that if a patient has been in congestive failure or has had an arrhythmia preoperatively, preoperative digitalization may be required. However, prophylactic digitalization is not without its complications and should not become a preoperative routine for patients who have normal cardiac function. Postoperative digitalization is discussed in a later section of this chapter.

Metabolic and nutritional preparation.—Most patients should have a screening BUN, electrolytes, and serum electrophoresis. If a significant degree of nutritional embarrassment has been a part of the patient's underlying disease, a period of time should be allowed to replace blood, electrolytes, and protein prior to any major extirpative surgery. This becomes extremely important in patients who have obstructing lesions of the esophagus, where nutritional depletion may have gone on for several months. The extra period of time used to prepare these patients with nutritional supplements parenterally, or by other alimentary means, will decrease the morbidity and mortality in the postoperative period. The specific methods whereby this can be accomplished are described in other chapters.

Autologous blood.—It was once thought that any patient undergoing thoracotomy would automatically require at least 1 unit of blood. Increased knowledge of anatomy and physiology, and greater experience with thoracotomy have markedly reduced blood requirement. Today it is quite feasible to perform major intrathoracic procedures, up to and including pneumonectomy, without requiring whole blood replacement. Only appropriate electrolyte solutions (e.g., lactated Ringer's) may be required. This does not mean that all patients who undergo these procedures can be so fortunate. In the presence of severe pleural disease, blood loss from the chest wall may be excessive even before the specimen has been removed. Despite the risks of multiple transfusions, blood under these circumstances must be replaced.

In most instances, however, patients approaching pulmonary surgery are in relatively good nutritional status with satisfactory blood counts. There is no reason why such patients cannot act as their own donors. Over the past 7–8 years, we have used a program of autologous transfusion for our patients undergoing major pulmonary resections. With judicious timing, it is possible to remove as many as 3–4 pints of the patient's own blood and store it under blood-bank conditions for use at the time of surgery. This program of autologous transfusion has virtually halved our requirement for commercial bank blood. Not only is such a program technically feasible and financially rewarding, but also it provides the patient's own blood for those marginal situations where a single transfusion is all that may be required. Autologous transfusion, thus, precludes the dangers of giving the so-called single transfusion. In addition, the patient's postvenesection blood volume is rapidly replaced with only a minimal decrease in both his hemoglobin and hematocrit. The patient then approaches surgery with an expanded blood volume and with bone marrow that is in a phase of reticulocytosis. We have found this program safe and economical, and have been able to accomplish even pleuropneumonectomy with utilization of only the patient's own (donated) blood.

Specific Preoperative Considerations

Pulmonary tuberculosis.—Once the diagnosis of pulmonary tuberculosis is confirmed bacteriologically, the basic form of treatment is chemotherapy. A whole host of chemotherapeutic agents are available for the appropriate medical treatment of pulmonary tuberculosis. The majority of patients are treated with a regimen of streptomycin, PAS and INH initially. If bacteriologic resistance develops, such other agents as ethambutol, cycloserine, viomycin, ethionamide, and even kanamycin and terramycin are available. On a controlled program of appropriate chemotherapy in correct combination and for appropriate periods of time, 80–85 per cent of all patients with pulmonary tuberculosis will require no additional surgical measures. At present, only 15–20 per cent of patients have such significant pulmonary residuals after chemotherapy as to warrant surgical consideration. This period of chemotherapy is somewhat variable, but no less than 5–6 months, plus conversion of sputum from positive to negative, should be considered before tuberculous residuals are assessed for the possibility of surgical intervention. In patients who are infected with atypical mycobacteria, where chemotherapeutic control may be somewhat variable and where the disease may be well localized but indolent, surgical intervention is considered earlier. In contradistinction, in some of the more advanced cases of tuberculosis, both pleural and parenchymal, patients may require inordinate periods of time on chemotherapy, ranging up to 1–2 years before it is felt that the maximum benefit of the drugs has been reached and that the residuals are now ready for and amenable to surgical excision.

Preoperative evaluation is as complete as possible, utilizing serial posteroanterior and lateral chest x-rays, anteroposterior and lateral laminagrams, and bronchograms in an attempt to localize anatomically the extent of residuals considered for surgical removal. Bronchoscopy is employed not only for those patients who have residual bronchial signs, but specifically to determine the presence of underlying endobronchial tuberculosis. Pulmonary function studies are carried out on all patients considered for surgery, especially when extensive pulmonary resections are considered. In selected instances, differential bronchospirometry and even right heart catheterization studies are made.

Surgical targets.—Chemotherapy has taken from surgical consideration most, if not all, of the minimal and moderately advanced lesions due to Mycobacterium tuberculosis. At the present time far advanced lesions are the prime surgical targets to consider. These include relatively large cavities, conglomerate nodular residuals, carnified and destroyed lobes or lungs, salvage cases with poor chemotherapeutic coverage, the diseases associated with atypical mycobacteria, the rare cicatricial residuals of endobronchial tuberculosis, and pleural and/or pleuro-parenchymal residuals of tuberculosis perhaps no longer affected by chemotherapy. In addition, there is a broad category of candidates whose potential chemotherapeutic coverage is poor, whose disease may be extensive, and whose behavior pattern is such that maintenance on long-term chemotherapy cannot be expected.

Postoperatively, chemotherapy is maintained on an individualized basis. Hospitalization ranges from 2 to 6 months after operation, depending upon the individual's medical and social circumstances.

Pulmonary emphysema.—In general, pulmonary emphysema can be considered in two categories: diffuse and localized. Diffuse forms of emphysema are in large measure a sequel of chronic obstructive disease, with the possible exception of a rare category of patients who have central major tracheobronchial obstructive disease associated with tracheomalacia. This type of diffuse process can be handled only medically at present. In contradistinction to this disease, localized bullous emphysema may be amenable to surgical consideration. The decrease in ventilatory and perfusion function in these cases is attributed to compression of normally ventilating and perfusing lung by greatly enlarged bullae. In large measure, those patients who have discrete, localized bullous emphysema, preferably unilateral, can become surgical candidates in an attempt to improve ventilatory function. Evaluation of this type prior to surgical intervention is again anatomic and physiologic. The plain chest x-ray only in part delineates the extent of the bullous emphysematous process. Bronchoscopy can assist in determining the presence of any underlying endobronchial disease, and a bronchogram affords visual evidence for the distensibility of peripheral compressed lung. Also, pulmonary scanning and angiography can confirm the presence of functional pulmonary vasculature. Physiologic studies, including simple pulmonary ventilatory functions and differential bronchospirometry, can highlight the extent of functional embarrassment.

Once anatomic involvement and functional status are assessed, medical preparation with antibiotics (based upon culture and sensitivity control), expectorants, bronchodilators and postural drainage will assist in clearing out the tracheobronchial tree. Functional improvement can be anticipated with the use of aerosols and positive-pressure breathing apparatus.

In those patients who are so assessed and prepared prior to surgical excision of blebs, the functional improvement postoperatively can be most striking.

NONTUBERCULOUS SUPPURATIVE LUNG DISEASE

1. *Bronchiectasis*
   A. *Types:* There are two basic types of bronchiectasis: congenital and acquired. *Congenital* bronchiectasis is an ill-defined entity whose subsequent clinical manifestations are indistinguishable from those of acquired disease. *Acquired* bronchiectasis includes:
      (1) Upper lobe cylindrical residuals (probably post-tuberculosis). These are usually not associated with copious secretions or with active tuberculosis but may on occasion produce bleeding. Ordinarily such residuals do *not* comprise a primary surgical target.
      (2) Saccular bronchiectasis. This entity is usually associated with a history of chronic respiratory infection, excessive secretions, recurrent pneumonitis, and frequent brisk hemoptyses. Anatomically, this is usually basal in distribution and associated with pyogenic infection with such gram-negative microorganisms as *Pseudomonas aeruginosa, Aerobacter aerogenes,* and *E. coli.* Most of the surgical candidates will have this type of bronchiectasis.
      (3) Kartagener's syndrome is a medical triad of sinusitis, saccular bronchiectasis and situs inversus (or dextrocardia). When symptomatic, it is managed in the same manner as saccular disease.

Clinical manifestations: Most patients with saccular bronchiectasis will experience excessive purulent secretions, recurrent pneumonitis and respiratory infection, and intermittent hemoptyses.

Diagnosis: The plain chest film does not confirm saccular bronchiectasis. Only a complete bronchogram can establish the diagnosis and map out anatomically the extent of involvement.

Management: For patients with multilobe scattered bronchiectatic disease only medical treatment is available. This usually consists of tracheobronchial toilet (aerosols, expectorants, postural drainage, humidifiers, IPPB, etc.), appropriate and repeated antibiotic therapy, bronchodilators, and prevention of respiratory infection.

Patients who have localized bronchiectatic disease with histories of repeated infections, excessive sputum production, and recurrent hemoptysis are prime surgical candidates. Surgery is considered preferably for those patients with unilateral bronchiectasis especially confined to one lobe. Involvement of the right lower lobe is frequently associated with right middle lobe bronchiectasis, and similarly left lower lobe bronchiectasis is frequently associated with lingular involvement. A complete bilateral bronchogram is mandatory before surgery, and if lingular or middle lobe bronchiectasis is present in association with lower lobe disease, these areas must be removed in conjunction with lower lobectomy. In a few instances, appropriately staged bilateral surgery, with removal of right lower and right middle lobes and left lower lobe and lingula has been accomplished.

For patients who are candidates for resection for bronchiectatic disease, adequate medical preparation as described above must precede surgical operation. Thoracotomy even in lateral position can be carried out safely if infection is controlled and expectorated secretions total less than 50 ml. per day.

2. *Lung abscess.*—Lung abscesses currently have a low incidence. The common causes include residuals of aspiration pneumonia, pneumonitis, septic emboli, penetrating wounds, obstructing lesions of the bronchus (e.g., carcinoma), and excavations of peripheral neoplasms. The latter lesion is usually associated with signs of infection; on x-ray, the lesion usually shows a thick, shaggy wall.

In contradistinction, patients with pyogenic lung abscesses present symptoms of infection (fever, chills, leukocytosis), expectoration of copious amounts of foul-smelling sputum, and occasional brisk hemoptysis.

X-rays of the chest usually reveal a well-circumscribed parenchymal lesion with an air–fluid level frequently located in the posterior segments of the lung (superior segments of lower lobe and posterior segments of the upper lobe), especially in association with aspiration pneumonitis.

Management: Lung abscesses can be managed conservatively for a time with appropriate antibiotics, using culture and sensitivity control. (The common microorganisms involved are Friedländer's bacillus (Klebsiella pneumoniae), and Staphylococcus aureus, and, as a late pathogen, Pseudomonas aeruginosa.) In addition, expectorants, aerosols, postural drainage and IPPB may facilitate drainage.

These patients should be bronchoscoped, not only to improve drainage but also to rule out the presence of obstructing foreign bodies or neoplasms.

In the main, most lung abscesses respond to this management, with improvement in symptoms and signs and decrease in the size of the cavity as seen on x-ray. If, after several weeks, the cavity persists, surgical excision as a segmentectomy or lobectomy can be carried out after appropriate anatomic and physiologic assessment. In rare instances, some patients with lung abscesses are so toxic that more immediate drainage may become necessary.

3. *Empyema.*—Empyemas are suppurative pleural sequelae to pneumonitis, penetrating wounds, septic emboli, or infradiaphragmatic complications. Diagnosis is established by thoracentesis. Appropriate antimicrobial therapy is based on bacteriologic culture and sensitivity studies.

The *sine qua non* of management of empyema is early adequate dependent drainage. Initially this is accomplished with thoracentesis or closed thoracostomy with an intercostal tube to water seal drainage. Definitive dependent drainage with rib resection is done early, as soon as the pocket is established and the ambient pleura is sealed. Further details of management are discussed in the section on postoperative complications.

Pulmonary neoplasms.—The lung is subject to invasion by a variety of neoplasms. Practically, however, about 95 per cent of all pulmonary tumors consist of malignant epithelial tumors (carcinoma).

Carcinoma: Clinical symptomatology of patients with carcinoma of the lung will vary according to the location of the neoplasm. They may occur either peripherally or centrally, the latter arising from one of the larger branches of the bronchial tree.

Peripheral lesions arise from a smaller branch of the bronchial tree in a peripheral location. They may be asymptomatic and be discovered only on routine roentgenographic surveys, often unfortunately attaining a relatively large size before that time. If the peripherally-placed neoplasm perforates into the free pleura, it may evoke an effusion of varying magnitude. If the pleural space is obliterated, direct invasion of the chest wall occurs (ribs and vertebral bodies) and usually severe pain ensues. If this invasion of the chest wall occurs at the thoracic inlet, the consequent invasion of the vertebral bodies and stellate ganglion along with the first or second rib and the lower portions of the brachial plexus results in a typical symptom complex, the Pancoast, or superior pulmonary sulcus, syndrome.

The centrally located neoplasms will manifest themselves by signs of obstruction and ulceration of the bronchus with subsequent distal suppuration. The symptoms include cough, hemoptysis, production of sputum, varying degrees of dyspnea, chills, fever, and signs of sepsis. Unilateral and selective wheezing is an early auscultatory sign of partially obstructing centrally located neoplasms.

With late disease, weight loss and disability are generally indicative of visceral metastases, particularly to the liver. In an occasional patient cerebral symptoms may be the presenting complaint in a patient with a pulmonary tumor.

MALIGNANT PULMONARY NEOPLASMS.—Bronchogenic carcinomas are of the epidermoid or squamous cell type in about 60 per cent of the cases.

Adenocarcinoma accounts for approximately 15 per cent.

The undifferentiated neoplasm, which may be referred to as an "oat" cell or a small-cell carcinoma, accounts for some 20 per cent.

Bronchiolar or alveolar cell carcinoma accounts for a small percentage of malignant pulmonary neoplasms.

Prognosis is in part related to cell structure, with the undifferentiated type having the worst ultimate outlook.

Diagnosis: After a complete and careful physical examination, the chest x-ray in posteroanterior and lateral projection is the principal means of diagnosis. This will identify either the peripheral lesion per se or the effects of bronchial obstruction, viz., varying degrees of atelectasis or superimposed pneumonitis. Selective laminagraphy may assist in ascertaining the location of a central neoplasm, outline hilar and mediastinal nodal extension, and define anatomically a peripherally placed lesion.

Sputum cytology and more recently bronchial brushing technics are valuable aids to diagnosis.

Bronchoscopic examination of patients with peripheral bronchogenic carcinoma is not apt to be diagnostically informative but may be useful to rule out other types of lesions and to collect bronchial secretions for cytologic examination. However, for patients with centrally placed lesions presenting with bronchial signs, bronchoscopy is mandatory. With this instrument, the lesions can be seen and biopsied directly or possibly be visualized with a telescopic lens.

Any recognized (supraclavicular) lymphadenopathy should be biopsied to obtain tissue for diagnosis, but, even more importantly, to ascertain whether extrathoracic metastases have occurred. When no palpable lymphadenopathy is present, resection of the scalene fat pad may be warranted, but the low diagnostic yield for positive nodes with metastatic carcinoma (6–8 per cent) does not justify this as a routine procedure.

The final step in establishing the diagnosis of bronchogenic carcinoma is at thoracotomy. If suspicion of neoplasm exists on clinical or radiologic grounds, and if the patient's physiologic status is satisfactory, definitive thoracotomy should not be deferred too long in attempts to obtain a preoperative tissue diagnosis.

Functional assessment: Pulmonary function tests with both clinical and laboratory evaluation of ventilation and perfusion and cardiac assessment are mandatory when extirpative pulmonary surgery is considered. Obviously, if pneumonectomy is required to remove the neoplasm and the patient cannot functionally sustain the loss of a lung, he must be considered inoperable.

Preoperative preparation: Patients awaiting pulmonary resection for bronchogenic carcinoma should have the same preoperative preparation as described earlier in this chapter. In general, pulmonary suppuration and underlying cardiac and metabolic diseases must be controlled with appropriate antibiotics and respiratory adjuvants. Preparation of the skin with germicidal soap is helpful.

Treatment

Resection.—The principal method of treatment of bronchogenic carcinoma is surgical excision. The extent of the resection will be determined by the anatomic location of the neoplasm but in general, lobectomy and pneumonectomy in conjunction with mediastinal and subcarinal nodal dissection are the procedures of choice. It is becoming increasingly evident that the most important prognostic factor in patients with bronchogenic carcinoma has to do with the viability of the hematogenously disseminated metastatic deposits. Local recurrences or massive mediastinal lymphadenopathy do not account for the bulk of deaths, whereas the presence of distant metastases to the brain, liver, and skeleton determine the ultimate outcome. In selected cases, local excision of parenchymal lesions or involved chest wall may be justified and even crowned with an occasional success.

X-ray therapy.—Roentgenotherapy has been the mainstay of treatment, in the hope of palliation for patients with extensive neoplasms not amenable to surgical excision or resection. The possible combination of preoperative x-ray therapy from a source such as cobalt followed by resection is currently being studied in the hope of improving survival rates from this disease. Some success has been demonstrated, particularly in tumors of the superior sulcus.

Chemotherapy.—A variety of agents have enjoyed minimal and transient success in controlling the primary and metastatic involvement from bronchogenic carcinoma. At present, no single chemotherapeutic agent has been so successful as to warrant its use as primary therapy for bronchogenic carcinoma.

Inoperability.—In general, criteria for inoperability include: extension of the neoplasm beyond the lung; superior vena caval obstruction; the presence of distant metastases; involvement of the left recurrent laryngeal nerve with attendant left vocal cord paralysis; the presence of malignant pleural effusion. Exceptions to these criteria do exist but discussion of them is beyond the scope of this presentation.

Prognosis and results.—In general terms, about one-third of the patients suffering from bronchogenic carcinoma are inoperable when first seen. An additional one-third of the original patients wiH be found unresectable at the time of surgical exploration. The final one-third of these patients will be candidates for resection. Of these and for average patients, a mortality rate of around 10 per cent for pneumonectomy and 2–3 per cent for lobectomy can be looked upon as acceptable. At the end of 3–5 years, it can be expected that some 20–25 per cent of the patients undergoing resection will be alive and free of their disease. It is, however, most discouraging to realize that this group represents only about 8 or 10 per cent of the total group of patients seen.

MISCELLANEOUS THORACIC PROBLEMS.—A host of other chest-wall, pleural, mediastinal, and benign pulmonary parenchymal lesions are encountered. Each has specific nuances of diagnosis and treatment, the details of which are beyond the scope of this chapter. However, adherence to the principles of bacteriologic evaluation, anatomic localization, and physiologic assessment is the keystone of management of any thoracic surgical entity.

Postoperative Care Following Thoracic Surgery

Regardless of the surgical procedure, certain problems are common to all during the postoperative period. The most common of these is pain.

The discomfort produced by the incision through the soft tissues of the chest is not particularly different from that caused by wounds of similar magnitude elsewhere. The most important factor is the pain produced by the incision through the costal chest wall, regardless of whether it includes resection of rib, is entirely intercostal, or involves multiple rib resections as in thoracoplasty.

Such pain may be classified arbitrarily as being of either psychologic or physiologic significance. Psychologically significant pain is of primary concern to the patient because it is objectionable and disturbing and "just plain hurts." When the pain, however, interferes with function, it is of physiologic significance; such far-reaching effects of thoracic pain are of tremendous importance.

First, pain of even mild degree results in some limitation of thoracic expansion, but it assumes great importance when marked splinting of the chest wall occurs. Patients with an injured hemithorax automatically restrict motion on the affected side, continuing, however, to make relatively full use of the uninvolved rib cage. Aggravation of pain, or failure to dissociate motion in the two hemithoraces, produces shallow, jerky respirations which often are grunting in character, because now both sides are being affected. This situation is obviously grave because ventilation is poor, cough is ineffective or even impossible, and secretions are retained in the bronchial tree.

This clinical picture often has its beginning in pain which leads to spasm of chest wall musculature, which in turn may become painful thereby perpetuating and aggravating the situation, completing the "vicious circle."

Second, even more subtle than these mechanical effects, pain can apparently produce pulmonary changes reflexly which tend to increase bronchial secretions and decrease the patient's ability to expel them, perhaps by producing some degree of bronchospasm and bronchorrhea. This condition of accumulation of fluid, known as wet lung, is a recognized clinical picture which often follows chest trauma.

Control of pain can be accomplished in various ways.

General measures.—A change of position in bed, a change in the elevation of the head rest, readjustment of pillows, readjustment of a lumpy or constrictive dressing, and proper attention to the possibility of tape or friction burns are to be considered by the thoughtful attendant, and their importance should not be minimized. Drainage tubes often contribute to the chest pain, but are a necessary evil in most instances. Tubes that are too large constitute an aggravating source of pain when placed intercostally. Tubes should be supported at the bedside by slings of some sort (pins or tape) so that they do not pull at the chest wall and, for obvious reasons, care should be exercised that the patient does not lie on them.

Narcotics.—Most patients require only moderate doses of narcotics, given every 3 or 4 hours. Our personal preference is for morphine; not only does this drug have a predictable effect as a narcotic but the sense of well-being it provides is often welcome.

Dosage should be guided by the patient's size, age, and tolerance to pain rather than by any preconceived schedule. Each dose must provide acceptable relief of pain, but should not unduly depress such other functions as respiration, cough, or the patient's ability to cooperate. It is better to use a small dose more often then to resort to a large dose at longer intervals. This is particularly true if the patient is allowed to develop pronounced splinting of the chest wall between doses, because the "vicious-circle" mechanism of pain followed by painful spasm is more difficult to break up than to prevent. Also, in patients who are unwilling to cough satisfactorily on demand, such an exercise will often be profitably engaged in after the narcotic has become effective. Such timing can minimize the undesirable side effects of narcotic administration.

Intercostal nerve block.—Since thoracotomy incisions through the costal chest wall involve the intercostal nerves, blocking of these pathways emerges as a logical approach to control of postoperative pain. Furthermore, in the event of severe pain, particularly if the patient has difficulty in expelling secretions, and if the presence of a wet lung is suspected or recognized, interruption of reflex pathways is mandatory. In fact, it is often the dramatic improvement in the status of the pulmonary bed following intercostal nerve block that argues strongly for the reflex basis of the development of wet lung.

Care of the Tracheobronchial Tree

Attention to the respiratory system is generally accepted as routine after any surgical procedure, but is particularly important following operations that interfere directly with the function of these organs. This is true especially following pulmonary operations for disorders characterized by more or less abundant tracheobronchial secretions. Not only can these secretions become dispersed throughout various portions of the tracheobronchial tree, but blood from the operative site may gravitate into the remaining portions of the system. Thus, it is clearly understood that such situations must be managed in the postoperative period if it has been impossible to eliminate them preoperatively or to prevent them during operation. In virtually all instances, the anesthesia, the presence of endotracheal tubes, and the manipulations required result in some increase of tracheobronchial secretions. Various approaches can be employed in the toilet of the tracheobronchial tree.

Adequate hydration and humidification.—The aim of humidification is to maintain a normal physiologic environment for the respiratory mucosa and to help liquefy any retained secretions. Obviously the best humidifier is the patient's intact airway. Dehydration tends to inspissate secretions. Water and electrolyte balance should be seen to, supplemented if necessary by aerosols.

A combination of heat and minimum water particle size is the most effective way of increasing the water content of inspired gas. Ordinarily the partial pressure of water vapor in expired air is 47 mm.Hg. In order to maintain this amount, the optimum droplet size should be 0.5 to 1.5 micra, which is large enough to minimize trapping of the particles during transit in the upper airway, yet small enough to insure deposition in the finer bronchi and alveoli. With this particle size the settling rate is slow and only minimum wetting occurs when the mist is directed against a smooth surface.

In general, water is an effective humidifying agent. Excessive washing of the lung with normal saline solution will cause a loss of surfactant, resulting in decreased compliance, increased interstitial edema and other microscopic alveolar changes. The details of aerosol humidification will be considered when mechanical respiration is discussed.

Several commercially available aerosols are effective in liquefying secretions. Similarly, bronchodilating aerosols, such as isoproterenol (Isuprel) (0.1 to 1 ml. of a 0.5 or 1 per cent solution) can liquefy secretions and reduce some of the bronchospastic effects of their retention.

Inducing the patient to cough.—During the first few hours after operation, spontaneous cough as well, probably, as the intrinsic bronchomotor mechanisms, including ciliary action of the lining epithelium, are obtunded. Later, pain makes the idea of coughing distinctly unattractive to the patient, so that those in attendance must insist on such performance. It is not enough merely to order the patient to cough. This should be firmly though sympathetically insisted upon until three or four good deep coughs have indicated a dry tracheobronchial tree or the secretions present have been delivered.

Most patients cough best in a sitting position. Instruct the patient to take two to three deep breaths and then cough. Sips of fluids, especially warm ones, such as tea or coffee, may help loosen secretions. Patients should not be allowed to cough until exhausted and should be given adequate rest before repeating the procedure.

Manual support of the operated side either by an attendant or by the patient's own hand, exerting gentle pressure timed to coincide with the expulsive effort of the cough will be helpful. There is no method of cleansing the tracheobronchial tree that approaches cough in efficiency, and insistence on its proper execution is mandatory regardless of the estimated amount of secretions present.

One other benefit derived from coughing is, of course, its effectiveness in promoting lung re-expansion when this organ or portion of it remains to be expanded after operation.

Nasotracheal suction.—Occasionally, a patient will resist the most persuasive and well integrated efforts to encourage effective coughing. In such cases, a more certain method of stimulating cough is required. To incite coughing, a urethral catheter is inserted through the nose and passed into the oral pharynx, using "clean" technic. When the tip of the catheter is estimated to be just above the level of the glottis, it is rapidly advanced during the inspiratory phase of respiration with the object of having it enter the trachea. If difficulty is encountered in effecting this maneuver, changing the degree of flexion or extension of the neck or applying various degrees of traction on the tongue may give the desired result. The entire maneuver is carried out as a blind procedure without preliminary preparation of the patient except to decompress a full stomach.

Once the catheter enters the trachea, coughing can hardly be restrained. Even though cough alone may produce secretions, intermittent suction of moderate degree applied to the catheter has the advantage of mechanically removing secretions. The catheter should be introduced into the trachea while disconnected from the suction apparatus, or, if connected, the suction should be turned off, because active suction at the catheter tip hampers its passage through the glottis. This interruption of suction may be very readily accomplished by inserting a Y tube into the system so that the suction can be broken at any desired time.

Suction should be applied to the catheter for short periods of a few seconds only, as severe drops in oxygen saturation can be produced by suction. Oxygen for administration should be available between periods of active suctioning. Irrigation of the airway with 5–10 ml. of sterile saline solution may further liberate secretions.

The tracheal catheter can usually be guided into either bronchus electively by turning the head away from the side to be catheterized. This is especially true if the catheter is passed through the nose instead of the mouth. Obviously, this maneuver must be initiated with the tip of the catheter above the tracheal bifurcation.

Principles and precautions in the use of intratracheal aspiration

a. Raise the backrest so that the patient is sitting upright in bed, and decompress stomach if necessary.

b. The procedure should be as "clean" as possible. Wash hands well, wear gloves, or use a sterile hemostat to grasp catheter.
c. A No. 14 or No. 16 sterile Coudé rubber catheter is attached to the suction machine, preferably with a Y-tube connector.
d. The catheter should be inserted without suction.
e. Suction is applied once the catheter is in the trachea by placing the thumb over the open end of the Y tube.
f. Suction should be applied for only 10-15 seconds at a time.
g. The catheter may be left in place without suction applied. Oxygen should be administered between periods of suctioning.
h. Suction should be applied as catheter is withdrawn, so that secretions will not be left in the oropharynx.

Bronchoscopy.—Should the previously described methods fail to produce the desired results, or if the patient has developed a recognized atelectasis, cleansing of the tracheobronchial tree under direct vision is indicated.

The procedure can be carried out in the recovery room or in the patient's own room without removal to an operating theater. Fully induced anesthesia, as for a diagnostic bronchoscopy, need not be insisted upon, and actually may be undesirable, since coughing is a beneficial result of the procedure. Control of the gag reflex by applying 1 or 2 per cent tetracaine (Pontocaine) solution or 5-10 per cent cocaine hydrochloride solution to the pharynx and laryngopharynx, and perhaps enough to the larynx to avoid the possibility of laryngeal spasm, is generally all that is required.

A preliminary dose of the currently used narcotic may be useful in minimizing discomfort to the patient and allaying apprehension. A convenient method of carrying out the procedure is to elevate the backrest bringing the patient to Fowler's or semi-Fowler's position. The operator mounts the bed frame behind the patient and introduces the bronchoscope from this position. Pillows are used to build up the shoulders so that the head falls back permitting easy exposure of the larynx for proper intubation. Oxygen should be administered through the side arm of the bronchoscope during the procedure.

Intestinal and gastric decompression.—Abdominal distention attending gastric dilatation or ileus (adynamic or dynamic) causes an elevation of the diaphragm and decrease in ventilation. In addition, vomiting and aspiration may occur. In the marginal respiratory patient, protracted nasogastric intubation is harmful because of the production of excess pharyngeal secretions. Temporary decompression of the stomach and intestinal tract will improve ventilation and prevent vomiting and aspiration. Plastic nasogastric tubes are fairly well tolerated in most patients. In patients who have undergone major gastrointestinal surgery, insertion of a gastrostomy tube may obviate the entire problem.

Oxygen therapy.—Oxygen is used to insure adequate tissue oxygenation, especially of the heart and brain, and to eliminate the compensatory responses to hypoxia. Postanesthetized, unconscious, anemic, hypovolemic, and acidotic patients require oxygen support irrespective of the level of hypoxia. Minor falls in arterial oxygen tension may be undesirable or dangerous in a patient with limited cardiac reserve.

The optimal concentration of oxygen is that which permits full use of the oxygen-carrying capacity of the arterial blood. In the sick or debilitated patient, increased physiologic shunting is present so frequently and to such a variable degree that it is impossible to predict the arterial oxygenation that can be achieved by any given concentration of oxygen in inspired air. A margin of safety is desirable and as a rule the optimal concentration of oxygen in inspired air is that which results in an arterial oxygen tension of approximately 100–150 mm. Hg at normal hemoglobin levels. Only in acute situations such as severe hemorrhage is a higher arterial oxygen tension desirable.

The presence of very severe pulmonary disease with large physiologic shunts may make it impossible at times to reach an arterial oxygen tension higher than 50–60 mm. Hg, even when 100 per cent oxygen is inspired. Since there is danger of overloading the vascular system in these patients, transfusion is seldom indicated. It becomes obvious that oxygen therapy by itself is never definitive treatment and that underlying physiologic derangements must be corrected.

Complications of Oxygen Therapy

1. *Respiratory depression* may develop when hypoxia is the principal stimulus to spontaneous respiration (carbon dioxide narcosis). This is likely to happen in patients who are under general anesthesia, heavily narcotized, or have been retaining carbon dioxide for long periods of time. Patients with profound respiratory depression and associated hypoventilation need some form of assistive or controlled ventilation to expel the carbon dioxide and, at the same time, to supply them with adequate oxygen. Patients who are given high concentrations of oxygen in an attempt to bring about satisfactory correction of underlying cyanosis may become increasingly drowsy while receiving such therapy. In addition, they may complain of headache or visual disturbances or become apneic. These symptoms indicate carbon dioxide retention with progressive respiratory acidosis.

2. *Circulatory depression* may follow oxygen administration. If the preceding period of hypoxia has led to pronounced sympathetic activation, the patient may undergo circulatory rebound upon correction of hypoxia and collapse will ensue. If airway obstruction or respiratory failure is treated promptly with endotracheal intubation, adequate ventilation, and oxygenation, severe circulatory failure may be avoided.
3. *Atelectasis* has been shown to occur more rapidly in a closed air space if it contains pure oxygen rather than room air. This concept is somewhat controversial, however. Suffice it to say that 100 per cent oxygen for protracted periods of time, for whatever reason, may be deleterious.
4. *Substernal pain* associated with high oxygen tensions may be attributed to tracheobronchitis, resulting from inadequate humidification of oxygen.

In general, oxygen toxicity is a vague term. It may be concluded that prolonged administration of oxygen under pressure has serious potential side effects. In some patients the danger of oxygen toxicity is secondary to the danger of tissue hypoxia; under those circumstances, 100 per cent oxygen should be given.

Technics of oxygen administration.—A variety of methods are available for administering oxygen. A nasal catheter is the most common and least expensive. The only precaution to observe with this technic is to insure that the tip of the catheter is kept just below the soft palate above the level of the uvula, to avoid undue drying of the mucosa or gastric distention by promoting the swallowing of oxygen. A 6–8 L. per minute flow provides oxygen concentrations of approximately 30–40 per cent.

Use of a disposable plastic face mask is simple and comfortable and is acceptable to most patients. The flows delivered through it must be equal to or larger than the patient's minute ventilation. With a reasonably tight fit, oxygen concentrations will be in the range of 60–80 per cent at a flow of 8–10 L. per minute.

A plastic face hood provides an open system that does not deliver as high a concentration of oxygen as other devices. Because of the effectiveness of high humidification, it is useful for short periods in treating laryngeal edema and thick tracheobronchial secretions.

Masks with reservoir bags should fit tightly and are indicated when administering 100 per cent oxygen. They may be used in conjunction with positive pressure and are useful in the treatment of pulmonary edema, asthma, and emphysema.

With the availability of newer devices, air-conditioned suites, and respiratory units, oxygen tents have become unnecessary.

The Cardiovascular System

General considerations.—A moderate increase in pulse rate and a moderate fall in blood pressure is all that need be expected in the recovery period in a patient whose blood losses at surgery have been properly replaced, who has a functionally intact chest wall, and has not been anoxic or hypercarbic during anesthesia.

The actual blood pressure readings are, of course, of relative importance only and should be evaluated on the basis of preoperative levels. Also, the patient who is lying still can be expected to have a lower level of blood pressure than one who is awake or has been moving about in bed. As a norm, it may be said that a systolic blood pressure of 100 mm. Hg or over in a quiet semiconscious patient who was originally normotensive is acceptable, particularly if the pulse rate is in the neighborhood of 100 beats per minute or less.

Falls in blood pressure require a check on the pleural drainage systems (if present) to determine that they are functioning. This will also indicate if there is evidence of bleeding from within the chest. If the result of this investigation is negative, possible airway obstruction by secretions must be determined, to ascertain that an adequate oxygen supply is being delivered to the lung.

After these areas have been checked, a reduced circulatory volume may be considered. The amount of blood lost as balanced against fluids given should be reviewed with an eye to determining the need for additional blood by transfusion. Laboratory studies, such as red blood cell counts and determination of hemoglobin and hematocrit values, are unreliable under early postoperative circumstances. It should be remembered that blood replacement in a 1:1 ratio to losses is not at all necessary, the patient being able to compensate adequately for 600–800 ml. losses without transfusion of homologous blood.

The risks of serum hepatitis and of transfusion reactions of various types dictate a conservative attitude toward giving homologous blood. However, the use of previously drawn autologous blood, when providently available, removes virtually all risks from blood transfusions and can be resorted to at the slightest indication that hypovolemia exists. Another source of autologous blood for transfusion is proper collection of blood spilled during operation. In the absence of autologous blood, transfusion of plasma carries less risk than homologous blood but is not entirely devoid of danger.

Even though blood volume may be readily determined by the RISA or other technic, such determinations under the changing clinical circumstances related to postoperative shock are unreliable as a practical guide to blood volume replacement. When sizable deficits are believed to have been incurred by large or continuous losses and sizable volume replacements are contemplated, particularly in patients whose cardiac reserve is doubtful or whose pulmonary vascular bed is compromised, danger of underreplacement or circulatory overload must be recognized. Monitoring of the central venous pressure by an indwelling catheter appears to afford the most practical method of charting a therapeutic course. However, extreme care must be taken in the placement of such a catheter in the superior vena cava, so that it correctly reflects central venous pressure; reliance upon a defective system may prove disastrous.

The use of vasopressors such as metaraminol (Aramine) or methoxamine HCl (Vasoxil) (3–5 mg. I.V. or 10–15 mg. I.M.) as a single dose may be considered, in the hope that a patient who is suspected of being hypovolemic may gain time during which readjustment of circulating volumes can occur. Return of the blood pressure to lowered or falling levels accompanied by tachycardia and other evidences of impending hypovolemic shock after dissipation of the physiologic effect of the administered vasopressor should be considered as a rather clear indication for support of the circulating volume by administration of blood or plasma.

The postoperative chest patient is best managed with the head of the bed elevated. The Trendelenburg position is particularly objectionable because of the reduction in vital capacity by the upward pressure of the abdominal viscera, encroaching upon thoracic volume. As soon as the vital signs are believed to be stable, elevation of the head of the bed is to be started and maintained at a point of comfort.

Arrhythmias and cardiac failure.—Cardiac irregularities are by no means uncommon after thoracic operations, particularly pulmonary resections. Right-sided operations seem to be more vulnerable than left-sided, and pneumonectomies more subject to this problem than lobectomies.

The irregularities range all the way from occasional extrasystoles to auricular fibrillation or flutter. The episodes may be transient and unnoticed by the patient or may produce palpitation, dyspnea, weakness, faintness, sweating and apprehension.

Transient episodes of irregularity documented by electrocardiography need no particular treatment. When persistent, and particularly if symptomatic, cardiac irregularities are cause for concern. Flutter or fibrillation that persists for 2–4 hours, even without complaint by the patient, probably requires action. The principal point of attack in management is the potential of cardiac failure rather than the mere disturbance of rhythm. Thus, emphasis has turned to digitalis rather than such drugs such as quinidine. It is probably best to prescribe a full digitalizing dose, to secure the full effect of the drug, rather than to temporize with small doses. Should this not bring about a return to sinus rhythm, quinidine may be added to the regimen.

Tissue Emphysema

Subcutaneous emphysema.—Escape of air from the pleural space through the thoracotomy wound into the fascial planes of the extracostal soft tissues constitutes an impressive situation when the volume of air is great. Once the air gains access to these superficial planes, it spreads along them and manifests its presence by distending the area, producing crepitation on palpation. Beyond discomfort to the patient, emphysema is not serious in and of itself. Its importance lies in the source of the air and its persistence or progressive character.

The air remaining in the pleural space around an incompletely expanded lung or lobe may be forced through defects in the costal portion of the thoracotomy wound when the patient coughs or strains or otherwise increases intrapulmonary pressure. If no significant amount of the air expelled from the pleura during these times is replaced by air leaks in the bronchus or the lung parenchyma through bronchial fistulae, the process is self-limited, since the expanded lung or lobe will finally displace all air from the pleura and no further increments can be added to the subcutaneous tissues.

If, on the other hand, air flows into the pleural space through large bronchial leaks or an aggregate of many small alveolar leaks, emphysema is serious, signifying actual or potential tension pneumothorax.

Closure of the costal portion of the chest wall is often not mechanically airtight and need not be so, because adequate decompression of the pleural space by drainage tube or tubes provides a ready exit for pneumothorax air. Supportive dressings applied so as to hold the extracostal tissues snugly against the costal line of incision generally complete a reasonable seal.

Evidence, however, that air is entering the pleural space at a rate greater than it is being decompressed through the provided exit (drainage tube), leading therefore to forced decompression into the soft tissues, is indeed serious. It is necessary under these circumstances to increase the flow rate for pleural decompression. This can best be done by adding suction to the system of drainage. Leaks and resultant emphysema not controllable by suction will require reoperation for control of the leaks at their source.

In the evaluation of emphysema, it is important to realize that once air has escaped into the soft tissues at any point, it can spread easily along fascial planes and, therefore, the mere presence of crepitation over a widening area of soft tissue need not mean worsening of the situation. Assessment at this point requires observation over a period of time to decide whether there actually is more air under the skin or whether the same amount of air has merely spread over a greater area. The tenseness of the tissues is a reasonably reliable guide in this matter.

Mediastinal emphysema.—Whereas occasionally enough air can escape into the mediastinum to interfere with venous return or breathing, perhaps in infants, in the adult this rarely, if ever, occurs. Such a tension pneumomediastinum can be decompressed by making an incision into the mediastinum through the suprasternal notch. The problem of mediastinal emphysema is fundamentally the same as that of subcutaneous accumulations of air.

Mediastinal emphysema is not fatal because the mediastinum cannot accommodate enough air under sufficient pressure to seriously interfere with vital functions. This does not mean that patients with mediastinal emphysema cannot die as result of the presence of air in this area, but the mechanism of death under these circumstances is disruption of the mediastinal pleura and the development of a pneumothorax which continues to pour air into one or both hemithoraces as the leak (which originally provided the air for the mediastinal emphysema) is perpetuated. Under these circumstances, a unilateral or bilateral tension pneumothorax, which progressively increases in amount can be set up and will result in fatality.

The dissemination of air in emphysema may not follow any predictable pattern based exclusively on anatomic arrangement of fascial planes, because most often there is air escaping into the subcutaneous planes as well as into the mediastinum. Thus, in advanced cases, air appears in the neck, producing a "bull-neck" effect, and perhaps also in the retropharyngeal tissues, producing the nasal quality of speech known as rhinolalia. Air may also pass along the vascular sheaths in the arms, along the femoral vessels in the upper thigh, or along muscular and subcutaneous planes over the thorax or the abdomen. Direct decompression of subcutaneous spaces by needle aspiration is possible but is not very helpful in the management of the overall problem and depends to what extent dissection of the subcutaneous layers has produced space capable of being aspirated.

Paradoxical Motion of the Chest Wall (see Fig. 4-1)

Respiration is termed paradoxical when a portion of the chest wall sinks on inspiration and rises on expiration, contrary to the movement

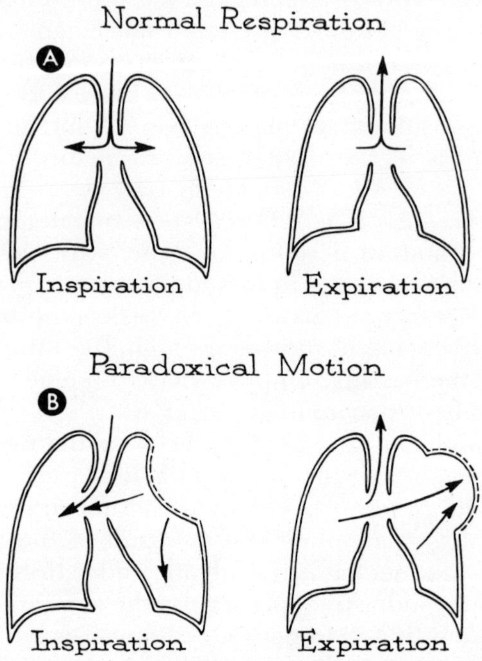

Fig. 4-1.—Normal respiration and paradoxical motion.

of the normal or intact portion of the wall. The term generally refers to such an occurrence in the costal chest wall, since this is the more obvious, but is applicable to the mediastinum and the diaphragm as well.

Paradoxical motion is possible at any time the rib cage loses its rigidity, as by resection of two or more ribs or by fractures involving two or more ribs both anteriorly and posteriorly. Likewise, fractures of ribs on either side of the sternum, for example, can render flail a portion or all of the sternum. Thus, the involved portion of the rib cage, being dissociated from the remainder of the rigid costal framework, is pulled in on inspiration by the negative intrathoracic pressure, sinking consequently as the rest of the rib cage expands. The reverse occurs on expiration. Such paradoxical motion renders breathing inefficient, cough ineffective, and, even more important, shuttles air back and forth between the lung underlying the flail portion of the chest wall and the other portions of the pulmonary bed. This latter feature results in rebreathing, leading to decreased oxygenation and retention of carbon dioxide. A small amount of paradoxical motion can be tolerated without serious consequences as, for example, in thoracoplasty.

Treatment is basically mechanical. Milder forms can be corrected by the use of sand bags, positioning the patient on the involved side, or applying pressure dressings to prevent the swinging motion of the chest wall. In some cases, the use of balanced traction attached to the flail segment of the chest wall by means of towel clips about the involved ribs may be sufficient.

A tracheostomy may be helpful in providing for tracheobronchial toilet as well as bypassing the laryngeal narrowing and to some extent reducing dead space in the tracheobronchial tree. Application of a mechanical respirator represents the ultimate in support.

Paradoxical motion of the mediastinum is usually corrected by adjusting intrapleural pressures and is not correctable by direct mechanical means. Paradoxical action of the diaphragm usually follows interference with the phrenic nerve, although it may occur without a recognizable cause.

PARENTERAL FLUIDS.—Since minimal dysfunction of the gastrointestinal tract is expected following chest surgery, early return to oral intake of food and water is to be encouraged. Generally, the patient arrives in the recovery ward receiving intravenous fluids. Fluid losses in the postoperative period are not expected to be large.

The intravenous setup should be kept open by a slow drip of 5 per cent dextrose in water until the patient has been able to accept oral intake with certainty. Lactated Ringer's solution may be used and blood replaced judiciously.

No limit to the volume of fluid to be administered need be set. The guiding principle should be to administer only that amount required to maintain adequate hydration. A reasonable amount is 2,000–3,000 ml. in the first 24 to 36 hours. Although the danger of overloading the circulation is real, it does not occur frequently except in patients with marginal cardiorespiratory reserves who have undergone extensive pulmonary resections.

DRAINAGE SYSTEMS

Water-seal drainage (Fig. 4-2).—It is almost universal practice to drain the pleural space after all operations except pneumonectomy. The purpose of drainage is to provide ready exit for accumulations of blood or fluid resulting from the surgical intervention and for the air remaining as a postoperative pneumothorax. Drainage provides a mechanism by which the remaining lung or portion thereof is favored in expanding to fill the hemithorax completely. Prompt filling of the chest cavity by lung is essential and provides the greatest assurance against the occurrence of pleural complications.

The drainage tubes should have walls sufficiently noncollapsible to assure a patent lumen. Currently, plastic tubes are preferred to rubber tubing.

A water seal is used to prevent free communication between the pleural cavity and the exterior. In simplest design, the chest tube is led from the pleura to a transparent (for ready visualization of its content) glass container, in which the end of the tube is submerged in water. This water bottle should always be at a level well below that of the patient's chest, and under no circumstances should the drainage or water-seal bottle approach the level of the patient's chest unless the tubes leading from the pleura have been clamped off. If a bottle is not placed at the appropriate level, the negative intrapleural pressure can pull or siphon fluid back into the chest.

Glass tubing replacing the rubber tubing inside the water-seal bottle permits visualization of the oscillation that accompanies respiration, as well as the character of the drainage. Also, a section of glass connector is useful in the system at some point near the patient, as a means of inspecting the character of the drainage and proving patency of the pleural tube when drainage flows into this "window" as the tubing distal to it is "milked" or "stripped." For best mechanical efficiency, each pleural tube should be connected to a separate water seal when more than one tube is used.

This system provides for egress of air and fluid from the pleural space and at the same time prevents ingress of air into it. The tip of the tube in the water seal should be just far enough below the surface of the water so that as water is drawn up into the tube on inspiration, the tip of the tube will still be below water level. If the tip is too far

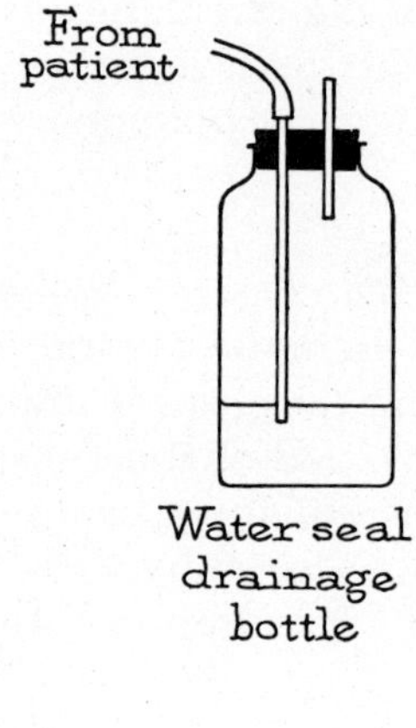

Fig. 4-2.—Simple water seal drainage.

below the surface of the water, an unnecessary increase will result in the degree of pressure required to expel air or fluid through the tube. A water-seal bottle providing ample surface area of water will be more efficient than a narrower one. Also, the container should be capable of accommodating a minimum of 400–500 ml. of drainage over and above the initial water content. If drainage is copious, the depth of the tube in the liquid may need readjustment. A mark should be placed on the bottle or some other means used to gauge the amount of drainage.

By carefully following the action of the fluid in the tubes and the amount and character of the drainage, much information concerning the progress of expansion of the lung can be deduced. This is especially true when an anterior (and usually superior), as well as the lower and posterior tube is in place. X-ray examinations of the chest in this period are generally limited for practical reasons to a portable frontal view. Under these circumstances any residual pleural space that may be unfilled by lung anteriorly or posteriorly may not be recognizable, yet if either or both drainage tubes still exhibit fluctuation, such a residual space is certainly present.

It is important to realize that the patient's position in bed can affect the behavior of the water seal and should be taken into account in any interpretation. With the patient semirecumbent, the remaining lower lobe or whole lung can be expected to drop into the posterior gutter and seal off the lower posterior drainage tube, stopping fluid fluctuations in the tube. If the lower lobe has been removed, the fluid in the lower tube can be expected to oscillate longer than in the upper tube.

Fluid should appear promptly from a lower tube. Appearance of some fluid in the upper tube generally signifies the imminence of complete re–expansion, as the fluid that remains in the pleural cavity is spread around by the expanding lung to come within the drainage field of the upper tube. Such illustrations are given merely as guides and can in no way be considered as absolutes.

Suction drainage (Fig. 4-3).—The water seal itself creates suction drainage, being a negative pressure system, sufficient to overcome the elastic recoil inherent in lung tissue, particularly when aided by periodic increases in intrapulmonic pressure such as produced by coughing, straining, and the like. Thus, if the air within the pleural space is not replaced by increments from bronchial or alveolar air leak, prompt and complete re–expansion of free lobes or lungs will occur by this mechanism alone.

If significant leaks are present, as may occur after segmental resec-

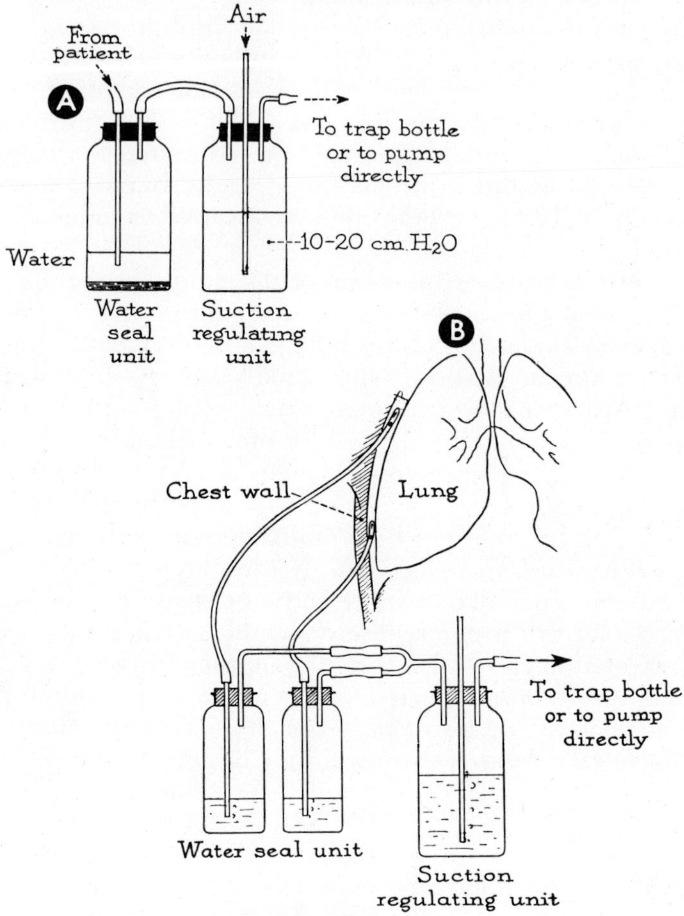

Fig. 4-3.—Suction drainage. *A*, single water seal; *B*, completely assembled unit.

tion, for example, the pneumothorax may be maintained beyond the ability of the water-seal system to eliminate it. Under such circumstances, increase in volume flow of pleural air to the outside is necessary in order to maintain a proper gradient of negative pressure within the pleura. Many surgeons resort to this increase in negative intrapleural pressure as a matter of routine.

Suction drainage has many modifications, but basically it includes a water seal next to the patient and a suction-breaking device next in line. The water seal is important in the event of a disruption in the system which would leave the patient's pleura open to the outside. The purpose of the suction-breaking device is to limit the maximum amount of suction applied to the water–seal bottle and, therefore, to the pleural space. The device consists of a portal for the application of suction and standpipe reaching nearly to the bottom of the bottle, but open to the outside. Water is placed in the jar and allowed to rise along the tube to a level, such that the distance between the lower end of the open tube and the surface of the water is the same as the degree of negative pressure desired (measured in centimeters of water). Thus, when suction is applied, the level of water within this open tube will sink in proportion to the amount of negative pressure created in the system. If a maximum of 15 cm. of negative pressure within the system is desired, the distance between the lower end of this tube and the surface of the water should be 15 cm. When such levels of negative pressure are reached, the level of water will have dropped to the lower tip of the tube and any increases of negative pressure beyond that will draw air into the bottle through the tube from the outside, automatically breaking the suction at this level. It is, therefore, apparent that when the breaker bottle fails to bubble at some time during the respiratory cycle, the desired degree of negative pressure or suction has not been achieved.

Reasons for this failure, which should be promptly investigated, include: (1) inadequate capacity of the pumping unit; (2) air leaks along the system of bottles or connectors; and (3) air leak into the pleura that is greater in volume per unit time than the volume of air that the pump can displace in the same period of time. It is important to distinguish between reasons (1) and (3) because (1) refers simply to a weak pump, incapable of producing the desired degree of negative pressure, whereas reason (3) implies a serious air leak within the pleura. These two situations can readily be differentiated by placing a clamp at the chest wall on the tube or tubes leading from the pleura to the water seal. If the pump can produce the desired degree of negative pressure, as evidenced by bubbling through the suction-breaker bottle, both the adequacy of the pump and the airtight nature of the system are assured up to the point of the clamp.

Evaluation of the extent of air leak within the pleura from bronchial or alveolar openings is a difficult problem, calling for mature judgment born of experience and can hardly be detailed here. It must be remembered, however, that a large amount of residual air within the pleura that is replaced slowly by small air leaks may cause the pump to work for some time before it can "catch up" with the situation. Also, it is not imperative that the suction-breaking mechanism bubble continuously to give assurance of adequate functioning of the system. The purpose of the method is to increase the intrapleural negative pressure and this need not necessarily be carried at all phases of respiration.

Beyond the two bottles described, a simple trap bottle may be placed between the pump and the suction-breaker to protect the pump from wetting, in the event of a spill-over from whatever cause. The final unit in this system is, of course, a source of suction.

Care of drainage tubes.—Tubes are to be securely anchored at the time they are placed. To prevent kinking (of rubber tubing) and to guard against undue traction by accidental tugging, they should be fixed to the dressing as well. It is also advisable to secure all connectors by a narrow strip of adhesive tape across them running from tubing to tubing. This will not reduce visibility at this "window," yet reduces the danger that the system may be pulled apart. A clamp of some type should be at hand to occlude each tube immediately should a disruption in the system occur.

Tubing should be just long enough to permit bed care, with room enough for the patient to turn or sit up with slight slack. Excess length is inadvisable because it merely increases the volume of dead space within the drainage system. The tubing should be supported at the edge of the bed in some fashion to reduce tugging by the mere weight of the tubing falling free.

Tubing should be checked for patency by observing oscillations within it or by the free passage of drainage. If these signs are not evident, or just as a matter of routine at each check of the patient's condition, the tube should be milked by stripping it toward the drainage bottle. It is also advantageous to do this with the patient sitting up as well as recumbent after the first few hours.

Since the desired direction of flow in the drainage tube is from pleura to water seal, we advise against reversing this flow by irrigations or instillations. Under certain situations, this may be a proper procedure, but in general efforts should be concentrated on maintaining patency of the tube and encouraging the impetus of flow from pleura to water seal.

Character and quantity of drainage.—The trauma of surgery and the blood that is spilled into the pleura at operation constitute irritants to which the pleura responds by an outpouring of fluid. This effusion is basically serous in nature and dilutes the blood. Although intervening factors, such as severe bacterial contamination and other less-well-understood influences may occasionally alter the character of this effusion, rendering it richer in fibrin and leading, perhaps, to clotting, this is not common.

The fluid evacuated from the pleural space during the first few hours following surgery is clearly bloody in character, tending to become serous by the end of 36 or 48 hours, as new increments of blood cease and the pleural reactive effusion predominates. The exact proportion of blood and serum and the speed of the transition vary widely; the important factor involved is the volume of whole blood in the drainage.

It is particularly important to note if a rather sudden increase in the amount of drainage, not accounted for by a change in position of the patient, occurs. This observation combined with signs of a reduced circulating volume, such as a falling blood pressure and rising pulse rate, tend to confirm the suspicion of continued bleeding into the pleura.

A difficult decision from the standpoint of management concerns the necessity to reopen the chest for hemostasis. The alternative plan is to retransfuse and observe further, on the assumption that there is no manageable source of bleeding upon which a direct surgical attack is justified. The vessel most commonly responsible for postoperative bleeding is either an unsecured bronchial artery or perhaps an intercostal vessel wounded during the closure. If a more-or-less accurate estimate of proportion of whole blood in the drainage is desired, determination of the hemoglobin content will generally suffice. Red blood cell counts may not be reliable because of laking. Detritus of various kinds may give a false hematocrit reading. Darkening of the color of the drainage to a brownish fluid or lightening of its color toward pink will likewise assure the observer, in the course of time, that active bleeding is probably not present.

Removal of tubes.—Thoracotomy tubes are ready for removal when their presence is no longer advantageous. This occurs when the lung or lobe is fully expanded. This is determined by x-ray examination and by the cessation of fluctuation in the system.

Further considerations include the amount of drainage as well as its character. Dark, bloody fluid lying in the tubing can generally be expected to be replaced by lighter or serous–type fluid over the next 12–24 hours and justifies leaving the tubes in place. Even though a clot may have developed in the tube, this further drainage can seep around it and the drain is, therefore, probably effective for a short while longer.

It is generally not desirable to remove tubes in less than 48 hours but they should certainly be removed in 5 to 7 days, ideally. A tube lying in the same tract for longer than 6 or 7 days seems to favor infection even though antibiotics have tended to increase this "period of grace."

To remove the tube from the pleura, the dressings and other anchors to the tube at the chest wall are freed, with the patient lying on the sound side. The operator stands at the patient's back. Before the final anchoring suture is cut, a ball of gauze some 2 in. in diameter is prepared, using two or three 4-by-4-in. gauze sponges. Also, in easy reach, three or four strips of adhesive tape 2 in. wide by 6 in. long are made available. The tube is then freed and held in one hand, the wad of gauze being grasped by the other hand. With a slight rotary motion to disengage the tube, it is quickly pulled from the chest while the gauze pack, which is being held firmly against the chest wall at the tube site, is pressed down to seal off the skin opening and tube tract. The gauze wad is then taped down snugly to maintain occlusion of the tube tract through the chest wall. No sucking of air should occur.

Care of the Wound

Properly made and closed thoracotomy wounds heal kindly and no special attention need be directed to them. They are inspected when the tubes are removed and, finally, when the sutures are removed. Antibiotics are used at the discretion of the surgeon and offer no special problem. Prophylactic use is not necessary.

General Nursing Routine

Posture of the patient.—Patients with thoracic disease or injury are most comfortable in Fowler's position. While unconscious, they are to be kept horizontal. The Trendelenburg position is not only unnecessary but undesirable because of the reduction in vital capacity produced by the encroachment of abdominal viscera gravitating upward.

When consciousness returns and the vital signs seem stable, a more vertical posture is sought. The patient should be turned frequently and may assume any position that is comfortable. It is perhaps best to encourage the pneumonectomy patient to lie on the operated side or in dorsal decubitus. This postural restriction is occasioned by the fear that, should the bronchus open when the operated side is uppermost, the fluid contained in that hemithorax might pour into the other lung. This fear may be somewhat exaggerated but the precaution seems reasonable. When lung tissue remains on the side which has been operated upon and drains are in place, the patient may lie on either side, but the presence of the tubes presents some hindrance to comfort in some positions.

Ambulation and mobilization.—Resumption of activity is indicated at the earliest possible moment. As soon as the circulatory system has become stabilized, the start should be made to the upright position. The position should be changed frequently from back to side, and the patient should be encouraged to undertake as much of this on his own power as seems reasonable. The arm on the operated side should be exercised actively as soon as the patient will co-operate. Sitting up in bed with help is desirable within the first 24 hours, and certainly by the end of 12 hours, the patient should sit up in bed and dangle his feet over the edge for periods of a few minutes at a time.

It is preferable to initiate early preliminary mobility in bed in any patient with indwelling drainage tubes, because attempts at more extended ambulation out of bed may result in complications involving the attached mechanical systems. After the tubes have been removed, full freedom may be allowed, even in patients having undergone resections for pulmonary tuberculosis. Patients without drainage systems attached may be allowed out of bed as soon as acceptable to the patient; this includes patients who have undergone penumonectomy. There seems to be little justification for preventing a willing patient from free mobilization except in cases where the mechanical restriction of drainage systems is involved. Reticent patients should be allowed a somewhat slower schedule, unless it seems certain that the reticence is due to timidity. This should be gently but firmly overcome by personnel giving assistance in demonstrating the safety and feasibility of ambulation.

Gastrointestinal disturbances.—Nausea and vomiting are absent or short-lived and cause only temporary inconvenience in the modern practice of anesthesia. Gastric distention is likewise rarely a problem in pulmonary or mediastinal operations. Air swallowing or the introduction of oxygen into the stomach consequent upon a poorly placed nasal catheter may, of course, require decompression by nasogastric tube.

If nausea persists, mild sedation with a barbiturate or the use of a drug such as prochlorperazine (Compazine), trimethobenzamide (Tigan), or dimenhydrinate (Dramamine) may be necessary. Belladonna should be used cautiously because of its undesirable effect in inspissating bronchial secretions.

Evacuation of the rectum need not be sought for 2 or 3 days. The use of milk of magnesia at bed time, ambulation out of bed, and a proper return to a full diet generally result in spontaneous evacuation in a reasonable time without resorting to more artificial means of inducing a bowel movement.

Urination.—Catheterization of the bladder may be required in some patients, but if the position in bed seems to be responsible for failure to urinate (in male patients) they may be allowed to stand by the bedside with assistance to accomplish this. Catheterizations of female patients is probably more expeditious in the first 24 hours than is utilization of a bedside or portable commode to achieve the advantage of the accustomed position. The quantity of urine, as well as its gross appearance, should be recorded for 2 or 3 days after operation. The first one or two voided or catheterized specimens should be analyzed chemically and examined microscopically. There are no urinary difficulties peculiar to the thoracic surgical patient.

Special Considerations

Specific Types of Thoracic Surgical Procedures

Operations on the chest wall.—Many of the operations on the chest wall have faded from practice because they were done for chronic empyema or for some forms of chronic pulmonary disease, such as tuberculosis. In such operations, the basic physiologic derangement to be considered in most or all patients was instability of the chest wall. When stiff-walled empyema spaces were unroofed, no appreciable problem was created because the degree of paradoxical motion under the resected chest wall was not significant. Excessive decostalization can, of course, produce this problem. The important features earmarked for attention postoperatively in a thoracoplasty patient therefore are: (1) control of paradoxical motion, and (2) careful insistence on expectoration of secretions by cough, particularly in a tuberculous patient, in whom this procedure will find its chief indication.

Should the pleura have been accidentally opened during the operation, attention must be directed to pneumothorax in the postoperative period. Most surgeons will have placed an intrapleural catheter connected to a water seal. Management of this phase then becomes similar to that of the thoracotomy patient in whom the lung remains intact. If a catheter has not been placed in the pleura, the extent of pneumothorax must be evaluated by x-ray examination and reduced by thoracentesis. Progress of the situation will require follow-up x-ray studies.

Operations within the Pleura

Simple thoracotomy.—When the chest is opened but no surgical intervention is carried out on the lung or other intrathoracic organ, postoperative management is elemental and will be described as a basic type into which variants may be introduced as the operative interventions become more complex.

The unconscious patient will be placed flat in bed. Oxygen inhalation will be started by nasal catheter at a flow of 6–8 L. per minute, the gas being bubbled through an appropriate humidifier. The drainage apparatus (usually one pleural drain tube will suffice) will be checked to insure against being kinked. It will be properly supported and the level of fluid in the water-seal bottle will be noted. The blood-pressure reading and pulse rate will be recorded. The color of the patient, the presence or absence of sweating, and the temperature of the extremities as determined by palpation will be noted. The amount and type of intravenous fluid received by the patient will be ascertained and any intravenous solutions currently being administered will be checked. It is well to inquire of the responsible surgeon or anesthetist as to any special problems to be anticipated or guarded against.

Postoperative observation continues with a check on pulse-rate and blood-pressure readings every 10–15 minutes for the first hour, and then at lengthening intervals as stability of the cardiovascular system is demonstrated.

When the patient regains consciousness, restlessness and/or pain may become a problem. Narcotics in moderate doses may be given. The dosage should be adjusted over the next several hours to provide adequate relief of pain, yet not produce any significant degree of lasting narcosis. Sleep or drowsiness resulting from the relief of pain is, of course, acceptable. When this stage of recovery is reached, routine coughing should be instituted. Every $1\frac{1}{2}$ or 2 hours, the patient should be told to cough, the attendant insisting that the effort be productive. The patient may be turned also at frequent intervals, particularly to obtain a position of reasonable comfort and convenience.

By this time, sufficient check on the blood pressure and pulse rate should have permitted recognition of the extent of their stability. When they have become stable, the head of the bed may be elevated to an acceptable level and kept there unless the blood pressure is adversely affected by the change in posture, in which case the move will be postponed and tried again some time later.

When the patient is fully awake, attention may be directed to weaning off the oxygen, as previously described. Unless otherwise indicated, intravenous fluids can be discontinued if the patient is no longer nauseated and has demonstrated the ability to retain water by mouth in appreciable quantity, or when the patient has voided urine.

Food and fluids may be offered as desired or tolerated. The temperature will have been taken at the first convenient opportunity postoperatively, preferably by rectum for the first 24 hours, and will be checked every 4 hours thereafter.

The speed with which these various steps are undertaken varies from individual to individual, but as a matter of routine should be carried on as speedily as circumstances permit.

By the end of 24 hours, minimal or no fluctuation is seen in the water seal, and the drainage should be serous or the entire system may be empty if complete lung expansion has occurred rapidly. The patient should have been sitting upright in bed and have dangled his feet over the side at least once. The chest should be checked by x-ray examination on the morning following operation (some surgeons check this on the day of operation). An x-ray picture taken with portable apparatus is preferable, thereby avoiding the hazard of transporting the patient with clamped-off drainage tubes, or transporting the drainage system along with the patient to a fluoroscope or the X-ray Department. The roentgenogram taken by the portable machine will provide all information necessary. The film should be exposed with the patient in the upright position. The most satisfactory method is to have the patient sit on the edge of the bed, dangling his feet over the side onto a chair while embracing the x-ray cassette in proper alignment. The x-ray machine is positioned so that a posteroanterior film is obtained. A lateral exposure can also be made but is not usually deemed necessary.

The x-ray film should be read promptly, so that any changes in management, indicated by the presence of atelectasis, failure of expansion, or significant accumulation of undrained fluid, can be made without delay.

The second day should see full freedom in bed. A generous range of motion for the affected arm is expected. Pain will be relieved judiciously and coughing insisted upon. The drainage tubes may be removed under ideal circumstances, but this is probably best delayed for another 24 hours because some output of fluid can still be expected. A daily check by x-ray examination is insisted upon by many surgeons as long as the drainage tubes are in place. Careful observation of the behavior of the water-seal bottles and a periodic check by x-ray film is, however, usually considered adequate.

When the tubes have been removed, out–of–bed ambulation may be allowed freely. Enemas may be given as indicated.

Lobectomy.—The basic approach is the same as for simple thoracotomy. A longer delay in filling of the chest cavity by the remaining lung tissue may, of course, be expected. If an upper lobe has been removed, the upper tube (two tubes are usual) will fluctuate longer, while the lower tube may fluctuate but little, evacuating principally the bloody pleural fluid. This is as might be expected, since the base can be filled more promptly by lung remaining in that area.

When a lower lobe has been removed, one tube only may suffice. At any rate, the principal functioning tube will be the lower one, evacuating both air and fluid as a rule.

Segmental pulmonary resection.—The basic management is again the same as for thoracotomy and lobectomy. Air leaks are more frequent and deposited clotted blood will lie along the raw segmental surfaces. Suction drainage will be required more often; some surgeons institute this immediately. It is the contention of others that immediate institution of high negative pressure to the pleural cavity may tend to keep open some of the air leaks which would seal if not placed under such stress. Therefore, some surgeons use gentler water-seal drainage for the first 24 hours. If the first x-ray examination does not show virtually complete re-expansion, or if important air leaks are still manifested at this time, suction drainage is instituted.

Pneumonectomy.—At the conclusion of the operation, after turning the patient to a recumbent position and during quiet breathing, the intrapleural pressure is determined *on the side operated upon,* and should have been adjusted to a physiologically negative or neutral state. This determination may be made by a pneumothorax apparatus. No provision for drainage is made in the average patient, the chest being closed tightly.

Postoperatively, the basic regimen is the same as that described for partial pulmonary resection with certain exceptions:

(1).—The amount of fluids and blood given intravenously should be more closely adjusted to avoid circulatory overload. Rales are generally heard over the remaining lung base and increased blood flow, manifested by prominence of the vascular markings, is seen on the x-ray films. This condition is commonly referred to as congestion. The increased blood flow lasts for 2 to 4 days, by which time the necessary circulatory readjustment has taken place and more nearly normal mobilization of the fluids in the pulmonary bed is taking place. Persistence of the increased flow for a longer period of time would suggest some failure of cardiac decompensation. If tachycardia and some dyspnea continue, control of the situation by diuretics and/or digitalization is to be considered. Salt intake should be restricted. The opinion of an experienced cardiologist is in order under these circumstances.

(2).—Since there is no lung to fill the hemithorax, this space is occupied by an effusion, and accumulation of fluid faster than the pneumothorax air is absorbed leads to increases in intrapleural pressure. This will shift the mediastinum toward the "good" side, thereby reducing the ventilation possible by that lung. Hence, the pressures in the pleural space should be checked whenever there is any suspicion of significant changes therein. Routine estimation and adjustment of intrapleural pressures need not be done at all if the subject remains comfortable and the mediastinum is in the midline.

(3).—In the absence of a drain, the patient may be allowed out of bed as soon as this is tolerable. The average well-compensated patient will be willing to sit in a chair by the second or third day.

(4).—The patient probably should not be allowed to lie on the unoperated side, with a vacated but partially fluid-filled hemithorax uppermost. In this position a sudden leak might cause flooding of the remaining lung.

Transpleural mediastonotomy.—Since the lung is intact, immediate postoperative management is the same as that following simple thoracotomy. The later problems that may arise in the area of operation within the mediastinum are beyond the scope of this work.

Sternal splitting incisions.—If the pleural spaces are not entered during the operation, the management is essentially the same as that following operations on the chest wall. If one or both pleurae have been entered, management will be determined by the existent circumstances and reference should be made to discussion of simple thoracotomy.

Thoracotomy and block resection of the chest wall.—This situation combines the problems of chest-wall instability with those of thoracotomy and to these may be added the problems caused by lung resection. One outstanding feature of such cases is that postoperative x-ray films are very difficult to interpret with certainty because of the distortion of the chest wall.

Fluid accumulations are confusing because they may occur in an extracostal plane, yet appear to be intrapleural. Such aspects of the problem must obviously be individualized.

Operations on the bronchial tree.—Except for the increased possibility of delay in pulmonary re-expansion or increased severity of air leak, the problems presented following bronchial-tree surgery are composites of the problems described following other and simpler chest operations.

Thoracotomy or lobectomy without drainage.—Even though in the minority, an occasional surgeon will prefer not to employ drainage following thoracotomy or lobectomy. Air or fluid in the pleura must be withdrawn by thoracentesis; the necessity for this, in most instances, will be determined by serial x-ray examinations.

Post-Thoracotomy Complications

Postoperative thoracic spaces.—Persistent air spaces following pulmonary resections have been attributed to bronchopleural fistulas and represented as a prelude to empyema. As such, they have been explored, drained, and collapsed in various combinations in attempts to prevent this complication.

It is contended that many of these situations represent merely seepage of gas from alveoli and, in other instances, simply reflect inability of the diseased underlying lung to overdistend sufficiently to obliterate the hemithorax, probably because of fibrosis. A few cases may well be due to small bronchial leaks, but most stabilize physiologically without infection.

In our experience spontaneous obliteration of these persistent postresectional spaces, even in tuberculosis, occurs in about 90 per cent of cases, the majority within 4 weeks. Late infections in such spaces have occurred in about 2 per cent of patients.

A "benign" postoperative space is a small one that is seen to be growing smaller on serial x-rays, is thin walled, and contains no fluid, or minimal and decreasing fluid; it is seen in a patient who is without fever, leukocytosis or major bronchial symptoms such as cough and expectoration.

Three basic categories of benign spaces are encountered: (1) closed noncommunicating spaces, (2) alveolar seepage spaces, and (3) spaces with persistent bronchial communications. Determination of intraspace pressures and O_2 and CO_2 gas content can assist in determining the type of space at hand, in the first-instance closed space (pneumothorax) air (4 per cent O_2 and 7 per cent CO_2); in the second instance, alveolar air (10 per cent O_2 and 5 per cent CO_2); and in the third instance, inspired air. Intraspace pressures are consistently negative unless a bronchial communication is present.

It is not meant to imply that *all* postresection spaces should be merely watched but not actively treated. However, by the application of appropriate criteria to each case, a decision can be reached which may preclude a mutilating and complicated surgical intervention and/or time-consuming convalescence. Overzealous and premature treatment may lead to complications.

In contradistinction to the "benign" space, a "malignant" space is more apt to be large and getting larger, have a thick wall, and contain fluid in increasing amounts. The patient usually has fever, leukocytosis, and is generally ill. In such spaces, early diagnosis of the incipient empyema and adequate treatment are mandatory.

1. Technical empyema.—Between the "benign" space on the one hand and the obviously suppurating process on the other can be recognized a space that must be vented, yet is essentially uninfected; this has been termed a "technical" empyema. This term describes the situation in which air continues to leak in amounts such that the drain tube cannot be removed within a safe period after partial pulmonary resection. The tube is therefore left in-lying as an open drain on the assumption that such a pleural space would be contaminated if not actually infected. If a decision is reached to retain such a tube, a sufficient time is allowed to insure pleural symphysis (over 14 days) and then the retained tube is connected to an empty water-seal bottle. If x-rays reveal some additional collapse of the pulmonary remnant, water can be added to convert the system to conventional water-seal drainage and additional time allowed to develop firm pleural adhesions. If, on the other hand, there are no significant x-ray changes, the tube can be cut and secured to the chest wall as an empyema drainage tube. This tube can subsequently be changed or cleaned weekly and replaced.

In most of these instances, the lung satisfactorily seals and expands and the tube can be permanently removed in several weeks. In some cases, however, the site of drainage of such retained tubes is not adequate or dependent and, as secondary infection ensues, revision of empyema drainage is carried out with rib resection if necessary.

2. Empyema.—This designates suppuration which complicates a surgical procedure. It may or may not be associated with a bronchopleural fistula. The clinical and radiologic signs include: fever, leukocytosis, anorexia, toxicity, excessive purulent sputum in the case of bronchopleural fistula, pleural exudation by x-ray, and later hypoproteinemia. Pus may be seen discharging through the patient's chest tubes or may be obtained on thoracentesis if chest tubes are no longer present.

Pathogenetically these may arise from operative contamination, associated suppurative parenchymal disease, or deep-seated wound infections which communicate with the pleural cavity rather than the outside. Examination of the pleural drainage or aspirate from the pleural space obtained by thoracentesis usually provides the diagnosis. Appropriate culture and sensitivity studies suggest the proper antibiotic. The microorganisms involved may be quite variable but the more common pathogens are Staphylococcus aureus, Hemophilus influenzae, E. coli, A. aerogenes, and Pseudomonas aeruginosa.

The *sine qua non* of management of postoperative empyema is early adequate dependent drainage—whether this is by thoracentesis, intercostal tubes (those present or those reinserted) or later by open drainage with rib resection. Appropriate antibiotic coverage may abort or limit the pyogenic process but is no substitute for drainage in established cases.

There are several categories of empyema to consider: (1) empyema following partial pulmonary resection without bronchial fistula; (2) empyema following partial pulmonary resection with a bronchial fistula; (3) empyema following pneumonectomy without bronchial fistula; and (4) empyema following pneumonectomy with a bronchial fistula.

1.—*Empyema following partial pulmonary resection without bronchial fistula.*—If the pleural content is thick pus and is rich in fibrin, it is unlikely that anything short of free drainage will suffice. When the pleural fluid contains 75 to 80 per cent sediment on standing, it can be assumed that sufficient fibrin is present to insure firm symphysis around the pleural abscess and that open dependent drainage can be used to hasten healing. This is best accomplished by a dependently placed rib resection. The tube can then be cleaned and changed periodically until the space obliterates.

2. *Empyema following partial pulmonary resection with a bronchial fistula.*—Since the empyema is being drained via the fistula and the pus is being coughed out, prompt drainage is necessary. Initially this can be accomplished by closed thoracostomy. Later rib resection is usually necessary.

3.—*Empyema following pneumonectomy without bronchial fistula.*—Here adequate dependent drainage, preferably by rib resection, is required: usually the mediastinum has become fixed by the time the empyema is evident. If there is any doubt of this circumstance due to the recency of the operation (3–7 days), temporary closed thoracostomy to water-seal drainage can be employed.

4.—*Empyema following pneumonectomy with a bronchial fistula.*—This dire complication is treated by open drainage with dependently placed rib resection after urgent evacuation of the pleural content via thoracentesis or tube thoracostomy. This is required to prevent drowning or other complication due to spill into the remaining lung.

Detailed discussion of the subsequent management of the stabilized infected spaces is not within the scope of this chapter but for completeness will be outlined.

A. When lung remains and is adjudged capable of expanding to obliterate the space, every effort to encourage this direction is justified. In absence of a bronchopleural fistula, decortication is indicated after assurance by sinograms and possibly laminagrams that good dependent drainage is in effect.

B. When a bronchopleural fistula persists, it is more difficult to be sure of the health of the lung remnant, so decortication is less clearly indicated but could be considered in conjunction with revision of the bronchial stump or further pulmonary resection.

C. If ultimately a space remains and offers no indication that it may obliterate, the space may necessitate thoracoplastic collapse and, in the case of a persistent bronchopleural fistula, ultimately a pedicled muscle implant.

D. When the hemithorax is empty, it is unlikely that spontaneous obliteration can ever occur. In absence of a bronchopleural fistula, sterilization of the cavity and closure of the drainage site is recommended. If this fails, or if the bronchopleural fistula persists, a thoracoplasty will be required to bring about closure unless it is elected to maintain drainage permanently.

Cardiac Arrest

The commonest cause of cardiac arrest is hypoxia and hypercarbia, whether associated with respiratory insufficiency, airway obstruction, or myocardial decompensation. Caridac resuscitative measures, either with closed-chest cardiac massage or open thoracotomy, with the use of oxygen and a variety of cardiac drugs and stimulants, are of no avail unless the airway is controlled. The *sine qua non* for successful cardiac resuscitation is immediate establishment of an adequate airway. Once the airway is secured, other resuscitative measures may be continued with greater likelihood of success. The respiratory acidosis that accompanies even momentary cardiac arrest must be corrected, as must the underlying electrolyte imbalances, particularly hyperkalemia. A definite system and routine for management of cardiac arrest is required so that nonproductive activity, panic, and inordinate delay can be averted. The details for this are presented elsewhere.

Respiratory Insufficiency and Failure

Respiratory insufficiency implies inability of the lungs to exchange gases adequately to meet the needs of the body during effort. Respiratory failure denotes inadequate ventilation and exchange at rest.

The former may be compensated for by reduction in activity unless there are superimposed stresses which can lead to respiratory failure and eventual death.

There are two types of respiratory insufficiency, acute and chronic. The former includes general problems which compromise pulmonary ventilation and perfusion; trauma leading to reflex bronchospasm, bronchorrhea, and loss of airway patency; acute congestive failure, overwhelming pulmonary suppuration, or inhalation of poison gases.

Chronic respiratory insufficiency with attendant cor pulmonale is often progressive over a period of years and is associated with degenerative pulmonary parenchymal changes in alveolar and capillary structures (e.g., pulmonary fibrosis, granulomatous disease, idiopathic diffuse pneumopathies). The loss of ventilation and/or perfusion leads to progressive failure of gaseous exchange and eventual pulmonary hypertension and combined cardiorespiratory failure.

This problem is of paramount importance after pulmonary resections. This loss of ventilatory surface coupled with emphysema in the pulmonary remnant may lead to chronic respiratory insufficiency and cor pulmonale. Because of the life-threatening nature of these derangements, the basis for therapeutic success resides in the early recognition of the problem.

Manifestations of Acute Respiratory Insufficiency

The most important manifestations of acute respiratory insufficiency are *hypoxia, hypercarbia, hypotension* and *dyspnea*. These abnormalities may occur singly or in combination.

Psychologic support of the patient with respiratory insufficiency.—As with any other critical illness, emotional support of the patient and the patient's family must be one of the prime considerations of the nursing and medical staff. The dyspneic patient is frightened. He often expresses a feeling of doom and desires constant attention. One of the main advantages of an intensive care unit is the constancy of attention and the reassurance to the patient of the presence of trained personnel. A simple explanation of the type of respiratory assistance being provided and its specific purpose should be given to the family. This is particularly helpful to the anxious and resistive patient who may rely on family support.

The majority of patients are conscious and alert during most of such illness. They are apprehensive and may be depressed and frustrated by their inability to communicate. Generally, encouragement of the patient and adequate explanations allay apprehension. The lack of sleep associated with constant care may be exhausting. Assurance that the patient is being watched at all times and adequate sedation are helpful. Mood-changing drugs, such as imipramine HCl (Tofranil), have been employed. Morphine, despite its potential depressant effect on respiration, relieves apprehension and fear of the numerous mechanical devices employed in the management of these patients.

Hypoxia.—Cyanosis is a manifestation of hypoxia. However, this is an unreliable index of the true state of arterial oxygenation. Ordinarily, cyanosis does not become apparent until the arterial oxygen saturation is below 85 per cent, although severe tissue hypoxia can occur with relatively high oxygen saturations and in the absence of cyanosis. Tissue hypoxia in the myocardium may lead to eventual hypotension and cardiac arrhythmia. Early and mild hypoxia leads to tachycardia. Late and severe hypoxia produces bradycardia, which is often a prelude to cardiac arrest. Hyperventilation is another major response to severe hypoxia. Cardiac output is increased because of the increase in cardiac rate, and associated sympathetic activity may lead to selective tissue vasoconstriction. This tends to increase peripheral resistance and eventually leads to elevated blood pressure. Thus, initial hypertension, tachycardia, and hyperventilation are common early signs of hypoxia. However, in the old, debilitated or narcotized patient there is a decrease in sympathetic response to hypoxia, and bradycardia, hypotension and ultimate circulatory arrest may occur early.

HYPERCARBIA.—Hypercarbia, or carbon dioxide retention, combines elements of both local circulatory depression and autonomic nervous system stimulation. The balance between the depressant and stimulant effects of carbon dioxide determines the clinical phase of respiratory insufficiency. The local effect of carbon dioxide is always depressant and that feature, associated with respiratory acidosis, depresses most tissue functions in the body, including cardiac and cerebral functions. It also causes general vasodilatation (with the possible exception of the pulmonary circulation). Thus, all degrees of circulatory failure may ensue and cerebral depression from mild sedation to deep anesthesia may occur.

An early sign of hypercarbia is increased cutaneous blood flow, with redness and sweating. The cerebral depressant effect of carbon dioxide is variable. The patient may remain conscious with carbon dioxide tensions in excess of 100 mm. Hg, provided the progression has been slow enough to allow time for the development of a compensatory metabolic alkalosis. Although the direct action of increased carbon dioxide on the respiratory center augments the respiratory drive leading to hyperventilation, central nervous system depression and muscular weakness may prevent any compensatory hyperventilation from materializing. Increased sympathetic activity leads to increased levels of circulating catecholamines (epinephrine and norepinephrine), resulting in increased cardiac output, hypertension and tachycardia. This response is evoked only in patients who are still capable of responding to sympathetic activation.

Other signs and symptoms of hypercarbia include muscle twitching, cardiac arrhythmias, visual defects and mental confusion. The skin may vary from warm and flushed to dry or sweaty. As the P_{CO_2} increases over 100 mm. Hg, the patient becomes progressively drowsy and will lapse into severe coma and eventual respiratory arrest.

Hypotension.—Hypotension obviously has many causes, of which hypoxia and hypercarbia are two of the most important. Arterial blood pressure depends on cardiac output and peripheral resistance. A mean arterial blood pressure of 100 mm. Hg may be obtained in a patient with normal cardiac output and peripheral resistance, or it may reflect either a low cardiac output with a high peripheral resistance or the reverse. The clinical picture accompanying hypotension differs according to the degree of peripheral vasoconstriction. Hypotension without vasoconstriction is characterized in general by warm and dry skin of natural color, and a pulse rate that is not increased. Ordinarily, if the patient is adequately perfusing his peripheral vascular bed, his urinary output remains essentially normal. This provides an excellent criterion of the seriousness of the hypotensive state. A hypotensive patient with peripheral vasoconstriction and increasing levels of retained carbon dioxide is cold, pale and sweaty, has tachycardia and a thready peripheral pulse and is oliguric or anuric.

Dyspnea.—Dyspnea is a subjective complaint of patients attempting to increase their ventilation without being able to do so. It may be caused by a variety of mechanisms, either singly or in combination, including: (1) increased work of breathing; (2) reduction of a functional residual capacity associated with atelectasis; (3) increased sensory inflow from respiratory muscle or pulmonary receptors; and (4) increased sensitivity to subjective phenomena. Regardless of the objective causes or mechanical defects associated with limitations of pulmonary ventilating and perfusing surfaces, dyspnea is one of the cardinal subjective criteria of respiratory insufficiency.

Pre-existing pulmonary disease appears to be a significant factor predisposing to respiratory complications, especially following major surgery. In particular, if such patients have undergone thoracic surgery with removal of functioning lung, they may develop respiratory insufficiency early. Degenerative diseases, such as pulmonary emphysema or chronic bronchitis, or suppurative lung disease, such as bronchiectasis or lung abscesses, may also predispose to respiratory insufficiency, culminating in an acute episode during the patient's hospital stay.

A variety of other factors have been indicted. These include age, obesity, smoking, pain and abdominal distention. In addition, analgesic agents such as morphine, meperidine (Demerol), and even acetylsalicylic acid, when given in excess, may cause ventilatory depression at both central and peripheral levels. Obviously, the barbiturate compounds are quite capable of depressing pulmonary ventilation and producing complications in patients with marginal respiratory reserve. With these features in mind, certain patients must be observed more closely in anticipation of difficulties.

In summary, certain general clinical criteria for respiratory insufficiency can be delineated. An elderly patient with underlying pulmonary or cardiac disease, who may be obese or is receiving sedative and/or analgesic drugs, and who perhaps exhibits a certain degree of ileus or abdominal distention, is a candidate for respiratory failure. As ventilatory and perfusion functions decrease and hypoxia and hypercarbia ensue, the patient will develop progressive anxiety, mild mental confusion and even tremors or frank convulsions. Tachypnea and tachycardia become apparent. Cyanosis will ensue if hypoxia becomes progressive. After initial hypertension, hypotension may occur, and, depending upon the degree of vasoconstriction, the patient will be cold, clammy, and sweaty. As respiratory insufficiency becomes progressive, the patient's compensatory mechanisms fail, hypotension becomes profound and irreversible, mental confusion progresses to stupor and coma, tachypnea leads to irregularity of respiratory effort, and tachycardia becomes bradycardia. Irreversible cardiorespiratory failure and death are almost inevitable.

Management of Acute Respiratory Failure

A patient, conscious or unconscious, whose airway becomes compromised requires immediate attention. Secretions must be aspirated quickly in the manner described previously. Insufflation of the lungs by mouth-to-mouth or mouth-to-nose technic is begun. An oropharyngeal airway is used to keep the tongue from falling back; this may incorporate an extension (S-shaped tube) for mouth-to-tube

TABLE 4-1.—MEANS OF VENTILATION BEFORE AIRWAY IS CLEARED

DEVICE	DRIVING FORCE	AIRWAY	GAS DELIVERED
Mouth-to-mouth	Thorax of resuscitator	Lift chin or resuscitation tube	Expired Air 13% O_2 3.5% CO_2
Bag (Ambu, etc.) Portable—best for emergency	Resuscitator's hand	Lift chin or oropharyngeal airway or endotracheal tube	Air 21% O_2, 79% N_2
Anesthesia bag + O_2 Better, but not as portable	Resuscitator's hand	Same as above	100% O_2
	AFTER AIRWAY IS CLEARED		
Gas operated respirators (Bird, Bennett, etc.)	O_2 under pressure	Any airway desired: mouth, endotracheal tube, tracheostomy	O_2, 40–100%
Electric-operated respirator, piston driven (Mörch, Emerson, Air-Shields, etc.)	Piston driven by electric motor	Tracheostomy, cuffed or uncuffed endotracheal tube. (Uncuffed patient may talk with air going by.)	Air (21%) or additional O_2

Devised by Ronald Rosenberg, M.D., Department of Anesthesia, University of Illinois, Tables 4-1 and 4-2 summarize our concepts of the diagnosis and management of respiratory failure; they are useful aids in training new personnel.

resuscitation. Once secretions are aspirated from the oropharynx and an airway is established, an elastic (Ambu) bag is used to carry out emergency ventilation.

These are only temporary measures. For better control of the airway, aspiration of secretions and ventilation, either endotracheal intubation or tracheostomy, should be performed (see Tables 4-1 and 4-2).

ENDOTRACHEAL INTUBATION

Whenever doubt exists about a patient's ability to maintain his airway, it is best to proceed with endotracheal intubation or to consider a tracheostomy, especially if prolonged respiratory support is anticipated. Such patients are marginal and unless ideal facilities are readily available for performing emergency tracheostomy, difficulty may be encountered and an airway which is critical to begin with may be entirely lost in the time that it takes to control bleeding and to introduce the cannula. A far safer method, even in experienced hands,

TABLE 4-2.—SCHEMA OF MANAGEMENT OF ACUTE AND CHRONIC RESPIRATORY FAILURE

	Diagnosis		Treatment			
Status of Patient	Clinical Findings	Laboratory Findings	Airway Control	Oxygen	Drugs	Miscellaneous
Conscious 1. Unobstructed Airway	Tachypnea (occ. hypoventilation) Tachycardia, bradycardia Dyspnea Cyanosis Hyper-, hypotension Mental confusion Somnolence Neurologic manifestations Warm, dry, cold, clammy, wheezing	P_{CO_2} ↑ > 40 mm Hg PO_2 ↓ < 90 mm Hg pH ↓ < 7.36 Hct ⇅ 40 Base deficit	Respiratory support Aspirate secretions PRN IPPB (pressure cycled)	Low flow, humidified; 40% or less	Liquefying agents: Alevaire Mucomyst Respiratory stimulants Digitalis, diuretics PRN for CHF Antibiotics Bronchodilators Vasopressors PRN Volume replacement	
2. Obstructed Airway	Same + noisy respirations Intercostal retraction	Variable	Secure airway Tracheal aspiration Bronchoscopy Endotracheal intubation Tracheostomy Respirator support PRN	Same	Same + sedate, once airway secured	
Unconscious 3. Partially Obstructed Airway	Same + irregular respirations, Cheyne-Stokes, Blots Hyporeflexia, areflexia Pupillary reaction Odors	Same as #1 Generally acidotic Rule out hyperventilation alkalosis	Maintain and secure airway Tracheal aspiration IPPB Respiratory support Endotracheal intubation Tracheostomy, if prolonged support necessary	Same	Same	Turning Feeding tube I.V. fluids Gastric decompression Foley cath. (monitor urine output) Cardiac monitoring
4. Completely Obstructed Airway	Same + stertorous respirations Intercostal retraction Severe cyanosis Apnea ±	Same as #1	Immediate: Endotracheal intubation Tracheostomy Continued ventilation necessary	Humidified <40%, especially if very elevated P_{CO_2}	Same	Same

is to introduce an endotracheal tube and then, if more prolonged respiratory support is indicated, perform elective tracheostomy later, at leisure.

INDICATIONS FOR ENDOTRACHEAL INTUBATION.—Endotracheal intubation is indicated for the following:

1. To establish and maintain a free airway.
2. To permit positive-pressure ventilation which cannot be done effectively by face mask.
3. To prevent aspiration of pharyngeal secretions or gastrointestinal content by sealing off the trachea from the digestive tract.
4. To permit effective removal of tracheobronchial secretions.

TECHNIC AND PRECAUTIONS.—In most hospitals the departments of anesthesia and surgery have personnel who can perform emergency endotracheal intubation. Ordinarily a tube 8–9 mm. in diameter is adequate to permit ventilation and aspiration of secretions. It should not be so long as to intubate either main stem bronchus and thereby occlude one lung. An oral airway (Guedel), to prevent the patient from biting down and occluding the tube, is placed and secured with adequate amounts of tape. The cuff on the endotracheal tube is inflated sufficiently to occlude the main tract and prevent air leak and aspiration around the tube. Adequately humidified oxygen may be introduced through the tube, once the secretions have been aspirated, and a variety of respirators can be attached to ventilate the patient.

Continued inflation of an endotracheal cuff cannot be allowed indefinitely because of the possibility of tracheal wall necrosis. We have adopted the policy that 24–36 hours of continuous cuffed intubation is maximal. After this time, if the patient does not have spontaneous return of respiration or requires additional support, tracheostomy is performed over the endotracheal tube, which is then removed. If a cuff is inflated longer than 24 hours and additional time is desired to decide on tracheostomy, the cuff should be deflated for at least 15 minutes every 2 hours and the tube slightly rotated to avoid any pressure points. The endotracheal tube can be changed periodically and thus 5–7 days may be allowed in which to decide on the necessity of tracheostomy.

COMPLICATIONS.—Complications of endotracheal intubation include vocal-cord damage and edema of the larynx and trachea. The latter is most often transient. Severe degrees of edema, however, with associated stridor and increased respiratory effort, requiring tracheostomy, may develop hours or even days after removal of the endotracheal tube. Milder forms of obstruction in an otherwise vigorous individual may be treated conservatively with very careful observation. High humidity and large doses of corticosteroids have been helpful in some patients. Tracheal slough and stenosis are rare complications and are caused by loss of blood supply and ulceration of the tracheal mucosa at the site of the inflated cuff. Complications arising while the endotracheal tube is in place may include one-lung intubation, with consequent obstruction and atelectasis of the contralateral lung. On occasion the tube may be inserted too close to the carina, causing inspissation of secretions and producing a bilateral bronchial plug. This is immediately life-threatening. With appropriate placement of the tube, gentle aspiration and adequate humidification, these complications may be avoided almost entirely. It is important that these patients be suctioned periodically to keep the airway patent. Suctioning is carried out in the same manner as that described below in tracheostomy care.

Tracheostomy

Indications.—Endotracheal intubation has replaced tracheostomy as the proper emergency procedure in the great majority of cases. Tracheostomy can then be done electively with the full benefits of an established airway. The indications for tracheostomy overlap those for endotracheal intubation: (1) to maintain a free airway; (2) to prevent aspiration; and (3) to permit comfortable and continuous use of positive-pressure ventilators.

A tracheostomy is needed whenever an endotracheal tube cannot be tolerated by a conscious patient, or if the passage of an endotracheal tube is impossible or undesirable. This may be the situation in certain cases of pharyngeal or laryngeal obstruction due to tumor, infection, vocal-cord paralysis or ankylosing spondylitis.

In patients with chronic respiratory insufficiency, permanent tracheostomy may be indicated. Only rarely should a tracheostomy be done in order to reduce the patient's anatomic dead space. Tracheostomy reduces anatomic dead space by about 50–100 ml. In patients with chronic lung disease the alveolar dead space is so large that reduction in the anatomic dead space is insignificant.

In burn patients where the oropharyngeal passages and even the trachea itself are damaged, endotracheal intubation may be quite hazardous. Tracheostomy is the procedure of choice in maintaining a patent and untraumatized airway.

Types of tracheostomy tubes.—A variety of tracheostomy cannulae are available. The Jackson or Hollinger silver tube is the most common. With the advent of respirators, however, numerous adaptations and modifications have been introduced. The Mörch tracheostomy tube is essentially the same as a Jackson silver tube except that it has a screw-on swivel adaptor on the inner cannula which serves as a connector to the respirator and allows suctioning without disconnecting the respirator. All these may have an endotracheal cuff attached to provide a closed system. A large cannula is preferred and, in most adults, one with an internal diameter of 6–8 mm. is suitable. When a cuff is used, it should fit the tracheostomy tube snugly. A 7 or 8 mm. endotracheal cuff on a no. 7 Jackson tracheostomy tube is average.

A malleable plastic tracheostomy tube with bonded cuff which inflates evenly has recently been developed. It is similar in design and construction to the classic tracheostomy tube but has the added advantage of a built-in cuff. More recently a double-cuff system has been employed on this tube, allowing the cuffs to be inflated alternately so that the two pressure points can likewise be alternated. These cuffs can be connected to a respirator in such a manner as to inflate the cuff only on inspiration.

TRACHEAL FENESTRATION.—Rockey has devised a technic of tracheal fenestration which provides the chronic respiratory cripple with a permanently available tracheal stoma which is, however, kept closed by ingeniously fashioned muscle and skin flaps. The principal feature is that it is a closed, not an open, stoma.

Hanlon has developed a plastic cannula with a detachable one-way flap valve for aspiration only. The flange on the plastic tracheostomy tube is sutured to the anterior wall of the trachea and is introduced in much the same manner as a routine tracheostomy. It has the advantage of simple aspiration without introduction of a hollow tube into the lumen of the trachea, and, in addition, with the detachable one-way flap valve, the patient can ventilate adequately and still cough and use the normal pathway for removal of secretions.

DANGERS AND COMPLICATIONS OF TRACHEOSTOMY.—With tracheostomy, the natural humidifying mechanisms are compromised. As a result, drying and crusting occur unless adequate humidification is provided. In addition, the patient loses the effectiveness of his cough and is largely dependent on tracheal aspiration for removal of secretions. Suctioning should be gentle to prevent damage to the ciliated epithelium and trauma to the trachea.

All patients who require tracheostomy should be cared for in a respiratory unit. This is particularly important when staffing on general wards is minimal. We unfortunately have seen catastrophic results in patients whose tracheostomies were inadequately managed.

CARE OF THE PATIENT WITH A TRACHEOSTOMY.—The nursing care of the tracheostomy patient is of prime importance. These patients are totally dependent on the personnel in attendance for assiduous care and reassurance.

PRINCIPLES AND PRECAUTIONS IN CARE OF THE TRACHEOSTOMY:

a. Sterile technic should be used and either sterile gloves or forceps employed when suctioning the tracheostomy.
b. Each time the trachea is aspirated, a new sterile suction catheter should be used. A separate catheter is used to aspirate the mouth or pharynx.
c. The method for suctioning is the same as stated in Principles *c*, *d*, *e* and *f* of intratracheal aspiration (p. 147).
d. The catheter should be inserted deep enough to stimulate coughing. This is usually in the range of 10–15 cm. In our experience, the nurse may be overcautious and limit her suctioning to the end of the cannula. This is inadequate and patients so suctioned may develop, just beyond the tip of the cannula, pools of secretion which become inspissated and obstruct the tracheostomy tube.
e. The catheter should be rotated 360° as it is withdrawn with suction on.
f. The catheter should be guided into each bronchus by turning the head away from the side to be intubated.
g. Patients should be turned from side to side at least every hour; this is particularly important in the comatose patient, to prevent pooling of secretions in dependent portions of lung.
h. Adequate humidification is mandatory. The ultrasonic nebulizer affords the most effective humidification. This nebulizer produces water particles of 0.8 to 1 micron in size and can deliver up to 3–6 ml. of moisture per minute. In addition to providing a greater degree of nebulization than any other method, the ultrasonic nebulizer does not require the use of oxygen (an asset in those patients where oxygen therapy is not desirable).

   Another efficient method is to provide humidity through a nebulizer that uses the Venturi principle. The nebulizer is attached by large bore tubing to a tracheostomy mask attached to a plastic collar which fits around the tracheostomy tube. This provides moisture at the rate of 0.5–1 ml. per minute.

   The addition of heat to the nebulization process will provide even greater saturation, since the aerosol is 100 per cent saturated at body temperature and will be delivered to the trachea at 98° F. or slightly above. This means the tracheal wall will not need to supply additional moisture to the air as it commonly does at lower temperatures.

Other methods of providing moisture include the instillation of sterile saline solution into the tracheostomy tube at frequent intervals. We commonly instill 5–10 ml. of saline solution into the tracheostomy tube just before suctioning, care being exercised to aspirate this immediately, especially in patients with an obtunded cough reflex.

i. The inner cannula should be removed at least every 2 hours for cleaning. It should be reinserted as soon as cleaned. Cleaning is effected with a test-tube brush, using detergent solutions and rinsing in sterile water.

j. The outer cannula should be changed only by the physician. An additional tracheostomy tube should be kept at the patient's bedside for emergency use. If reinsertion of the inner cannula becomes difficult, the physician must be notified at once. (We change tracheostomy tubes every 7 days unless more frequent change is indicated.)

k. There is no prescribed timetable for suctioning the tracheostomy tube, frequency of suctioning depending entirely on the amount of secretions present. Some patients may require suctioning every 15 minutes; most are suctioned at 1–2 hour intervals. Suctioning will be most effective following change in position or after aerosol treatment with mucolytic agents.

To avoid hypoxia, the patient should not be suctioned for more than 10–15 seconds without being allowed to take a breath. If repeated suctioning is necessary, the patient should receive oxygen, preferably 100 per cent, for a few minutes between aspirations.

l. The catheter should be of such size as not to occlude the stoma. Ordinarily a no. 14 or no. 16 French catheter is adequate.

Removal of tracheostomy cannula.—The following criteria serve as a guide to the proper time for removal of the tracheostomy cannula:

1. The patient must have demonstrated complete independence of respirator support over a 24-hour period and be able to breathe deeply and cough effectively. Physiologically expressed, this requires a vital capacity of approximately three times the predicted normal tidal volume.
2. The patient must possess adequate cough, gag and swallow reflexes.
3. The patient must be able to bring up secretions well enough so that intratracheal aspiration has not been required for at least 24 hours.
4. The tracheostomy tube may be "corked," so that the patient has

essentially a normal airway around the tracheostomy tube with normal glottic function. If he tolerates such intermittent occlusion, gradually being increased in length of time, the tracheal cannula can be removed and a dry sponge placed over the stoma. Ordinarily the tracheal stoma heals without secondary closure.

In most patients it is desirable to remove the tracheostomy tube as early as is consistent with safety to avoid the complications of protracted tracheal intubation. Early removal, even perhaps 4 to 5 days after introduction of the tracheostomy, can be accomplished in a few patients who are not in chronic respiratory insufficiency but required only short and temporary support.

Mechanical Respirator Therapy

Many makes of mechanical respirators are commercially available. They are classified either as pressure-cycled or volume-controlled ventilators and may be used intermittently or continuously for assistance or control of ventilation. To be acceptable, a respirator must be easy to maintain, clean, and sterilize, in addition to having an adequate humidifying system.

1. *Pressure-cycled or pressure-limited ventilators.*—This type of respirator will inflate the patient's lungs until a preset pressure has been reached, at which time the inspiratory phase stops and expiration begins. With the use of a pressure-limited ventilator, the tidal volume produced by the preset pressure will be a function of the resistance of the patient's lungs and of the inspiratory flow rate. Since pulmonary compliance and airway resistance may change considerably in a given patient from day to day, or even from hour to hour, the expired minute and tidal volumes should be monitored frequently to insure that pressure settings are adequate.

The Bennett and Bird machines are pressure-controlled ventilators. There are several models of each available. Most models can be used intermittently or continuously. A small Bennett machine without controls for automatic cycling is available solely for treatments. The usual force for both the Bennett and Bird respirators is oxygen under pressure. However, both are available in an electric model which uses compressed air instead of oxygen.

2. *Volume-controlled ventilators.*—The Mörch, Emerson, Air-Shields, Bennett MA-1, and Engstrom respirators are volume-controlled ventilators. These automatic respirators are used only for patients in acute respiratory distress and not for IPPB therapy. They are most effective in patients who require continuous respiratory support.

Volume-controlled ventilators differ from pressure-controlled ventilators in that they deliver a predetermined volume of air, which can vary from 0 to 3 liters with each inspiration. The volume used is determined by the patient's estimated or measured normal tidal volume. The volume must be great enough to overcome airway resistance and decreased pulmonary compliance, and to compensate for leaks in the system, especially when the respirator is used with an uncuffed (open) tracheostomy tube. Volume-cycled respirators maintain relatively constant minute and tidal volumes regardless of changes in pulmonary compliance and airway resistance. The accuracy of tidal volume administration depends on the size of the air leak between the respirator and the trachea. A volume-limited respirator should have incorporated in it a safety valve that will bleed the system when a preset pressure has been reached, especially if a closed (cuffed tracheostomy tube) system is employed.

The Bennett MA–1 ventilator is one of the most versatile of our present volume ventilators. This unit employs a compressor-bellows, double-circuit system and delivers a preset volume of gas with variable pressures. Manually adjustable pressure limits are available from 20 to 80 cm. H_2O as safety and warning devices. Humidification is supplied with the Cascade humidifier. The unit is equipped with a monitoring spirometer which monitors tidal and/or sigh volumes on the exhaled-air principle. Expiratory negative pressure is an optional system. A well-equipped control panel allows tailoring tidal volume, respiratory rate, maximal pressure limits, maximum flow rates from 10 to 100 L. per minute, O_2 concentrations from room air to 100 per cent, mechanical sighs from 2 to 15 times per hour with separate volume and pressure-limit controls, and expiratory resistance.

The MA–1 may be used as either an assistor or controlled mode. As a controlled ventilator, inspiration is initiated by a timer adjusted to the desired rate per minute and is volume-limited at end inspiration unless the preset pressure limit is reached first. Inspiratory: expiratory ratios may be tailored by adjusting the inspiratory flow rates. In the assistor mode, inspiration is initiated by the patient's spontaneous inspiratory effort. Sensitivity of the unit to the patient's inspiratory efforts may be manually adjusted over a wide range. When the sensitivity control is completely off, no amount of patient effort will cycle the unit, and ventilation will be completely controlled.

This unit is equipped with warning systems that activate if spontaneous ventilation has occurred, pressure limits have been exceeded, inspiratory:expiratory ratios are less than 1:1, a sigh cycle has occurred, proper O_2 concentrations are not being delivered, or the preset tidal volume is not being delivered.

In many hospitals, the Department of Inhalation Therapy or the Department of Anesthesia has direct control of this equipment. Despite this hierarchy of administration, all medical and nursing personnel, both within and outside of the Intensive Therapy Unit, should be familiar with this equipment. Only continued experience with these machines in clinical cases will impart the knowledge and confidence that is required for their use in critically ill patients.

MANAGEMENT OF PATIENTS UNDERGOING PROLONGED ARTIFICIAL VENTILATION.—No patient should be maintained on continuous respirator control unless superior technical and medical supervision is available. Obstruction to the airway and mechanical failure of the respirator are disastrous complications. A respirator is no substitute for assiduous mechanical cleansing of the tracheobronchial tree. It is indeed unwise to attempt to clear out the lower recesses of the lung by using positive-pressure respirators alone. The drying effects of positive pressure in the face of obstructive secretions will tend further to impact and inspissate those secretions, leading to progressive segmental or subsegmental atelectasis. The prime prerequisite for successful use of respirators is a clean and patent airway.

Periodic monitoring of physiologic parameters, including blood gases, serum electrolytes, tidal volume and vital capacity, is an integral part of the management of patients undergoing continuous and prolonged artificial ventilation. Patients with CO_2 retention who are suddenly placed on respirators in order to improve ventilation may rapidly reverse these high CO_2 tensions. Gordon and others have shown that rapid reversal of P_{CO_2} may lead to sudden ventricular fibrillation and death. Patients should gradually be brought to optimum levels of volume-pressure flows by use of O_2 concentrations that are just adequate to maintain normal O_2 saturation.

Systemic circulatory effects of protracted artificial ventilation are well documented. Cournand and others have shown that mean airway pressure must be as low as possible in order to avoid interference with circulation. A low mean airway pressure can be maintained when the duration of positive airway pressure on inspiration is less than or equal to the expiration phase when no positive pressure is applied. It is obvious that an increased mean airway pressure may impede venous return to the right heart. When this occurs alternately in patients on continuous controlled ventilation, a paradoxical pulse and blood pressure results.

Ordinarily about 15 respirations per minute is the optimal rate of ventilation. If this frequency in combination with a desired tidal volume (e.g., 500 ml.) is inadequate to maintain CO_2 removal, the rate is adjusted upward. If a rate of more than 20–25 breaths per minute is required to accomplish this, the tidal volume also must be increased. In addition, it is important to produce periodic hyperinflation to simulate the normal sigh mechanism in respiration. In some volume-cycled ventilators, such as the Bennett MA–1, the frequency of the sigh and the volume increment increase that it imparts to ventilation can be programmed into the respirator system.

COMPLICATIONS OF PROLONGED ARTIFICIAL VENTILATION

Tracheal necrosis.—For patients in respiratory failure who require prolonged controlled ventilatory assistance, a closed airway affords in most instances the most efficient use of ventilators. A cuffed tracheostomy tube is usually used to accomplish this. If the patient is able to ventilate adequately without respirator support, the cuff need not be inflated. Should controlled ventilation become necessary, a closed system using a cuffed tracheostomy tube is most efficient for both pressure- and volume-cycled ventilators. Excessive inflation of such cuffs for protracted periods of time can produce tracheal wall necrosis. For these patients, therefore, the cuff should initially be inflated only sufficiently to prevent significant air leak around the cannula or through the mouth. Under ordinary circumstances, 5–7 ml. of air will be sufficient to accomplish this, depending, of course, on the size of the tracheostomy tube and the caliber of the trachea itself. In addition, the cuff should be deflated every hour for 5–10 minutes, depending upon the patient's ability to ventilate with an incompetent system.

Prior to deflation of the cuff, the pharynx and mouth should be aspirated of all retained secretions to prevent their entering the trachea. More recently, systems have been devised to inflate these cuffs on inspiration alone and deflate them on expiration. This simple attachment may run off the pressure system of the respirator to provide a closed system on inspiration and an open system on expiration, thus decreasing the amount of pressure on the tracheal wall. Once tracheal wall necrosis has occurred, antibiotic and adrenal steroid therapy may help prevent stricture formation.

Diffuse atelectasis.—Diffuse atelectasis occurs commonly during constant-volume ventilation with normal or smaller than normal tidal volumes. It is obvious that the prevention of diffuse air space collapse requires a correct ventilatory pattern. Patients who are not attuned or adapted to controlled ventilation and cannot cycle with the machine may require sedation, reassurance, and even 100 per cent

O_2 to block their respiratory drive. In the latter situation, the patient should be observed closely for CO_2 accumulation attendant upon high O_2 tensions. All the therapeutic adjuvants, including adequate aspiration, humidification of the inspired gases, chest physiotherapy, hourly to 2-hourly turning and periodic hyperinflation are mandatory. If the atelectasis cannot be remedied, therapeutic bronchoscopy is required.

Gastrointestinal complications.—Gastric dilatation and ileus are common sequelae among comatose patients maintained on respirators. Such distention leads to elevation of the left hemidiaphragm with subsequent reduction in ventilation and may cause hypotension and hypokalemia in extreme cases. Vomiting with aspiration can be disastrous in this circumstance and gastric decompression should be used to prevent this catastrophe. When the airway is protected with a tracheostomy, or by an endotracheal tube, a nasogastric tube may be kept in place with relative safety. Without a tracheostomy, periodic insertion and subsequent removal of the nasogastric tube for gastric decompression is desirable. The problem may be minimized by the use of a cuffed tube and by decreasing the inspiratory pressure on the respirator.

Alveolar capillary block.—Patients who require controlled respiration for indefinite periods of time (upward of several months), may develop increasingly "stiff" and noncompliant lungs.

In one instance of which we were aware, a patient developed an increasingly severe alveolar capillary block, probably due to hyalinization of the alveolar capillary membrane, and required progressive increases in the rate and volume of ventilation. Despite all ventilatory maneuvers, the patient could not adequately exchange gases and eventually succumbed both to the underlying disease and no doubt to the therapy used to treat it initially.

Hyperventilation.—Hyperventilation and resultant respiratory alkalosis occasionally occur in patients receiving continuous respirator assistance and control. This condition is suggested by chest pain, syncope, tingling and numbness of fingers and toes, vertigo, carpopedal spasm and even tetany. To avoid the hyperventilation syndrome, the respiratory rate of the machine should be periodically decreased by 6–8 respirations per minute.

Excessive adrenergic response to bronchodilating drugs.—When palpitation or nervousness occurs during or immediately following positive-pressure treatment with bronchodilating agents such as isoproterenol (Isuprel), excessive absorption of the drug is suggested. When administered, these agents should be appropriately diluted and, because of their sympathomimetic effects, should not be given more than every 3–4 hours.

Bronchospasm and paroxysmal cough.—The development of bronchospasm may indicate hypersensitivity to some of the aerosol medication being employed in conjunction with the respirator. In other instances it may represent an inefficient humidifying system with attendant drying. In the first instance treatment with these aerosol agents should be stopped, and in the second situation, humidifying systems must be improved.

Weaning from respirator support.—As a rule, weaning from the respirator should start as soon as possible in an attempt to return the patient to his normal mechanisms for ventilation and humidification. This is of importance to prevent secondary infection, to restore normal tone more quickly to the muscles of breathing and also for the psychologic benefit to the patient as he recognizes his improvement.

On the other hand, premature attempts at weaning are inadvisable. To determine the precise time for weaning requires considerable judgment and experience. In general, the average patient can be taken off the respirator when his vital capacity is greater than two or three times his normal tidal volume. When weaning is first tried, a patient should be taken off the respirator for 3–4 minutes every half hour; if this is tolerated, the periods can then be increased.

Adequately humidified oxygen should be provided when the patient is off the respirator. This progressive removal from respirator control may require mild sedation to allay the patient's anxiety. Few patients become independent of respirator support until their vital capacity has increased to 30–35 per cent of predicted normal values. It is quite obvious that chest physiotherapy, postural drainage, tracheal toilet, antibiotics, and oxygen support should be maintained even when weaning appears complete. Patients (particularly those who are old and debilitated) should remain under close observation for several days after weaning is completed. Generally speaking, the longer the period of respirator support, the slower the weaning process.

Tables 4-1 and 4-2 summarize the management of patients maintained on prolonged artificial ventilation.

Special Guidelines for the Care of Patients on Respirators

A. Pressure-Controlled Ventilators:

1. Ensure airtight system. When a face mask is used, it must fit

securely; in unconscious patients, an oropharyngeal airway may be necessary. With a cuffed tracheostomy tube, an adaptor is attached, making tracheal suctioning possible without disconnecting the respirator.

2. Respirators make a characteristic sound on inspiration and expiration. Once personnel have learned to identify the normal sounds, they can be alert for any changes that indicate difficulty. This is especially important in patients on automatic cycling. An obstructed airway should be suspected any time the respirations become noisy. In addition, the rate of the ventilator will increase as airway resistance increases. If there is complete obstruction, the inhalation valve will "chatter." When there is a leak in the airway, the machine will *hiss* or the pressure-gauge dial will fail to reach the preset level.
3. The time of the inspiratory phase of respiration should not exceed that of the expiratory phase. During IPPB administration, the intrathoracic pressure is increased and right atrial and ventricular filling is reduced, leading to decreased stroke volume and cardiac output. Thus, the expiratory phase needs to be long enough to allow the stroke volume and cardiac output to increase before inspiration begins again. We attempt to maintain a ratio of $1-1\frac{1}{2}$ seconds inhalation to 3 seconds exhalation. In patients with any underlying problem already decreasing cardiac output (shock, hemorrhage, acute pulmonary edema, congestive heart failure), the pressure administered should be in the range of 10–15 cm. of water. Pressure higher than this tends to compromise cardiac output and increase hypoxia.
4. Pressure-controlled ventilators can deliver 100 per cent O_2. The dilution valve on the machine, however, allows for mixture of room air with the O_2 to a concentration of 40 per cent. As 100 per cent O_2 may be extremely hazardous in some patients, it should never be administered indiscriminately. In patients with chronic respiratory disease such as asthma and emphysema, O_2 should be diluted to 40 per cent; 40 per cent O_2 is twice the concentration in room air and is probably sufficient except in situations of severe hypoxia.
5. Since these ventilators operate on O_2 under pressure, an auxiliary gas supply should be available to maintain the patient on continuous ventilation in case the wall O_2 supply fails.

B. VOLUME-CONTROLLED RESPIRATORS:

1. These machines are used with a tracheostomy (cuffed or uncuffed) or an endotracheal tube. Face masks cannot be used.

2. The intensive care unit must have an auxiliary electric power source for emergencies. In case of a power failure, the patient should be disconnected from the respirator and ventilated by mouth-to-mouth or mouth-to-tube technic, Ambu (or similar) bag, or hand bellows until the respirator is connected to the auxiliary power source. Personnel should be taught to push the bag or bellows slowly and to count out a normal respiratory rate. In an emergency, some people push the bag so rapidly that the patient is receiving little effective ventilation. Once the patient is reconnected to the respirator, 100 per cent O_2 should be given for a short time to overcome hypoxia which may have developed during the power failure.

CRITERIA CONFIRMING ADEQUATE VENTILATION:

a. Absence of cyanosis or improvement in skin color.
b. Rhythmic expansion of the chest with expiratory phase longer than inspiratory phase.
c. Normal pulse: a drop in pulse rate may indicate decreased cardiac output due to increase in intrathoracic pressure.
d. Stationary blood pressure: a drop in blood pressure may indicate decreased cardiac output.
e. Absence of neurologic signs.
f. Audible rhythmicity of respiration.
g. Normal functioning of respirator.
h. Absence of hyper- or hypoventilation.

CRITERIA INDICATING INADEQUATE VENTILATION:

a. Impaired ventilatory excursion on respirator, caused by—
    1. Kinking of connecting tubes
    2. Occlusion of tubing with water, blood, mucus
    3. Low volume flow, and/or pressure settings
    4. Obstructed tracheostomy
    5. Bronchospasm
    6. Pulmonary edema
b. Prolonged expiratory phase with delay in inspiratory cycle, caused by—
    1. Connection leaks
    2. Excessive pressure setting
    3. Low rates
c. Absent inspiratory cycle, caused by—
    1. Failure to connect respirator to O_2 supply or electric outlet
    2. Sensitivity control set too low
    3. Leak between the patient and the machine
    4. Incorrect respiratory rate

d. Absent expiratory cycle, caused by—
   1. "Sticky" or malfunctioning exhalation valve
   2. Air leak in system
e. Hyperventilation, caused by—
   1. High respiratory rate
   2. High pressure control
   3. High volume control
   4. High flow rate
f. Hypoventilation, caused by—
   1. Low respiratory rate
   2. Low pressure control
   3. Low volume control
   4. Low flow rate

BRONCHODILATORS.—Intravenous, oral, and rectal aminophylline is valuable. Isoproterenol (Isuprel) administered sublingually and as an aerosol is effective in relieving bronchospasm. In conjunction with this, expectorants such as potassium iodide, ammonium chloride, and a whole host of commercial preparations can assist adequate liquefaction of secretions, thereby preventing bronchospasm. The continued use of expectorants may cause bronchorrhea. Water is still a most effective liquefying agent.

VENTILATORY STIMULANTS.—Nikethamide (Coramine) and caffeine sodium benzoate have been used in the past to stimulate respiration but in most instances have only limited value. Newer agents such as vanillic acid diethylamide (Emivan) have also been tried for this purpose; however, their true efficacy remains uncertain.

ADRENOCORTICAL STEROIDS.—Steroids have proved valuable in the treatment of inflammatory pulmonary and bronchospastic diseases. In those patients who have alveolar-capillary membrane thickening, the inflammatory process may be arrested or even reversed with this regimen. The dangers of adrenal cortical steroid therapy are well documented, and patients must be followed closely while on these drugs. Adequate antibiotic and chemotherapeutic agents are administered to patients with respiratory infections who are also receiving steroids.

Other drugs, such as digitalis and diuretics, necessary for associated cardiac decompensation and cardiac arrhythmias, are discussed elsewhere.

PULMONARY INFECTION.—Prevention of pulmonary infection in patients with protracted controlled ventilation requires: (1) meticulous removal of secretions; (2) prevention and prompt treatment of atelectasis; (3) aseptic and atraumatic tracheostomy care; (4) frequent sterilization of IPPB equipment, humidifiers, tubes, valves and tracheostomy implements (either by cold or gas sterilization); (5) prevention of cross-infection with isolation precautions; (6) maintenance of maximum host resistance to infection by insuring an adequate state of hydration and nutrition with adequate blood volume, tissue perfusion, and oxygenation; (7) antibiotics specifically employed with bacteriologic culture and sensitivity control.

Resistant strains of Staphylococcus aureus, Proteus, Pseudomonas aeruginosa and Klebsiella are the predominating pathogens encountered. On occasion, aerosol antibiotics may be employed. Aerosolized polymyxin B sulfate, which is toxic when given parenterally, may be used in doses of 50 mg./3–5 ml. every 6 hours for the treatment of Pseudomonas respiratory infections.

RESPIRATORY DRUGS.—Many drugs are available for use in respiratory failure. These include (1) antibiotics, (2) bronchodilators, (3) ventilatory stimulants, and (4) steroids. Choice of antibiotics should be based on culture and sensitivity control whenever possible; however, prophylactic antibiotics, without culture and sensitivity, can be used in emergencies to protect against superinfection. Prolonged use of antibiotics may produce bacteriologic resistance, complicating fungal diseases, and systemic reactions, such as enteritis. These drugs should be used in well-controlled therapeutic regimens, with adequate doses and for finite periods of time, with bacteriologic culture and sensitivity rechecks at frequent intervals.

Minor Surgical Procedures During the Postoperative Period

1. THORACENTESIS (FIG. 4-4) —Thoracentesis is used to remove air or fluid from the pleural cavity and consists of introducing a needle attached to a syringe into the pleural cavity. The site of the puncture is determined by the location of the material to be aspirated. Since fluid is generally found in the dependent portions of the pleural cavity, the usual site of puncture is the 7th or 8th intercostal space in the posterior axillary line. In pleural disease, because of the elevation of the diaphragm, no appreciable extent of the pleural cavity is apt to be found below this level posteriorly or below a line running to the corresponding nipple. Within an area of the chest where the presence of fluid is suspected by the appearance of the x-ray film, it is usually advisable to place the needle at the spot where the absence of, or greatest decrease in, transmission of tactile fremitus is found on physical examination.

The patient may be placed in any convenient position, but generally the sitting position is most advantageous. By elevating the head of

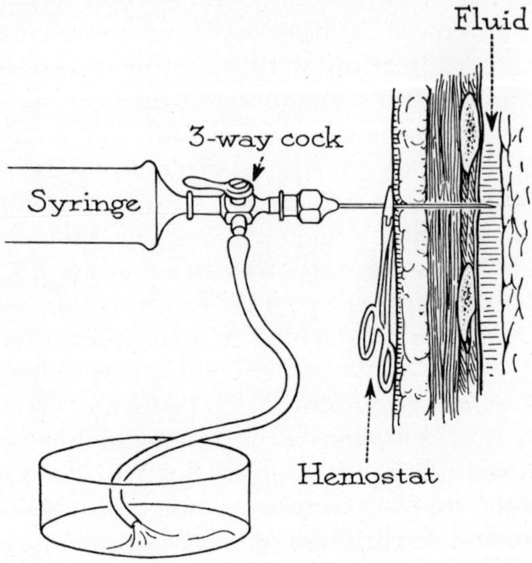

Fig. 4-4.—Thoracentesis performed with syringe, needle and stopcocks.

the bed, this can be achieved easily and the anterior or lateral portion of the chest can be aspirated without further displacement of the patient. For posterior aspiration, without moving the patient from his bed, he may be turned so that his feet dangle over the edge of the bed and are supported on a chair, with the sound side of his chest against the elevated head of the bed or further propped up by pillows.

Steps in thoracentesis are as follows:

(1) The appropriate field is selected for the site of puncture.

(2) An adequate skin field is prepared around the site selected for puncture.

(3) Utilizing a 5 or 10 ml. syringe and a 1% or 2% solution of procaine (Novocain) or lidocaine (Xylocaine), a skin wheal is produced at the site of puncture (by a small needle), being centered over the selected intercostal space.

(4) Changing to a larger needle (2 in., of greater caliber) the skin wheal is pierced and the needle advanced to the level of the rib cage. Additional amounts of procaine or lidocaine should be injected as the needle advances. A rib may be encountered, or may actually be sought with the needle point for determination of level.

The intercostal muscles are entered with the needle and well infiltrated with the anesthetic to insure adequate anesthetization of the pleura. The needle is now advanced slowly, with further injections of the anesthetic. When it is estimated that the pleura is being approached, traction can be maintained on the plunger of the syringe. With traction on the syringe, pleural fluid or air will appear in the syringe as soon as the pleura is entered.

(5) If any appreciable amount of fluid is believed to be present, it is advisable to remove the anesthetizing syringe and needle. A larger syringe of 30 or 50 ml. capacity is now connected to a 3-way stopcock and the needle is placed on this in turn, so that the syringe and needle are in a straight line. The side arm of the stopcock will be used to discharge the aspirated material. A length of rubber tubing properly fitted to the side arm will transport the fluid to a suitable container. It is well to test the assembled apparatus beforehand to ascertain the position of the stopcock control to connect needle and syringe and syringe and discharge tube. Also, all connections should be airtight.

The needle is now inserted into the pleura along the previously anesthetized tract, with traction on the syringe plunger, to again determine the moment of entry into the pleural cavity. At this depth, it is convenient to secure a hemostat to the needle flush with the skin. This tends to stabilize the apparatus and avoid the undesirable advancing and withdrawing of the needle that might be produced by the pulling and pushing of the syringe as it is filled and emptied. Needless to say, all apparatus must be sterile and the entire procedure carried on under strict asepsis.

Fluid may be withdrawn until the space is evacuated. If large amounts are present, however, the procedure should be stopped when the patient shows discomfort. The onset of coughing should be a signal that sufficient fluid has been removed for the moment, as coughing indicates that the lung has not been able to expand to compensate for the volume of fluid withdrawn and that negative pressure is being created within the pleural space, causing displacement of other intrathoracic organs. Air can be replaced to equilibrate intrapleural pressures under these circumstances, but this defeats the purpose of the procedure, which is to obliterate the pleural space by emptying it.

Another method of thoracentesis, which avoids the need of the rigid needle-stopcock-syringe system, consists of introducing the needle into the pleural space with a length of rubber tubing connecting the needle to the syringe. Each time the syringe is to be emptied, the tubing is clamped by a hemostat and the syringe disconnected and evacuated into the proper container. In order to stabilize the depth of needle, a hemostat is placed on the needle flush with the skin. However, the rigid system is much more efficient than the flexible.

A vacuum bottle connected to the system and ultimately to the pleura will provide aspirating force for the evacuation of pleural content; however, this method may aspirate fluid so rapidly that patient discomfort results.

2. INTERCOSTAL NERVE BLOCK (SEE FIG. 4–5).—The block should be carried to the nerve involved by the incision and extended to at least one or possibly two nerves above and below this level to assure adequate control of overlapping innervation. Attempts to block the intercostal nerve at a point medial to the angle of the rib are not recommended because of the danger that the solution may enter a prolongation of the dural sheath, which occasionally extends out to this point. This could result in an intrathecal injection of the agent. Also, since the nerve runs obliquely across the intercostal space medial to the angle of the rib and is not, therefore, in juxtaposition to the rib, no satisfactory landmark is present to insure accuracy in the procedure. Attempts to block the nerve anteriorly are generally unsatisfactory because the principal trunk of the nerve is being broken up into its various branches. The direct infiltration of a fractured rib at the site of fracture may occasionally be justified.

Fig. 4–5.—Technique of intercostal nerve block.

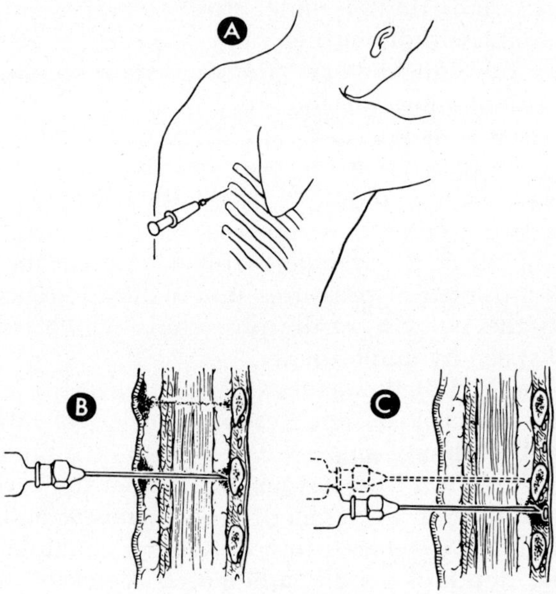

The patient is rolled onto the unoperated side and the paravertebral area prepared. Skin wheals are produced by a fine, short needle over the appropriate interspaces along the lateral edge of the paraspinal mass of muscle. A longer needle is then used to infiltrate the back muscles as the needle seeks the rib. The needle then sloped under the inferior edge of the corresponding rib and less than 4 ml. of anesthetic is injected, after being certain that the needle has not entered an intercostal vessel.

Long-acting agents seem to offer no consistently superior results over procaine or lidocaine, and some of them may be dangerous. Local anesthetic blocks may be repeated as required. The first attempt may bring relief that lasts for the expected period of pharmacologic action of the drug, but the second or third injections may result in prolonged periods of relief.

3. Determination of intrapleural pressures.—This is carried out essentially in the same manner as a thoracentesis except that the site of puncture should be selected where fluid, if present, will *not* be encountered, because if fluid enters the system, fluctuations and pleural pressures may not be transmitted to the manometer. Thus, the second anterior intercostal space is the site usually selected for puncture with the patient in semi-Fowler's position. The skin is prepared and the skin and pleura are anesthetized as for thoracentesis.

A separate needle, syringe, and 3-way stopcock are connected to the manometer and attached to a pneumothorax apparatus, the rubber tubing on the discharge vent of the stopcock serving as the connection. The tubing to the stopcock is sterile, but connections can be made by an attendant so long as the operator remains sterile. The needle, syringe, and 3-way stopcock are assembled and the needle is inserted into the pleura. If the needle and syringe are connected through the stopcock, the entrance of the needle into the pleura will be indicated when air is pulled into the syringe as the plunger is kept under traction. If the needle is connected to the stopcock through the side vent and, therefore, to the manometer, entry of the needle into the pleura is heralded by the onset of fluctuation registered on the manometer. If the former connection was in use, the stopcock control should be turned to connect needle and side vent, at which time manometric fluctuations will occur.

For accuracy, manometric readings should be taken during quiet breathing.

Intrapleural pressure can be adjusted by injection or removal of air, using the pneumothorax apparatus or by the syringe. Since small amounts of air withdrawn and delivered will often suffice to bring about the proper level of intrapleural pressure, a 30 ml. syringe is usually used, although a 10 ml. syringe may occasionally be adequate. This adjustment is made by switching the stopcock control to connect needle and syringe for the withdrawal of air, when appropriate repositioning of the control will again permit taking pleural pressure readings. To inject air through the syringe, the syringe can be detached and filled with room air while the needle is connected to the manometer. When the syringe is replaced on the stopcock, the control is properly turned, and measured amounts of air can be injected from the syringe. If large amounts of air are to be injected or withdrawn, this can best be accomplished by using a pneumothorax apparatus.

An obvious precaution calls for complete familiarity with the pneumothorax apparatus at hand before initiating this operation.

4. INSERTION OF AN INTERCOSTAL CATHETER (SEE FIG. 4–6).—Two methods are in general use for placing a catheter within the pleural space for the purpose of removing air or, on occasion, fluid from the intercostal cavity.

The neatest method involves the use of a thoracotomy trocar. The area through which the catheter will be inserted is selected by review of x-ray films, even though in most instances the catheter will be inserted into the second anterior intercostal space or through the fourth intercostal space in the axilla. The procedure can be carried out with the patient in his own bed.

The skin is prepared about the proper site and the chest wall is anesthetized as described for thoracentesis. A small incision is made in the skin with a knife blade, so that the trocar shaft will not be gripped by the skin. The trocar, with its in-lying sharp-pointed stylet, is then inserted into this skin incision and advanced along the anesthetized tract, passing between the ribs. A rotary motion will aid in the steady advance of the instrument. Entry of the trocar into the pleural cavity is readily recognized. The trocar is advanced sufficiently to insure that the shaft of the instrument and not merely the point of the stylet is inside the pleura. The stylet is now fully withdrawn and the catheter is passed into the pleura, whereupon the trocar is removed as the catheter is fed into it. When the trocar shaft emerges from the skin, a hemostat is clamped across the catheter flush with the skin and the catheter is pulled completely through the trocar. The catheter is then anchored to the skin either by suture or adhesive tape and the area is covered by a suitable dressing. A water-seal device is connected to the catheter and the system can then be opened by removal of the hemostat. Though sucking of some air

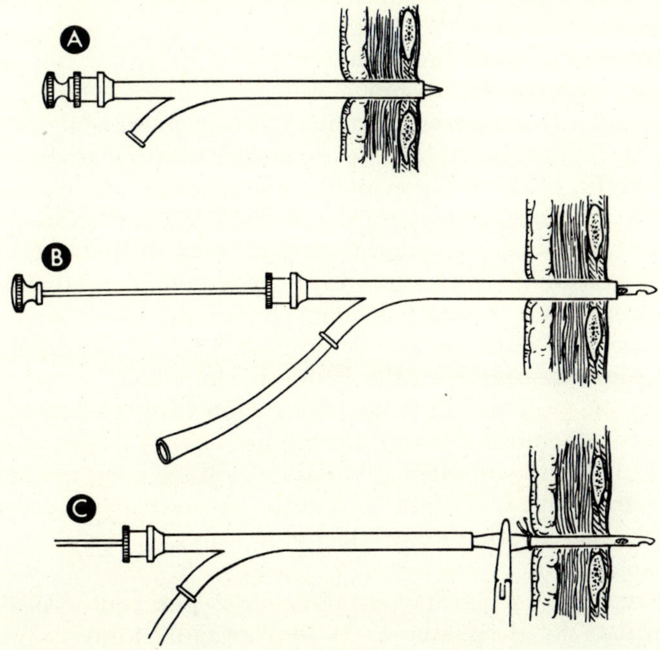

Fig. 4–6.—Insertion of thoracotomy trocar into pleural cavity.

is not of serious consequence during the period of catheter insertion, this should be kept to a minimum.

Certain precautions should be taken before the trocar is inserted. The catheter to be inserted should be passed through the trocar to make sure it will pass easily and especially that the funnel end of the catheter will not hang. An ordinary urethral catheter is best suited for this purpose. Two or three additional fenestrations are made in the catheter an inch or so apart, increasing the available openings for ingress of drainage into the system. When this is done, the distance that the catheter must be fed beyond the trocar to insure that all fenestrations lie within the pleura should be clearly determined while testing the respective sizes of trocar and catheter, as outlined above.

The other method for placing a catheter within the pleural space is that of direct insertion of the catheter, a hemostat or similar instrument being used as a guide.

In this method, preparation and anesthetization of the appropriate site is the same as described above. The skin is cut with a small knife blade. A medium or large hemostatic forceps is used to open the tissues by blunt dissection. When the pleura is entered, the jaws of the forceps are spread and the catheter is fed between the separated jaws for the appropriate distance into the pleura. The hemostat is then removed. The catheter is connected to a water seal and secured to the chest wall as previously described. A plastic catheter carrying a pointed stylet is currently available as a packaged commodity.

Other instruments have been devised for the insertion of decompressing systems into the pleural cavity. One, an S-shaped metallic needle (Clagett needle), can be inserted through a small stab wound in the skin, pushed through the muscles of the chest wall and the intercostal space, entering the pleura, and being positioned to lie along the pleural surface on the inside of the chest cavity and along the skin on the outside. This needle is then directly connected to a water seal for decompression of the pleura.

The use of similar devices of smaller caliber, such as the Buffalo needle or Intracath catheters, generally applied in intravenous positions, are also available for decompression, particularly of thin effusions and air.

5. Tracheostomy technics.—One or 2 per cent procaine provides adequate local anesthesia. A high tracheostomy is preferable in order to position the tip of the cannula well above the carina. Either a midline and vertical or a curved collar incision can be made. Cosmetically, a curved collar incision is preferable; however, the limited exposure gained may reduce the speed with which the tracheostomy can be performed, especially in emergencies. When the patient's airway is controlled by endotracheal intubation, this incision can be used. In urgent cases, and particularly in patients with thick, heavy necks, a midline vertical incision provides extension of the incision upward or downward, as may be required. An emergency tracheostomy is best performed using a vertical incision.

To avoid aspiration of blood, it is important that hemostasis be obtained prior to opening the tracheal wall. If the pyramidal lobe of the thyroid overrides the area for tracheostomy, it should be dissected off and/or transected with adequate hemostasis before opening into the tracheal lumen. It is preferable to expose and enter the pretracheal fascia, which is relatively avascular, and identify the third tracheal ring, a portion of which is excised to provide an adequate opening. The fragment of cartilage to be removed must be gripped firmly to prevent its slippage into the tracheal lumen. Prior to incision of the trachea, a tracheal hook is used to grasp the trachea and elevate it so that its position will not vary with respiration or swallowing. A Jackson dilator spreads the tracheal opening so that a cannula (no. 7 or 8), with or without an attached cuff, may be readily introduced and immediate aspiration begun. If a bacteriologic specimen is desired, a Luken's tube is spliced into the aspirating system to trap secretions.

The incision is loosely closed around the tracheostomy tube. Usually, a single silk suture suffices to approximate the skin so the tracheostomy tube rests evenly without abutment against the posterior tracheal wall. The tube is firmly secured with ties around the neck. An appropriately folded, uncut 4×4-in. gauze pad, inserted around the flange of the tube, makes a neat and safe dressing.

NEGATIVE PHASE OF IPPB RESPIRATORS.—The Bennett PR-2 and the Bird Mark VIII and IX have negative-pressure and positive-pressure phases, permitting their use for both inspiration and expiration. The negative pressure gauge should not be set at more than 3 cm. H_2O. Increase in negative pressure on exhalation is helpful in reducing residual volume in severe obstructive ventilatory defects such as emphysema.

BIBLIOGRAPHY

Bates, D. V., and Christie, R. V.: *Respiratory Function in Disease* (Philadelphia: W. B. Saunders Company, 1964).

Bendixen, H. H., Egbert, L. D., Hedley-Whyte, J., Laver, M. B., and Pontoppidan, H.: *Respiratory Care* (St. Louis: C. V. Mosby Company, 1965).

Langston, H. T.: The Thorax Pleura and Lungs, in *Christopher's Textbook of Surgery*, Loyal Davis, M.D. (ed.) (9th ed.; Philadelphia: W. B. Saunders Company, 1968).

Meltzer, L. E., Abdellah, F. G., and Kitchell, J. R.: Concepts and Practices of Intensive Care, in Wilma J. Phipps *et al.*, *Respiratory Insufficiency and Failure* (Philadelphia: The Charles Press, 1969).

Pace, W. R.: *Pulmonary Physiology in Clinical Practice* (Philadelphia: F. A. Davis Company, 1965).

Sadove, M. S., and Cross, J. H.: Recovery Room, in H. T. Langston, M.D. (ed.), *Immediate Postoperative Management* (Philadelphia: W. B. Saunders Company, 1956).

CHAPTER

5

Artificial Mechanical Respiration in the Postoperative Period

E. TRIER MÖRCH, M.D., PH.D.

RESPIRATION IN THE POSTOPERATIVE PATIENT is affected by so many factors that it probably is never "normal" and very often is insufficient. Thus, respiratory failure is probably the most common and serious complication in the period immediately following major surgery. The more important factors influencing respiration include residual anesthesia and/or muscle relaxants; loss of fluids and heat during surgery; the trauma of manipulation of the tissues, organs and blood; plus alterations in the electrolytes and acid-base balance. Usually, it is not possible or even logical to pinpoint one single reason for inadequate ventilation but rather to suspect a multitude of varying known and unknown causes, which could vaguely, but justifiably, be called "exhaustion."

The work of breathing in normal life accounts for 5–10% of the total metabolism, which means that 5–10% of the work of the heart is done for the purpose of breathing. Following thoracotomies, the lungs, chest wall and other components of the respiratory apparatus are no longer normal, so the work of breathing, and with it, the work of the heart, will often be increased by 20–40%. Thus, one of the main indications for the use of mechanical artificial respiration following major surgery is to take over this extra work, thereby reducing the load on the heart and preventing exhaustion.

Assisted or Controlled Respiration

Assisted respiration is a supplement to a patient's active but insufficient respiration. The patient initiates the inhalation phase, and the respirator blows until a predetermined pressure is attained and then allows passive exhalation.

Controlled respiration is a more powerful form of artificial ventilation, in which the patient is not breathing spontaneously and the respirator is doing all the work of breathing for him. In the majority of postoperative patients, controlled respiration is preferable because it guarantees sufficient ventilation and prevents exhaustion.

Weaning from the respirator should not be attempted before the clinical and laboratory findings indicate that the patient is able to breathe adequately. Moderate respiratory alkalosis with hypocarbia, ideally around 25–35 mm. Hg Pa_{CO_2}, is intentionally maintained to keep the patient in apnea while on the respirator. By gradually reducing the alveolar ventilation, the CO_2 will increase in the alveolar air, in the arterial blood and in the respiratory center. The patient will begin breathing when the Pa_{CO_2} approaches the normal level of $\pm$ 40 mm. Hg. In the majority of cases, normal Pa_{CO_2} can be restored in 3 to 5 minutes, and only in extremely rare instances will this take 10 minutes or more.

The patient must be followed closely for the first several hours after use of the respirator is terminated, and both clinical and laboratory findings must be assessed repeatedly. The dangers are related to inadequate ventilation and exhaustion. Hypoventilation can result in hypoxia, hypercarbia or both (asphyxia). Hypoxia may cause cyanosis, but only if the hemoglobin count is fairly normal. Moderate to severe hypoxia may develop without cyanosis in the anemic patient, since cyanosis is visible only when at least 5 Gm. of hemoglobin is present as reduced hemoglobin in 100 ml. of blood. Hypoxia will also result in cerebral depression, with the potential dangers of permanent brain damage. Blood-gas analysis is the most reliable way to determine the amount of O_2 in the blood. The normal value for PaO_2 is around 100 mm. Hg; less than 80 mm. Hg should call for vigorous therapy.

On the other hand, hypercarbia will cause tachycardia, an increase in blood pressure and peripheral vasodilation. This may predispose to misinterpretation of the clinical picture, as some of the first warning symptoms of shock (hypotension and peripheral vasoconstriction) are masked. Under these conditions, the situation may become so grave that the overt manifestations of shock may abruptly appear. Had the CO_2 level been normal or low, the symptoms and signs of impending shock would have occurred earlier. Here, too, blood-gas determinations are the safest and most reliable way to diagnose hypercarbia (respiratory acidosis).

Respirator treatment should be reinstituted immediately if symptoms indicate, or even if in doubt. It will not harm the patient to be kept on a respirator a little too long or even to be reconnected to the machine, and this is often the best way to prevent hypoxia or asphyxia.

Summary.—Assisted respiration is supplementation of a patient's respiration; controlled respiration is a complete substitution of the patient's respiration. Weaning from the respirator should be done gradually; if in doubt, continue positive-pressure ventilation.

Blood-Gas Interpretation

Although acid-base balance has been discussed in a previous chapter, the subject is so intimately a part of the management of respiratory problems that repetition is justified. Although O_2 and CO_2 can be expressed in many different units, e.g., partial pressure, content, volume %, saturation, carrying capacity, millimoles, etc., this multitude of expressions is neither necessary nor practical for a clinical understanding and application of blood-gas analysis.

The most practical and simple unit of measurement for O_2 and CO_2 is the pressure [tension] of these gases in the body. For example, venous blood with an oxygen tension (Pv_{O_2}) of 50–70 mm. Hg is exposed to a much higher pressure of O_2 in the pulmonary capillaries, approximately 100 mm. Hg. Since any gas must follow the pressure gradient, i.e., flow from high to a lower pressure, O_2 diffuses into the blood until equilibrium is attained, which occurs at approximately 100 mm. Hg. The arterial blood transports O_2 at this pressure to the tissues, where the O_2 is lower. Thus, O_2 must diffuse out of the blood into the surrounding media. In the following discussions, these gases will be expressed only as "mm. Hg partial."

The most important physiologic measurements in the clinical treatment of patients with respiratory problems are:

1) Pa_{CO_2} (partial pressure of arterial CO_2)
2) Pa_{O_2} (partial pressure of arterial oxygen)
3) Base Excess
4) The pH of the arterial blood.

1. Arterial Carbon Dioxide

The normal Pa_{CO_2} is 40 ± mm. Hg. A Pa_{CO_2} above 45 mm. Hg represents respiratory acidosis and is invariably the result of insufficient ventilation. Since CO_2 diffuses very rapidly from the pulmonary capillaries into the alveoli, it is usually possible to keep the CO_2 at or below normal level by alveolar ventilation. For a patient on a respirator, the ideal Pa_{CO_2} level is slightly below the normal, i.e., 25–35 mm. Hg, which is low enough to maintain hyperventilation-apnea.

A Pa_{CO_2} below 35 mm. Hg represents respiratory alkalosis, which

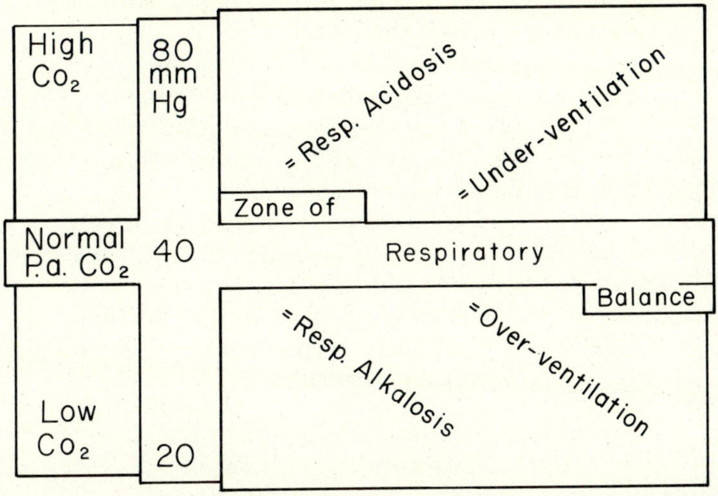

Fig. 5-1.—Pa_{CO_2} of 40 mm. Hg ± 5 represents the "Zone of Respiratory Balance." Respiratory acidosis means higher CO_2, respiratory alkalosis lower CO_2.

seems to have little, if any, harmful effects. While this represents the present author's opinion on a most controversial topic, it is based on a rather extensive experience. While respiratory alkalosis seems to have little ill effect, even minor acidosis is very upsetting for most organ functions, probably due to interference with enzymatic processes. Respiratory acidosis may cause cardiac arrhythmias, hypotension and disturbances in the functions of the brain, liver and kidneys.

The present author believes that CO_2 can be compared to garbage, to the exhaust from a gasoline engine or fumes from a stove or fire, and that it is useful to remove as much garbage as possible. The most important normal effect of CO_2 is stimulation of the respiratory center. With hyperventilation, the CO_2 can be reduced, often with great ease, to below 35 mm. Hg; apnea results, but this is exactly what is desired in an attempt to unload, especially from the heart, the heavy burden of breathing with impaired respiratory machinery (see Fig. 5-1).

Overenthusiastic hyperventilation may cause the Pa_{CO_2} to drop to 15 mm. Hg, which is an unnecessarily low level. However, even this excessive hyperventilation and respiratory alkalosis seems to have few harmful effects. One possible exception has been postulated, and this is in patients who are receiving such large doses of digitalis that they are on the verge of digitalis intoxication. As mentioned in Chapter 1, respiratory alkalosis may shift the K^+ from the plasma to the intracellular fluid and also into the urine. A small shift of K^+ from the plasma may possibly change the situation from potential to manifest digitalis intoxication. However, this is a postulate, and there are no reasons to maintain such extreme levels of Pa_{CO_2}; the situation is easy to correct, simply by reducing ventilation until the Pa_{CO_2} is about 25–35 mm. Hg, and by giving enough supplementary K^+ to keep the blood potassium level normal.

Summary.—Hypercarbia (abnormally high CO_2 levels) is synonymous with respiratory acidosis; it is nearly always caused by hypoventilation and can be corrected in a few minutes by increasing the ventilation. Respiratory acidosis is dangerous, whereas respiratory alkalosis is associated with little if any danger. The ideal Pa_{CO_2} is 25–35 mm. Hg; *if in doubt, overventilate.*

2. Arterial Oxygen

Oxygen in arterial blood can be expressed and measured as saturation (Sa_{O_2}) and tension (Pa_{O_2}). Saturation is an expression of the amount of O_2 available in the blood chemically combined with the hemoglobin, while the O_2 tension is the pressure of the physically dissolved O_2. This measurement is important because it is the pressure at which oxygen is offered to the tissues.

In normal life, O_2 in the alveolar space is separated from the blood in the pulmonary capillaries by only two microscopic layers of cells; this permits its rapid diffusion into the blood. In the postoperative period, however, we often encounter the "heavy," wet lung, with poor compliance, because fluids have accumulated in the potential space between the alveoli and the capillaries. This interstitial edema interferes with the diffusion of O_2 inward and CO_2 outward. Oxygen, however, diffuses 20 times more slowly than CO_2, so a reduced diffusion shows up earlier and more dramatically in O_2 than in CO_2 tension.

The normal Pa_{O_2} is approximately 100 mm. Hg, the ideal range in the postoperative period being 80–150 mm. Hg, which is an extremely narrow range. An oxygen tension below 80 mm. Hg may result in tissue hypoxia, while a Pa_{O_2} above 150 mm. Hg may cause oxygen toxicity, which has an adverse effect on the lung. However, if the oxygen tension is below 80 mm. Hg after surgery, the concentration (and the tension) of O_2 in the inhaled atmosphere should be increased, taking the calculated risk of exposing the patient to higher oxygen tensions and resultant oxygen toxicity. The latter is a lesser evil than the rapid and lethal aspects of hypoxia.

Ideally, diffusion should be expressed as the difference between the oxygen tension in the alveolar air and in the arterial blood, and should be measured in both places. However, in most instances, only the arterial oxygen tension is known. This can be altered by increasing or decreasing the oxygen concentration in the inhaled atmosphere.

Summary.—The Pa_{O_2} is an expression of diffusion, while the Pa_{CO_2} reflects ventilation. The ideal tension for oxygen is 80–150 mm. Hg, and for CO_2 it is 25–35 mm. Hg. *If in doubt, keep the O_2 high and the CO_2 low.*

3. Base Excess

Base Excess (BE) is the third factor of clinical importance. (This very practical term, introduced by Siggaard-Andersen, of Copenhagen, is discussed in detail in Chapter 1. Base excess is the *change* or deviation of buffer base from its normal value, or the observed buffer base minus the normal.

The buffering ability of the blood is complex and depends upon several factors, some of the more powerful being the buffer pairs, i.e., a weak acid and its conjugated base (its highly dissociated salts, e.g., $H_2CO_3 + NaHCO_3$). The most important buffers in the blood are bicarbonate/carbonic acid, hemoglobin, the plasma proteins and organic and inorganic phosphate. Bicarbonate/carbonic acid is by far the most important of all the buffers and accounts for more than 50% of all the buffering in whole blood.

The buffers in the body have one purpose: to dampen and reduce the harmful effects of the changing amounts of acids or bases (alkali). Expressed in another way, they pacify the largest amount of acids or bases with the least change in acidity of the blood:ion concentration. To illustrate mechanism, let us see how the most important buffer pair, the sodium bicarbonate/carbonic acid ($NaHCO_3/H_2CO_3$) can pacify, or at least buffer, the harmful effects of a deadly acid such as hydrochloric acid (HCl) and of a deadly base such as sodium hydroxide (NaOH). $HCl + NaHCO_3 = NaCl + H_2CO_3$:

$$H^+ + Cl^- + Na^+ + HCO_3^- = Na^+ + Cl^- + H_2CO_3 \begin{cases} \nearrow CO_2 \text{ blows off.} \\ \searrow H_2O \text{ remains.} \end{cases}$$

In this example, we started with a deadly acid and ended up with a harmless or even beneficial salt (NaCl) and carbonic acid, which the body can eliminate by blowing CO_2 off via the lungs and producing water, which the body needs.

Or consider a strong base, sodium hydroxide: NaOH + carbonic acid = sodium bicarbonate + water:

$$Na^+ + OH^- + H^+ + HCO_3^- = Na^+ + HCO_3^- + H_2O.$$

In this example, we started with a deadly base and ended up with a harmless or even beneficial salt ($NaHCO_3$) and water, which the body needs.

For the sake of simplicity, the blood buffers can also be classified in two groups:

1) The bicarbonate system (HCO_3^-), located primarily in the plasma and *2) the nonbicarbonate system* (Buf^-) located primarily in the erythrocytes (hemoglobin being the most important).

A base is a substance which can combine with H^+ formed by acids. A great number of acids are produced during normal metabolism, whereas excess blood can create acids in the form of H_2CO_3 in a few minutes, whereas it cannot create bases. For these reasons, most of the buffer systems are concerned with neutralization or elimination of acids (which is the same as conservation of bases). The different bases involved in buffering of the blood are often called Buffer Bases (BB).

The *Buffer Base* is the sum of all the bases in 1 liter of whole blood, normally 48 mEq./liter, or $BB = HCO_3^- + Buf^-$. If, for example, 8 mEq. of a base is added to 1 liter of normal blood, the BB would be $48 + 8 = 56$ mEq./liter, or 8 mEq. in EXCESS of the normal 48; thus the base excess (BE) would be +8. If acid is added (which would be equivalent to the subtraction of base because acid ties up base), then the BB would be $48 - 8 = 40$ mEq./liter, or 8 mEq. in deficit of the normal 48; thus the base excess (BE) would be −8.

Base excess is a very practical term to express the total acidity (or alkalinity) of the blood. A negative BE is an expression of metabolic acidosis, which is dangerous and should be corrected as early as possible, although metabolic acidosis can be caused by a multitude of pathologic processes, one of the most common of which is hypoxia, which interferes with normal metabolism of glucose and glycogen.

Metabolistic implications.—Most of the dietary carbohydrates are polymers of glycogen (glucose, fructose or galactose), which are all hexoses (i.e., containing 6 carbon atoms per molecule). The principal circulating sugar is glucose. The breakdown of glucose to CO_2 and water is called *glycolysis*; through a series of complicated chemical reactions, glucose is the most important source of energy for the body. Glucose is degraded to pyruvic acid and other tricarboxylic acids (containing 3 carbon atoms per molecule). This part of glucose metabolism is anaerobic. Normally, when an adequate amount of O_2 is present, pyruvic acid is metabolized through a series of chemical reactions called the Krebs cycle (citric acid cycle or tricarboxylic acid cycle). This is the common pathway for oxidation to CO_2 and water. It is by far the most important source of energy, but it does not function under anaerobic conditions.

Whenever circulation is reduced, generally or locally, deficient O_2 supply may interfere with the tricarboxylic acid cycle. This is often observed in the postoperative period, in low cardiac output state or whenever peripheral vasoconstriction exists—be it from hypovolemia, pain, hypothermia or any other cause. As a result, tricarboxylic acids will accumulate, with resultant metabolic acidosis. This has a deleterious effect on the heart, liver and kidneys, probably by interfering with enzymatic processes which are extremely sensitive to changes in acids or in pH. The acids present can easily be neutralized by $NaHCO_3$, but acidosis will soon recur unless the underlying cause is removed. This may be very easy in case of isolated peripheral vasoconstriction but may be very difficult or even impossible if the etiology is insufficient cardiac output.

The respiratory centers in the medulla oblongata are sensitive primarily to CO_2, but also to other acids and changes in pH. Any acid, e.g., the metabolic acids, will stimulate, or rather irritate, the respiratory centers, cause dyspnea, and made it impossible to take over respiration by hyperventilating.

Both metabolic and respiratory acidosis are dangerous conditions, and behave as two completely different entities. Therefore, they should be treated differently—respiratory acidosis by increased ventilation, and metabolic acidosis by a symptomatic neutralization of the acids with $NaHCO_3$, concomitantly with removal of the cause.

Calculation of the dose of $NaHCO_3$ is often described in a complicated way and based on facts that may or may not be known; for example, in emergency cases it may not even be possible to weigh the patient, and body weight is one of the fundamental factors in this calculation. Body water is approximately two thirds of the body weight. One third of this water is extracellular, in the plasma and in the interstitial fluid; this amount of the water can and must be corrected for metabolic acids. The intracellular water will shift more slowly and should therefore only partly be included in the calculation for correction of metabolic acidosis.

"Dynamic Water."—The present author has simplified the calculations necessary for determining the dose of $NaHCO_3$ by substituting a series of approximations resulting in figures so simple that

"kitchen mathematics" suffice and has coined a new term, "Dynamic Water," for the water which changes rapidly and therefore must be neutralized rapidly. The "Dynamic Water" consists of the extracellular water and a small fraction of the intracellular water, or approximately half of the total body water; it is therefore equivalent to one third of the body weight. (Approximation #1).

Since the body weight is not always known, this calculation assumes the weight of male patients as 75 kg. and of females as 60 kg. These figures are chosen because they are easily divided by 3 and result in round numbers that are easily multiplied. Thus, the Dynamic Water of a male patient is 25 liters (1/3 of 75 kg.) and of a female, 20 liters (1/3 of 60 kg.). (Approximation #2).

The base excess (BE), when negative, expresses acidosis in mEq. per liter, or, for Dynamic Water, the absolute amount of bicarbonate necessary to neutralize would thus be the BE multiplied by the Dynamic Water. An example will illustrate:

Let us assume that the laboratory results show a BE of −10, which means that each liter of Dynamic Water has an excess amount of acids of 10 mEq., which require 10 mEq. of base, i.e., of bicarbonate, for neutralization. If the patient is female, she is assumed to have 20 liters of Dynamic Water, each with a deficit of 10 mEq., or a total need for $10 \times 20 = 200$ mEq. of sodium bicarbonate. In the U.S.A., the most common commercial preparations of $NaHCO_3$ contain ±44 (aver. 44.6) mEq. per ampule of 50 ml. Since the figure 44.6 is inconvenient for our use, let us approximate and call it 50 mEq.; thus, 4 ampules would contain the required 200 mEq. (Approximation #3.)

At this time we must look at the patient. If she is a thin, frail female, then 3 ampules should be given; if normal size, 4 ampules; and if a large, heavy female, 5 ampules might be given. If the patient is a male, it must be assumed that the Dynamic Water is 25 liters; with a BE of −10, the total need for bicarbonate would be $25 \times 10 = 250$ mEq. =5 ampules. By looking at the patient, we can decide whether he should receive 4, 5 or 6 ampules.

The author is fully aware of the fact that this calculation is based on three approximations: 1) that the Dynamic Water is one third of the body weight, 2) that males weigh 75 kg. and females 60 kg., and 3) that an ampule contains ±50 mEq. of $NaHCO_3$. However, combined with a little common sense, the results are the same as those obtained by much more complicated methods, requiring slide rules, computers or a pad of paper and half an hour of hard work. The proposed use of "kitchen mathematics" will give the result in 2 seconds without any complicated machinery.

Another "rule of thumb" requires even less calculation: one ampule of $NaHCO_3$ (44.6 mEq.) will raise the BE approximately 2 mEq./liter in the average adult patient. However, the first calculation is superior because it can be used for Na^+, K^+ and other electrolytes.

Summary.—Metabolic acidosis can be measured by the base excess (BE), and must be treated in a dual way: 1) by $NaHCO_3$, which neutralizes the acids present, and 2) by removal of the cause of the acidosis, which is usually tissue hypoxia due to insufficient circulation.

4. Blood Hydrogen Ion Concentration

The *pH* of the blood has not even been mentioned in the previous discussion of respiratory and metabolic acidosis because it is a confusing and an often unimportant factor which might even be directly misleading if too much clinical importance is placed upon it.

The pH is a distracting negative logarithm of the hydrogen ion concentration of acids, respiratory and/or metabolic. One liter of neutral water contains approximately 1:10,000,000 Gm. of H^+ and the same number of OH^- ions:

$$H_2O \rightleftharpoons H^+ + OH^-$$

This small amount of H^+ can also be expressed as $1:10^7$ or 10^{-7} Gm. The logarithm of a figure is defined as the exponent that must be placed over the base figure of 10 to obtain the figure in question. Since $1:10,000,000 = 1:10^7 = 10^{-7}$, the logarithm of this figure is -7. In 1909, Sorensen, of Copenhagen, suggested that the hydrogen ion (H^+) concentration or tension could be called the pH and could be expressed as the negative logarithm of the concentration. Thus neutral water would have a pH of 7 (the negative of -7 is $+7$).

Carbon dioxide is produced continually by the metabolism of all living cells. The concentration will therefore increase inside the cells and CO_2 will diffuse out, into the plasma and into the erythrocytes, where carbonic anhydrase is present. This enzyme facilitates the reaction of CO_2 with water to form carbonic acid, which then dissociates to H^+ and bicarbonate ions:

$$CO_2 + H_2O \rightleftharpoons H_2CO_3 \rightleftharpoons H^+ + HCO_3^-$$

This is probably the most important chemical reaction in all the production, excretion and regulation of acids in the red cells, the kidneys and the acid-producing cells of the stomach. As the CO_2 increases, so does the H^+.

The pH of the blood can be calculated by means of the Henderson-

Hasselbalch equation, described in detail in Chapter 1:

$$pH = pK + \log \frac{HCO_3^-}{\text{dissolved } CO_2 + H_2CO_3}$$

This complicated equation is necessary for the calculation of pH but is not necessary for understanding the relationship between pH and CO_2. The pK is the negative logarithm of the equilibrium constant for several chemical reactions; in the case discussed here, for the reaction:

$$H_2CO_3 \rightleftharpoons H^+ + HCO_3^-, \text{ or to be more specific:}$$

$$K = \frac{H^+ \times HCO_3^-}{H_2CO_3}$$

This fraction, however does not change very much or very fast, so for the present discussion we can ignore it. The amount of dissolved CO_2 and H_2CO_3 is proportional to the P_{CO_2} (the pressure of the CO_2), and the sum of these two items can therefore be expressed as a function of P_{CO_2}:

$$\text{dissolved } CO_2 + H_2CO_3 = P_{CO_2} \times 0.0314.$$

A logarithm is difficult to understand, but when a figure increases, so does its logarithm, so for the present discussion, it can be ignored also. In this way, the Henderson-Hasselbalch equation can be simplified to

$$pH = \text{something} + \frac{HCO_3^-}{P_{CO_2} \times 0.03}$$

or

$$pH = \frac{HCO_3^-}{CO_2}$$

Now, an equation, or rather an approximation, is available which is much simpler and easier to understand. In underventilation, the CO_2 increases, the denominator increases, the divisor is a larger figure, and the value of the fraction decreases, yielding a lower pH. Vice versa, overventilation causes the CO_2 to be blown off, the CO_2 decreases, the divisor is a smaller figure, so the pH increases. This relationship is still somewhat complicated, but Siggaard-Andersen has made it much simpler by an ingenious arrangement of his nomogram (see Fig. 5-2). He plots the CO_2, which is a linear function, on a logarithmic scale (the ordinate in Figure 5-2), and the pH which is a logarithmic function on a linear scale (the abscissa). In this way, the relationship between CO_2 and pH will fall on a straight line.

It is neither necessary nor practical to remember too many figures,

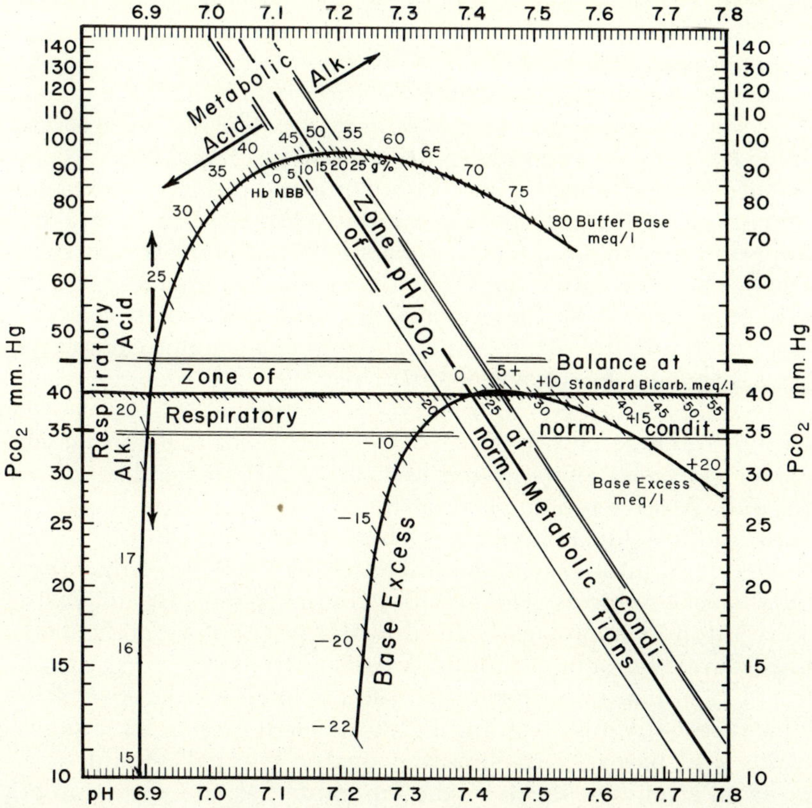

Fig. 5-2.—Siggaard-Andersen curve nomogram with two zones added. The zone of respiratory balance separates respiratory acidosis from alkalosis. The zone of metabolic balance (the slanted zone) separates metabolic acidosis from alkalosis. (Modified from drawing, courtesy of Radiometer, Copenhagen, Denmark.)

but three points on this line are easy to remember: the normal P_{CO_2} in arterial blood is 40 mm. Hg, which corresponds to a normal pH of 7.40. A Pa_{CO_2} of double the normal (i.e., 80 mm. Hg) would result in a pH of 7.20, and a Pa_{CO_2} of half normal (i.e., 20) would give a pH of 7.60. (Pa_{CO_2} of 80–40–20 mm. Hg would give a pH of 7.2–7.4–7.6). Therefore the slanted line, or rather zone around the line, is the area of expected CO_2/pH relations when all the metabolic compounds are normal; it could also be called the zone of normal metabolic conditions. If the patient is overventilated to a Pa_{CO_2} of 20, the pH should be 7.6. If the pH is anything other than 7.6, there must be *other* acid-base influences on the pH, i.e., metabolic acidosis/alkalosis. Any point to the left of this slanted zone (a lower pH) is indicative of metabolic acidosis, and any point to the right indicates metabolic alkalosis.

Summary.—The pH of the blood depends on the amount of CO_2 present (the respiratory acid-base condition) and on all the metabolic acid-bases present. The present author uses the pH only as an academic check on the reliability of the blood-gas laboratory.

"Compensated acidosis" is a confusing and dangerous expression, common during the postoperative period. Often a respiratory alkalosis is superimposed upon a metabolic acidosis and the pH may even be normal. This, however, does not mean that the metabolic acidosis has been removed or "compensated"; it simply means that an unimportant figure, the pH, has been forced back to a normal and meaningless number. For example, in a patient with diabetic acidosis, the pH can be returned to normal if the individual is hyperventilated with a respirator. However, this does not mean that the metabolic acidosis has been compensated and that the diabetes does not need treatment. Always remember that the patient is still in danger until the metabolic acidosis is treated. The acidosis is a warning of serious pathology and interferes with vital functions, such as cardiac rhythm.

Summary.—Acidosis can not be "compensated" by alkalosis but is very often "camouflaged" by the pH. Respiratory and metabolic acidosis are two separate entities and must be treated separately. The pH is *not* an indicator for treatment, since it is an expression of the balance between acids and bases and will be normal if an excess of acids and bases exists simultaneously. The pH should be used only as an academic check on the laboratory, as an expression of the combined effects of metabolic and respiratory conditions.

Pressure- and Volume-Depending Respirators

Respirators can be classified into two groups: *pressure* and *volume* depending [or "controlled"] respirators. A pressure-depending respirator blows the air (or any mixture of air, oxygen, other gases or vapors) into the patient until a predetermined pressure is attained; it then allows the air to escape. A volume-depending respirator blows a predetermined volume into the patient and then lets it escape. The pressure created depends both on the volume and the compliance. Although there are numerous technical differences between different machines, this is unimportant for the basic understanding. In the U.S.A. today, the respirators commonly used in the postoperative period are: pressure-depending respirators: Bennett and Bird; volume-depending respirators: Mörch, Emerson, Air-Shields, Engström and the two newly introduced, Bennett MA 1 and Ohio 560.

It is important to realize that pressure and volume cannot be separated. When the lungs are inflated to a certain pressure, a certain volume will be introduced into the lungs. A larger volume will enter when a higher pressure is applied, and vice versa. Conversely, when a certain volume is pushed into the lungs, a certain pressure is created. A larger volume will produce a higher pressure and vice versa.

Compliance.—The relationship between volume and pressure is called *compliance.* Compliance depends on a multitude of factors, the most important of which are the elasticity of the lungs, the chest and abdominal walls, the muscle tone and/or degree of relaxation of the smooth muscles of the bronchi and lungs, the striated muscles of the diaphragm and abdominal wall and the resistance to air flow in the respiratory tract.

Compliance can be defined as the "stretchability" of the lungs and chest wall, or the change in lung volume per unit change in airway pressure ($\Delta V/\Delta P$). In young individuals, the normal value is about 0.1 liter per cm. H_2O pressure, or the normal tidal volume of 0.5 liter is moved by a change in airway pressure of 5 cm. H_2O.

In the postoperative period the compliance may remain constant, improve or deteriorate. If a pressure-depending respirator were adjusted perfectly, it would create the ideal tidal volume; if a volume-depending respirator were adjusted ideally, it would create the same pressure, so there would be no difference as long as the compliance remained the same. But compliance does not remain the same, and most hospitals do not have enough highly trained people to observe these changes in compliance and to adjust the respirators accordingly. Thus, the various respirators perform much differently, as shown in Figure 5-3.

Compliance will improve or deteriorate. When *compliance improves* and the patient is on a *pressure-depending respirator,* the same pressure will cause a larger volume to enter the lungs during each stroke. This stretches and thereby traumatizes the lungs, stimulates the Hering-Breuer reflex to an unnecessary degree and increases the ventilation beyond the ideal. When the patient is on a *volume-depending respirator* and the compliance improves, the same volume will maintain the same ventilation but will create less pressure in the lungs, with less stretch and less trauma, which supports and accelerates the improvement.

When *compliance deteriorates* and the patient is on a *pressure-depending respirator,* the same pressure will blow a smaller amount of tidal air into the patient, with a decrease in ventilation and the danger of hypoxia. When the patient is on a *volume-depending respirator* and the compliance deteriorates, the volume will remain

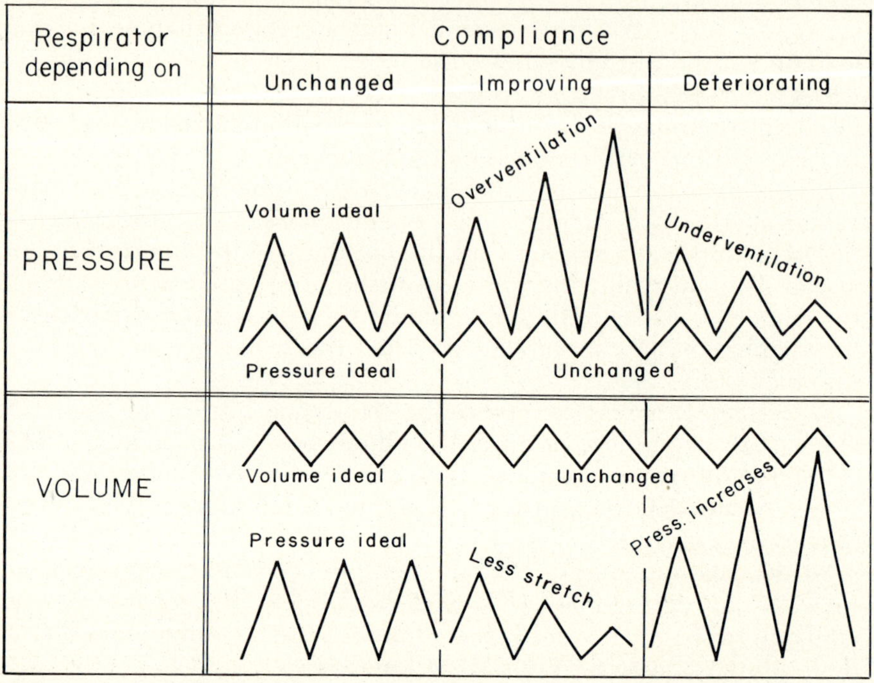

Fig. 5-3.—Compliance may stay unchanged, improve, or deteriorate. An unattended patient on a pressure-dependent respirator may develop a life-threatening asphyxia if compliance deteriorates, whereas a volume-dependent respirator would be much safer in a similar situation.

essentially the same. The only disadvantage would be an increase in intrapulmonary pressure. Thus, for long-term controlled respiration during the postoperative period under actual working conditions, which are ordinarily optimal, the volume-depending respirators are safer. The pressure-depending respirators are indicated during anesthesia, for brief periods in the postoperative period when the patient is not breathing satisfactorily, and for the repeated treatment of asthma and emphysema where humidity, bronchodilators, antibiotics and drugs can be used to dilute the bronchial secretions.

Summary.—Mechanical respirators can be divided into two classes: volume-depending and pressure-depending. The volume-depending respirators are safest for long-term use; the pressure-depending respirators are indicated for brief medical treatment of respiratory diseases, where the patient is still breathing adequately but needs some medication in the airways.

Cuff or No Cuff on Tracheostomy Tubes

Artificial respiration through a tracheostomy tube is usually administered with an airtight system using an inflatable cuff on the tube. An airtight system is necessary when a pressure-depending respirator is used, whereas most volume-depending respirators can be used with or without a leak.

The cuffed tracheostomy tube (see Fig. 5-4) has two advantages: 1) it is easy to measure the tidal volume and thereby the ventilation and 2) it is easy to keep the humidity high. However, the *disadvantages* are many and severe:

1) The cuff is unreliable, and the situation is critical and often fatal when it ruptures.

2) The cuff may slip down over the end of the tube and act as a one-way valve, so that air can enter the lungs but cannot escape. This situation is also likely to become fatal.

3) It is difficult to sterilize the cuff and to keep it sterile while attaching it to the tube.

4) The cuff is expensive.

5) The uneven surface of the cuffed tube makes insertion more difficult and painful.

Fig. 5-4.—Tracheostomy tube with cuff inflated creates an airtight system.

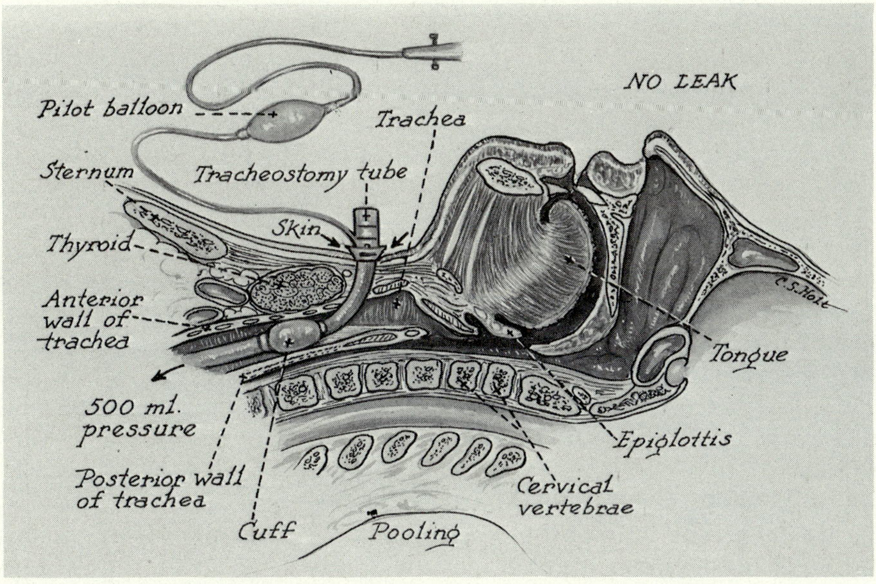

6) The pressure of the cuff upon the tracheal mucosa will always cause irritation and inflammation and may compromise the circulation in the mucosa enough to produce necrosis.

7) Tracheocele has been caused by the prolonged pressure.

8) Tracheal stenosis or septa have developed as the tracheal scars shrink, and represent extremely serious complications which may require surgical resection of the trachea.

9) Secretions, saliva, food and liquids can accumulate in the trachea and larynx above the cuff and create an ideal medium for bacteria, so that a foul and dangerous infection may result.

10) The patient cannot talk because no air passes the vocal cords. This is a very unpleasant and sometimes dangerous predicament for extremely sick patients.

Many advocates of the cuffed tube deflate the cuff for about 5 minutes every hour. This, however, is not enough to prevent damage to the mucosa, and the ventilation is likely to be insufficient while the cuff is deflated. If ventilation can be maintained at a sufficient level during this period, why can it not be maintained all the time with the cuff deflated? The inflated cuff is rarely if ever necessary, in the present author's experience. If the user insists on an inflated cuff, great care must be taken to prevent overinflation. The ideal would be a microscopic leak between the tracheal wall and the cuff, big enough to prevent pressure on the mucosa and small enough for sufficient ventilation. Some users have a cuff on the tube but do not inflate it; it is there only in the event of difficulties with ventilation. This might be justifiable for the first day or so, until one is satisfied with the patient's condition; subsequently an uncuffed tube can be used.

The uncuffed tracheostomy tube (see Fig. 5-5) for artificial respiration was first used by Trier Mörch at the University of Kansas Medical Center during a polio epidemic in 1951 and described by Trier Mörch, Saxton and Gish in 1956. At the outset, it seemed unreasonable that such an open, leaking system could be effective, but it has worked satisfactorily in the majority of patients. Compensation for leaks is the basic principle. If air under pressure has a choice between two routes with different resistance, most of the air will follow the route of least resistance, but some air will still escape through the other avenue. If, for example, the desired tidal volume is 500 ml. but the leak is so great that 1000 ml. escapes, then a total volume of 1500 ml. will satisfy the tidal volume and at the same time compensate for the leak. The ratio of the outer diameter of the tracheostomy tube to the inner diameter of the trachea is important and determines the

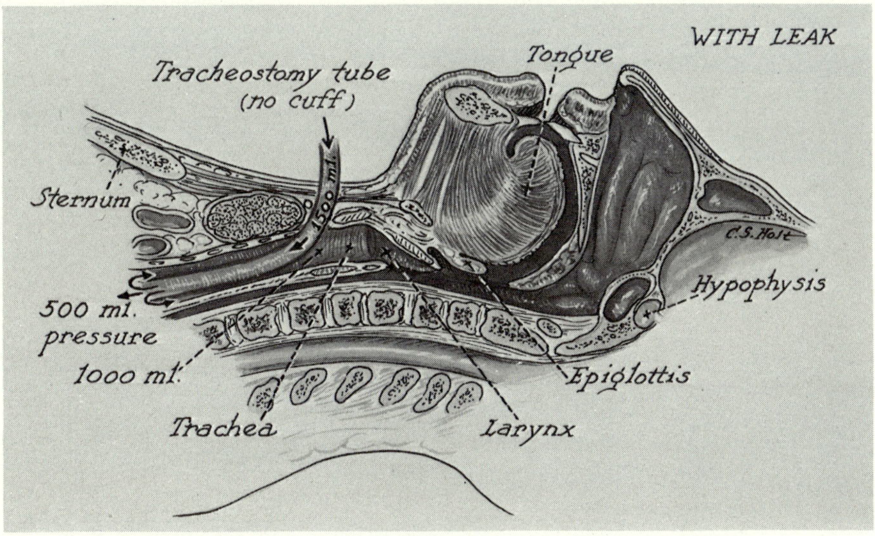

Fig. 5-5.—Uncuffed tracheostomy tube creates a leaking system.

leak. The system works best when the tracheostomy tube is relatively large; this reduces the leak and at the same time makes aspiration easier.

The *advantages and disadvantages* of the uncuffed tracheostomy tube are opposite to those of the cuffed tube. There are only two *disadvantages* to the uncuffed tube (and they correspond to the advantages of the cuffed tube):

1) It is difficult, if not impossible, to measure the tidal volume and thus the *ventilation.* The volume can be only estimated from the movements of the chest and abdomen and adjusted until these movements are slightly greater than for normal breathing. However, as a rule, the patients are overventilated to an unnecessary degree. Thus, the arterial CO_2 tension is the best for ventilation, maintaining this between 25 and 35 mm. Hg. This should be checked frequently, for it is surprising how fast a ventilatory equilibrium is reached, usually in 3–5 minutes. Very often the Pa_{CO_2} is found to be 20 mm. Hg or less. This can easily be raised by decreasing either the volume or the rate of ventilation or both.

2) *Humidification* of the inspired air must be kept high. Until recently, this was very difficult, and the large volume of air had a tendency to dry the secretions in the airways, and crust formations were often found on the tracheostomy tube. These crusts were especially troublesome and dangerous when present on the outside of the

outer tube where they could not be observed easily and early. In some cases, crusts broke off and caused partial or complete obstruction of the distal airways. In recent years, however, many highly efficient humidifiers have been developed, such as the heated nebulizers and the ultrasonic humidifiers, so that humidity no longer is a problem.

The ideal humidity varies from patient to patient and with climatic conditions. Most patients are comfortable and maintain liquid secretions when the inhaled air is approximately saturated with humidity at room temperature. Only rarely is it necessary to go higher. With the common use of blood-gas determinations and the modern, efficient humidifiers there are really no serious disadvantages to the use of uncuffed tracheostomy tubes. There are, however, several important *advantages:*

1) There is no cuff to rupture and occlude the airway.

2) Sterilization is easier.

3) It is less expensive.

4) The tube is easier to insert over the sensitive surfaces of a fresh tracheostomy and is less traumatic and painful.

5) There is no mechanical or chemical irritation of the tracheal mucosa from pressure, thus no danger of tracheal stenosis.

6) Liquids in the upper trachea, above the tip of the tracheostomy tube, be it secretions, saliva or food, will be blown up into the mouth or pharynx from where they can easily be removed or swallowed. (It is surprising to see how early the patient can learn to take food and liquids by mouth. The trick is to swallow during expiration. If swallowing is attempted during inspiration, while the machine is blowing, the leaking air may blow the food out of the mouth.)

7) The leaking air passes upward between the vocal cords and will thus enable the patient to talk, which is an enormous relief for the patient and makes nursing care easier and better. It is very frustrating for everybody involved to watch a patient with an inflated cuff frantically attempt to talk and to watch the nurse try to understand, and then finally, to see one or both parties give up in utter despair. Most patients will learn very fast that it is possible to talk only while the machine is blowing, but it may be necessary to explain this to the patient by . . . talking to him . . . while . . . the machine . . . is blowing only!

Summary.—Tracheostomy tubes can be used with or without a cuff. The airtight system created by an inflated cuff has two advantages, but many and serious disadvantages. In the acute phase, the cuff may cause damage to the tracheal mucosa, pressure necrosis, infection and perforation. Tracheal stenosis or septa caused by shrinking scar formation are not uncommon as a delayed complication. The leaking system without a cuff is far simpler, safer and more economical and has only two unimportant disadvantages.

BIBLIOGRAPHY

Avery, E. E., Mörch, E. T., and Benson, D. W.: Critically crushed chests. A new method of treatment with continuous mechanical hyperventilation to produce alkalotic apnea and internal stabilization, J. Thoracic Surg. 32:291–311, 1956.

Ayres, S.: Treatment of acute and chronic respiratory acidosis with a volume cycled respirator, Ann. Int. Med. 62:1096, 1965.

Bjork, V. O., and Engstron, C. G.: The treatment of ventilatory insufficiency by tracheotomy and artificial ventilation, J. Thoracic & Cardiovas. Surg. 34:228–241, 1957.

Block, A. J., and Ball, C. B.: Acute respiratory failure. Observations on the use of the Mörch piston respirator, Ann. Int. Med. 65:957–975, 1966.

Dobkin, A. B. (ed.): *Ventilators and Inhalation Therapy:* International Anesthesiology Clinics (Boston: Little, Brown & Company, 1966.)

Feldman, S. A. (ed.): *Tracheostomy and Artificial Ventilation in the Treatment of Respiratory Failure* (Baltimore: Williams & Wilkins, 1967.)

Heironimus, T. W.: *Mechanical Artificial Ventilation* (Springfield, Ill.: Charles C Thomas, Publisher, 1967.)

Mörch, E. T., Saxton, G. A., and Gish, G.: Artificial respiration via the uncuffed tracheostomy tube, J.A.M.A. 160:864–867, March 1956.

Mörch, E. T., and Saxton, G. A.: Tracheostomy tube connectors, Anesthesiology 17:366–367, 1956.

Mushin, W. W., Rendell-Baker, L., and Thompson, P. W.: *Automatic Ventilation of the Lung* (Oxford, England: Blackwell, 1969.)

Safar, P.: *Respiratory Therapy* (Philadelphia: F. A. Davis Company, 1965.)

Siggaard-Andersen, O.: *Acid-Base Status of the Blood* (Baltimore: Williams & Wilkins, 1964.)

Spencer, F. C., Benson, D. W., Liu, W. C., and Bahnson, H. T.: Use of a mechanical respirator in the management of respiratory insufficiency following trauma or operation for cardiac or pulmonary disease, J. Thoracic & Cardiovas. Surg. 38:758, 1959.

CHAPTER

6

Thoracic Trauma

BERNARD J. LEININGER, M.D.

THE MANAGEMENT OF PATIENTS who have sustained trauma to the thorax is one of the more challenging aspects of surgery. It does not require extraordinary ability, yet prompt decisions together with appropriate actions may spell the difference between death and survival. Perhaps it is this consideration that appeals to the surgeon's ego and makes it so rewarding to successfully care for these patients.

The giving of detailed instructions on management of thoracic trauma is somewhat akin to giving instruction on making love. No set formula will apply to every situation and a good deal of personal initiative is required. In short, the exigencies of thoracic trauma preclude a cookbook type of response; yet we will attempt to set forth general principles to serve as a guide for individual application.

Resuscitation

In these days of specialization, it is not unusual for a patient admitted to a medical center emergency ward to be surrounded by five or more surgical subspecialty groups. While there is no doubt that this may represent the ultimate in medical advancement, the well-being of the patient may suffer from the fragmented interests of the various disciplines. It is imperative, therefore, that one physician assume the responsibility for the over-all care of the patient. While other surgical subspecialists may be involved in more extensive procedures in caring for these patients, the thoracic surgeon, by virtue of his training, is usually best qualified for the supervision of the resuscitative measures. Successful resuscitation of a severely injured patient requires an awareness of the priority of the different organ systems.

The major responsibility is to sustain the O_2 exchange and blood transport systems, upon which all organs of the body are dependent. Effective ventilation is paramount to resuscitation. Once proper ventilation is established, the causes of circulatory failure can be dealt with.

Ventilation

It has long been the custom to have rather elaborate tracheostomy trays in the emergency suites. The establishment of an airway meant the performance of an emergency tracheostomy upon a struggling, often anoxic, patient in a poorly-lighted area, with the surgeon asking for equipment and assistance that were usually not available. A laryngoscope, endotracheal tube, and Ambu bag are the *sine qua non* in equipment of any area in which resuscitative measures may need to be carried out. In short, it is far more expeditious to insert an endotracheal tube and thereby establish effective ventilation in a matter of seconds. Small amounts of topical anesthesia instilled through the endotracheal tube will decrease the discomfort of such a tube in a conscious patient. Attention can then be directed to the next step of therapy. If a tracheostomy is needed, it can be carried out later with the endotracheal tube in place and usually under optimal operating-room conditions.

The next consideration is the integrity of the pleural cavities. Is there a tension pneumothorax that causes further embarrassment of ventilation with each inspiratory effort? The shifting of the trachea to the contralateral side or the rapid development of subcutaneous emphysema may suggest such a condition. The restriction of lung expansion secondary to a massive hemothorax is less likely to be the cause of acutely impaired ventilation. Auscultation of the lung is not passé; it can give much information simply and rapidly. In a respiratory emergency, it is both poor and timorous judgment to await confirmation of tension pneumothorax by a portable x-ray machine before treatment is begun. If a question arises concerning the integrity of the pleural cavities, it is far better to err by unnecessarily instituting closed drainage of one or both pleural spaces than by permitting impaired ventilation to go untreated.

Circulation

The next consideration in insuring proper tissue oxygenation is effective circulation. The causes for circulatory failure are multiple; however, the most likely and remedial cause in acute trauma is hypovolemia. An effective method for intravenous administration of fluids, drugs, blood and blood components is essential. A plastic catheter inserted through a peripheral vein and passed into the superior vena cava is ideal for both intravenous infusions and monitoring of the central venous pressure. In profound shock the peripheral veins are collapsed and even a cutdown on a peripheral vein may not work, due to intense venous spasm. Insertion of an intracatheter or a large-bore needle directly into the femoral vein by simply placing a finger over the femoral artery and directing the puncture medially will save valuable time and many frustrations.

Obviously, every attempt to correct hypotension should be promptly made. Insufficient coronary, renal, and cerebral perfusion associated with hypotension is poorly tolerated, especially in the aged and the severely injured patient. Hypotension following trauma generally has a definite cause, and that cause must be sought. To attribute decreased blood pressure to head trauma or neurogenic shock risks overlooking a remedial situation. In blunt trauma, the loss of blood into the pleural spaces, abdominal cavity, within organs and tissue spaces can be most subtle. The diagnostic pleural or peritoneal aspiration with a needle and syringe may expeditiously identify the presence of hemorrhage so that blood volume replacement may be promptly initiated.

The blood specimen for type and crossmatch (compatability testing) should be obtained at the time the intravenous infusion is established. The use of plasma expanders or albumin while awaiting blood typing and crossmatching is most acceptable. The administration of O negative unmatched blood is rarely needed and may lead to a complicated hematologic picture. The rapid infusion of one or more liters of sodium lactate solution or similar fluids is most effective in improving tissue and organ perfusion and in bringing the patient out of shock; however, if blood or colloid is not subsequently administered, the patient will revert into shock within a few hours. The continued, rapid loss of blood indicates a need for surgical intervention.

Circulatory failure may be aggravated by metabolic acidosis caused by a prolonged period of inadequate tissue perfusion. This can beget vasomotor collapse. The use of intravenous sodium bicarbonate will help to repair the base deficit and counteract the deleterious effects of metabolic acidosis on the myocardium. Finally, the pump mechanism itself may fail. Cardiac tamponade, myocardial contusions, and coronary artery lacerations are discussed elsewhere in this chapter.

Acute Cardiac Tamponade and Penetrating Heart Wounds

Penetrating trauma to the heart and acute cardiac tamponade will be discussed together. It is now more than 70 years since Rehn's historic cardiorrhaphy. Resuscitation from almost certain death of a patient with cardiac tamponade still remains one of the most dramatic and rewarding acts in surgery. Mechanical interference with the return of blood to the atria of the heart is lethal. When the pressure within the pericardium equals that of the vena cava and pulmonary veins, diastolic filling of the atria cannot occur, cardiac output falls and death ensues.

The exact sequence of events producing cardiac arrest is not clearly known. When cardiac output falls, compensatory tachycardia and peripheral vasoconstriction help initially to maintain blood pressure in spite of decreased tissue perfusion. An increase in intrapericardial pressure would, as a matter of simple physics, seem to exert its greatest effect on the low-pressure, thin-walled chambers such as the atria and veins. Almost complete circumferential attachment of the pericardium to the veins would seem to prevent collapse of these structures with distention of the pericardium. This is mentioned because it has been postulated that venous return at the entry to the right atrium is the point of obstruction.

Acute cardiac tamponade may adversely affect the myocardium in a number of ways. In addition to coronary blood flow being reduced by low cardiac output, mechanical interference may also be a factor. Furthermore, the endogenous release of increased amounts of catecholamines upon an acidotic, anoxic myocardium may prematurely induce cardiac arrest.

Cardiac tamponade must be suspected and given priority of treatment in all patients with penetrating trauma in the region of the heart. The concomitant findings of venous distention, paradoxical pulse and muffled heart sounds are diagnostic when they can be elicited. Distended neck veins associated with hypotension should strongly suggest cardiac tamponade. Muffled heart sounds and paradoxical pulse frequently cannot be assessed because of extreme restlessness, which in itself is perhaps the most diagnostic and yet misinterpreted sign. These patients are usually agitated and often combative unless cerebral perfusion is so low that coma has supervened. The concomitant odor of alcohol on the breath may give the false impression that the restlessness is due to an inebriated patient, whereas, in reality, a life-threatening situation is present. It has been observed that these patients are more comfortable in an upright, slightly forward position and will violently resist efforts to place them supine; however, we are unaware of a physiologic explanation for this phenomenon.

Dependence upon x-rays of the chest to diagnose cardiac tamponade is hazardous. The amount of blood in the pericardium required to produce tamponade depends upon the speed with which it forms. If the bleeding into the pericardium occurs rapidly, as little as 100 ml. can produce tamponade, whereas, as the pericardium has the ability to stretch tremendously, as much as 400–500 ml. of blood can accumulate over an 18–24-hour period without cardiac tamponade.

Cardiac tamponade may be present with a normal cardiac silhouette. An associated left hemothorax is perhaps the most frequent abnormality seen in the chest x-ray. Fluoroscopy will demonstrate decreased cardiac pulsations; while usually the patient's condition will not permit complete x-ray examination, the procedure is worth while in some diagnostic problems.

One of the simplest yet most informative parameters to monitor in cardiac tamponade is the central venous pressure (CVP.) Elevation above 15 cm. of H_2O or a rising CVP of a patient in shock with penetrating trauma in the region of the heart should be considered to be cardiac tamponade until proved otherwise—"proved otherwise" being a properly-performed negative pericardicentesis or pericardiotomy. Except for patients in extremis requiring immediate thoracotomy, such as for gunshot wounds of the heart, diagnostic and therapeutic pericardicentesis should be performed in all patients suspected of having cardiac tamponade.

Pericardicentesis can be performed by either the paraxyphoid or the left fourth intercostal space approach. We have favored the paraxyphoid because clots of blood will frequently form in the posterior pericardium, displacing the heart anteriorly and making the myocardium and coronary vessels more vulnerable to the intercostal approach. A short skin incision in the left paraxyphoid area will allow a large-gauge, short-beveled needle to make perceptible contact with the chondral arch. The needle is then slightly withdrawn and directed beneath the arch into the pericardium. Constant aspirating pressure on the barrel of the syringe will help to gauge the depth necessary for removing pericardial fluid. If the tip of the needle is pointed in the direction of the left ventricle, a definite thrust with each cardiac systole can usually be felt; however, if pointed toward the right ventricle or atria, cardiac impulse may not be perceptible. Frequently, too, cardiac action is weak due to a depressed and anoxic myocardium. Such hearts are extremely irritable and prone to go into ventricular fibrillation. The amount of preparation for performing pericardicentesis is wholly dependent upon the condition of the patient and the facilities, equipment and personnel available. A sterile ECG precordial lead attached to the aspirating needle will show a current of injury pattern (elevation of the S-T segment) when the tip of the needle touches the ventricle. This is helpful in averting intracardiac aspiration or injury to the myocardium and coronary vessels. The exigency of cardiac tamponade, however, would generally preclude such a sophisticated maneuver. When time permits, the patient's ECG should be constantly monitored, as the myocardium may be extremely irritable. Cardiac drugs and defibrillation equipment should be readied in anticipation of arrhythmias and ventricular fibrillation. Ideally, the procedure should be performed in the operating room.

The axiom that blood aspirated from the pericardial cavity has the fibrin removed and therefore will not clot is not completely true. Lacerations of the atria of the heart may allow the pericardial cavity to serve as a common chamber freely communicating with the atria. We have seen this occur in a case of blunt trauma causing a rupture of the right atrial appendage. Cardiac lacerations that bleed profusely, while decompressing through the pericardium into the mediastinum or pleural space, may yield pericardial blood that clots. Usually half of the blood removed from the pericardium at the time of surgery is clotted. Clots have a greater tendency to form around the atria and right ventricle, presumably because of less motion in those areas. One must be aware of the fact that because blood in the pericardium can clot, a negative pericardicentesis does not rule out cardiac tamponade. The quantity of blood aspirated in cardiac tamponade is inconstant, varying from 10 to 200 ml.; however, dramatic clinical improvement has been documented with removal of as little as 15 to 30 ml.

The ECG tracing for the most part is not very specific in the early diagnosis of penetrating trauma to the heart. It may be normal, show an injury pattern, or show changes compatible with pericarditis. Almost invariably a pattern of pericarditis develops after several days.

Differences in effects of gunshot and stab wounds.—Gunshot wounds usually produce a more extensive disruption of the wall and practically always result in two cardiac wounds. In stab wounds the sternum and ribs protect the heart somewhat, whereas a missile injury can penetrate any chamber and in any direction. Almost every bullet wound, particularly when there is no exit wound, raises the possibility of cardiac penetration. We recall a bullet that entered the right midthigh, traveled up the leg, across the abdominal cavity, and produced a through-and-through perforation of the left ventricle.

The larger holes in the pericardium produced by gunshot wounds favor decompression of the pericardial blood into the pleural space.

This is why left hemothorax is practically always associated with missile wounds of the heart and, by the same token, cardiac tamponade is much less likely to occur. These patients are more apt to succumb acutely from hemorrhage than from cardiac tamponade; as a result a large number do not reach the hospital alive.

Controversy has raged between proponents of routine and selective surgical exploration. In some centers, all cases of penetrating cardiac injuries are explored; others explore only those with signs of recurrent cardiac tamponade. It is fair to say that the number of proponents of the early exploration camp has grown considerably over the past 5 years. Certainly all cases of gunshot wounds of the heart should be operated upon as soon as possible. Pericardicentesis should be performed only as a therapeutic maneuver to relieve cardiac tamponade. There have been cases in which gunshot wounds of the heart have sealed off, only to have a blowout of the sealed hole occur 1 to 3 weeks later, resulting in sudden death. The disruption of myocardial fibers that occurs from a bullet injury is too great to expect healing of a wall subjected to contractions and internal pressures.

A stab wound of the heart, on the other hand, may seal, and there is no doubt that a number of these patients can be managed without surgery. However, there is too little risk at present attendant upon thoracotomy to allow the uncertainty of continued observation, particularly in a compromised situation. The burden of responsibility is on the surgeon who elects to follow these patients. As a consequence, they should be observed in intensive care units or an area of comparable surveillance where subtle changes can be assessed by competent personnel. The most reliable single parameter to monitor is a change in the CVP. The operating-room personnel should be alerted and a surgical team readily available. If observation by competent personnel cannot be assured, it is far better to proceed with thoracotomy.

The anesthesiologist and surgeon should be cognizant of the effects of positive-pressure breathing (PPB) on patients with cardiac tamponade. The increase in intrathoracic pressure from PPB may be sufficient to further compromise or abolish the venous-atrial gradient. Cardiac arrest may occur following institution of PPB and the necessity for immediate decompression, and resuscitation by pericardiotomy should be anticipated. Closed-chest cardiac massage is usually not effective in penetrating cardiac wounds.

Preparations for surgical repair of a wound of the heart must be expeditiously carried out. Details for this depend upon the condition of the patient, equipment and personnel available and the type of injury anticipated. Theoretically, a number of injuries could be best handled by cardiopulmonary bypass—e.g., disruption of either the aortic or mitral valve, large septal defects, aorto-cardiac fistulas and coronary artery injuries. Practically, few patients with these injuries reach the hospital alive, and those who do are sufficiently compensated as not to require immediate repair of the intracardiac defect. Most traumatic intracardiac defects that have been successfully repaired have been repaired on an elective basis. Cardiopulmonary bypass to aid in resuscitating a moribund patient should have increasing application in severe cardiac trauma. Surgical management of cardiac injuries should not be deferred or delayed while awaiting cardiopulmonary bypass; however, most injuries can be managed without it.

Hypovolemia.—This frequently is a major factor, particularly in gunshot wounds of the heart, and volume replacement is important. Even in cardiac tamponade when hypovolemia is not the primary problem we have found the rapid infusion of fluids and colloids salubrious. The infusion of fluids further increases venous pressure and thereby aids in cardiac filling.

Surgical exposure for penetrating cardiac trauma may be dependent upon equipment available, location of the injury and preference of the surgeon. In the majority of circumstances, an anterolateral approach through the left 5th or 4th interspace is, in our opinion, best. The pericardium is opened anterior to the phrenic nerve. Injuries to the posterior aspect of the left ventricle can be repaired by placing a laparotomy pad in the pericardium and elevating the apex of the heart for short periods. Added exposure can be gained by extending the incision transsternally, usually up one interspace into the right 4th or 3rd interspace, or by cutting with scissors the chondral portions of the cage along the left side of the sternum. If the injury is localized to the right atrium or vena cava, a right anterior 4th interspace incision can be used. If cardiopulmonary bypass together with instruments to split the sternum rapidly are readily available, a median sternotomy offers the advantage of good exposure for both repair and bypass.

Suturing.—Many technics for suturing cardiac wounds have been advocated. We have found direct pressure by use of a small wet sponge will control the hemorrhage and best stabilize the heart to allow placement of sutures with relative ease. Stab wounds inflicted with a penknife or icepick into the left ventricle will usually seal the bleeding from the cardiac chamber spontaneously by virtue of a thick, contracting myocardium. Bleeding may continue into the pericardium from the epicardium or coronary vasculature; superficial epicardial stitches are usually sufficient to stop the bleeding. Missile wounds, lacerations of the right ventricle and particularly wounds in a previously diseased myocardium are best repaired using mattress stitches with Teflon pledgets on double-armed sutures. These sutures are placed deep in the myocardium. A vascular clamp can frequently be placed over atrial lacerations and closure with a 000 or 0000 permanent suture leisurely accomplished.

Hemorrhage.—Bleeding from cardiac wounds may be so profuse as to obscure the bleeding site. Much has been written about the Sauerbruch's grip and inflow occlusion to gain control of the situation; however, usually about the time these maneuvers are considered, the heart conveniently arrests. Repair can then be carried out and hopefully the heart resuscitated. Fibrillation of the heart for 3 minutes is another way to gain control when equipment is available.

An attempt should be made to repair major coronary artery disruptions. Autogenous vein grafts may be necessary to replace destroyed segments in missile injuries, whereas a direct anastomosis may be feasible in a stab wound. Again, the majority of these patients will not survive to reach the hospital, and one is more likely to be confronted with a laceration to a distal branch. Hemorrhage from partial lacerations in the coronary vessels can frequently be stopped by direct pressure over the hole, accomplished by sewing an autogenous graft of muscle or fat over the vessel. This may obviate ligating a coronary vessel. Perforation into the underlying cardiac cavity can usually be managed by placing mattress sutures beneath the more superficial coronary vessel.

Penetrating cardiac injuries to the conduction bundle with heart block obviously require provisions for cardiac pacing.

Blunt Trauma of the Chest

Approximately 55,000 people in the United States are killed annually in automobile accidents. With the increase in population and automobiles it is reasonable to expect the yearly mortality to continue to increase in spite of recent interest in auto-safety legislation. Forty per cent of automobile fatalities are said to be associated with major thoracic injuries, of which the majority are a result of blunt trauma to the thorax. The diagnostic subtleties of these lesions are attested by the frequently encountered late sequelae. In the past, radiographic mediastinal widening was commonly ascribed to "venous bleeding." Arteriography has now identified many such to be major arterial disruptions. The surgical literature is replete with accounts of both aneurysms of the third portion of the aortic arch and strangulation of abdominal viscera through a diaphragmatic hernia months to years after patients had sustained blunt trauma. For clarity of presentation we will discuss the different types of injuries as single anatomic entities, whereas in reality we are frequently confronted with a combination of such injuries.

Thoracic Cage

The bony thorax is a semirigid structure housing the cardiopulmonary system, great vessels and esophagus. Respiration is dependent upon both an airtight chest wall and maintenance of the three-dimensional contour of the rib cage to permit negative pressure and the necessary lung volume within the chest. Osseous and cartilaginous components afford some protection to the heart and lungs. In the young, the rib cage is pliable, allowing an extreme degree of compression, whereas in the elderly, rib fractures occur from rela-

Fig. 6-1.—Chest x-ray of 51-year-old male, taken 3 hours after he had sustained blunt trauma to the chest in an automobile accident. Arrow in apex of left chest points to border of partially collapsed lung. Bilateral rib fractures, both anteriorly and posteriorly, resulted in a flail chest. Note area of pulmonary contusion in lower portion of left lung.

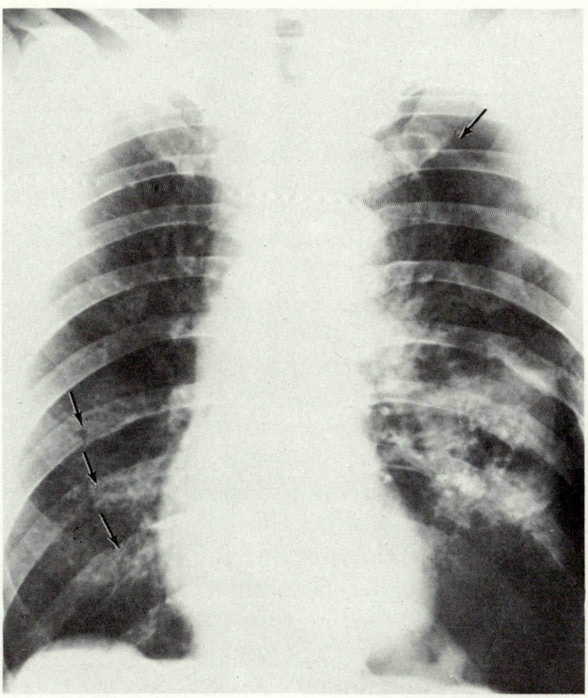

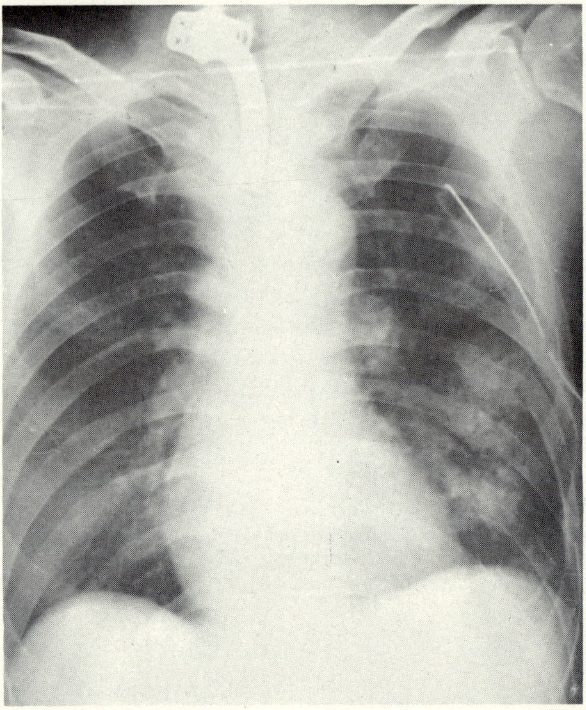

Fig. 6–2.—Same patient as Figure 6–1. X-ray taken 6 hours later, showing lung to be expanded and a cuffed tracheostomy tube in place. The large bore (number 28 F) chest tube, in addition to air, drained 900 ml. of bloody fluid. Mechanical ventilation was necessary for 9 days.

tively minor trauma. Major intrathoracic injuries such as ruptured bronchus, cardiac contusion and disruption of the thoracic aorta may occur, particularly in the young, without loss of the structural integrity of the rib cage.

FLAIL CHEST (See Figs. 6-1, 6-2, and 6-3).—By flail chest is meant the paradoxical respiratory movements of the rib cage caused by instability of one or more portions of the chest wall. The unstable portion of the chest wall moves inward on inspiration and outward on expiration. During inspiration the intrapleural negative pressure increases and the atmospheric pressure acts to push in the flail segment. During expiration the intrapleural pressure exceeds atmospheric pressure and the flail segment is pushed out. Hence the respiratory movements are said to be paradoxical or in a direction opposite to that of the involved segments.

Car accidents in which the body strikes the steering wheel or is hurled from the car commonly result in a flail chest. The immediate effects on ventilation may be well tolerated, as the work of tidal ventilation is minimal in a normal lung. The need for assisted ventilation in the immediate post-trauma period may not be apparent. A second physician evaluating the same patient a few hours later may be utterly amazed that mechanical ventilation was not instituted, for the patient may then be hypoxic, restless and exhibit a severe degree of paradoxical motion. The sequence of events of ineffective cough, pain, retained secretions and possibly contused or atelectatic lung soon causes an increase in the work of ventilation, reflected by a decrease in pulmonary compliance. Increased effort causes more paradoxical movements and a vicious cycle ensues. The harder the patient tries to breathe, the more ineffective is the ventilation. Associated injuries such as hemopneumothorax, hypovolemia and head trauma may contribute significantly to the ventilatory problems. While certainly not all patients with a flail chest require treatment with a mechanical ventilator, frequent assessment of the ventilatory status is mandatory

Fig. 6-3.—Same patient as Figures 6-1 and 6-2. X-rays taken 14 days later, showing multiple rib fractures more distinctly. The left lung parenchyma and pleural space show satisfactory clearing. Chest and tracheostomy tubes were removed. Patient was discharged 15 days after injury.

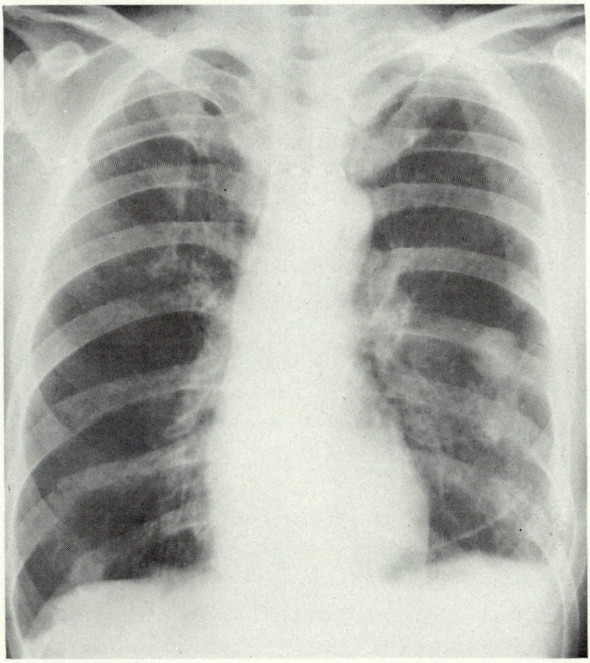

to avert insidious, progressive respiratory insufficiency leading to hypoxia and cardiac arrest.

Methods of management.—There is still considerable controversy over the treatment of flail chest. Historically, the first effort to stabilize the chest wall was by splinting the flail segment, usually with circumferential compression dressings or a sandbag. While these methods helped to prevent paradoxical movements from interfering with ventilation, both chest-wall deformity and compression of the underlying lung are the sequelae. External stabilization by use of skeletal traction is designed to maintain the structural integrity of the rib cage. Its main limitation is in the severely traumatized thorax.

There is no doubt that the mechanical ventilator has revolutionized the treatment of flail chest. It affords a means of overcoming decreased compliance of a traumatized lung and eliminates the work of ventilation. In spite of these advantages there are a number of at least theoretic disadvantages, most of which have to do with proper equipment, trained personnel and cost. The need for a tracheostomy, exposure of the tracheobronchial tree to contamination from ventilators and tracheal aspirators, and the driving of bronchial secretions down into the lung radicals are hazards that are real but for the most part can be successfully managed. Often the treatment is predicated upon the equipment, facilities and trained personnel available. Therefore, one should be familiar with the different methods of management.

Internal stabilization (ventilator).—One of the great advances in management of flail chest was the demonstration that chest-wall fractures could be internally splinted in quasi-inspiration by a ventilator. This allows restoration of the thoracic contour while at the same time taking over the work of ventilation. The original volume-controlled ventilators understandably had shortcomings and many complications were encountered. A high flow of air with a floating type tracheostomy tube allowing excess air to escape back into the oropharynx was used. Since the early ventilators did not have a humidifier, the irritation and drying effect of high-velocity air flow to the bronchial mucosa caused mucus plugs to form. Many of these patients died before the need for endoscopic aspirating and lavage to prevent obstruction of a major bronchus by a mucus plug was recognized.

Improvement in equipment and experience in its proper use have since accrued. Built-in humidifiers on the ventilators and use of a cuffed tracheostomy tube have reduced the irritation to the bronchial mucosa caused by excessive air flow. Space does not permit a detailed discussion of merits and disadvantages of all ventilators currently available, yet selection of proper equipment needed in a given situation is vital. Ventilators with sufficient volume and pressure to push the chest wall out and to overcome anticipated respiratory resistance must be used. We are frequently asked to see patients on whom treatment for flail chest has been initated with a ventilator that is pressure controlled, or the patient is having pain and respiratory distress because the ventilator is set on assisted ventilation. *Pressure-controlled ventilators* shut off when a preset airway pressure is reached. Changes in compliance and airway resistance would require almost constant monitoring of the pressure setting to insure adequate ventilation.

A *volume-controlled ventilator* maintains a constant volume regardless of airway pressure changes. Respirations should be controlled by automatic ventilation, thus eliminating the negative pressure required to initiate inspiration. Particularly when fractures of the rib cage are unstable, the inspiratory effort causes motion of the fractures, resulting in pain. Although the combination of restlessness, pain and altered sensorium may render control of respiration difficult, breathing against the ventilator should not be permitted. Once the airway is controlled and a means of taking over ventilation available, the necessary amounts of sedatives, narcotics, and even muscle relaxants can be given.

The objection to using narcotics with associated head injuries is valid; however, hypoxia superimposed on brain trauma is more deleterious than the effects of narcotics. Use of muscle relaxants presupposes attendance by qualified personnel until the muscle-paralyzing effect has worn off. Once the patient has been sedated and ventilation control effected, hyperventilation is helpful in depressing the respiratory center, thus enabling control to be maintained.

It has been said that hyperventilation producing a drop of the Pa_{CO_2} to 30 mm. Hg or below will produce apnea, thereby eliminating asynchronous respiration. This, unfortunately, we have not found to be true. These patients generally require sedation. Inhalation therapists should be available at all times to service and help regulate the ventilators. Any question as to the effectiveness of treatment should be answered by determination of blood-gas studies. Severe respiratory alkalosis should be avoided as well as hypoventilation. Inability to bring the blood-gas studies into normal range should initiate an investigation as to the cause.

Flail chest injuries are commonly accompanied with space problems such as hemothoraces, pneumothoraces and hemopneumothoraces. Positive-pressure ventilation can, of course, cause tension pneumothorax in a previously expanded lung. When pneumothorax is present in a patient receiving positive-pressure ventilation, the pleural space should be decompressed with a chest tube. This is no place for thoracentesis. Daily chest x-rays for the first few days after injury are needed to assess the pleural spaces and lung parenchyma. If bronchial obstruction is suggested by atelectasis, bronchoscopy can be performed through the tracheostomy stoma. Oxygen administered through the side arm of the bronchoscope increases alveolar Po_2, affording some increase in safety; nonetheless, endoscopy should be expeditiously carried out.

Supervision of tracheostomy care is extremely important. Particularly in areas where the nursing staff is unfamiliar with proper tracheostomy care, it is wise to write detailed instructions. Proper fitting of the cuff placed on a tracheostomy tube is mandatory. An inflated cuff that is too big may slip off or over the end, producing an airway obstruction. Rubber and plastic tracheostomy tubes with built-in dual cuffs for alternate inflation are now available. Single cuffs are deflated for several minutes of each hour to prevent ischemic changes in the tracheal wall. The oropharynx is aspirated prior to releasing the tracheostomy cuff to prevent the secretions in the oropharynx from being aspirated into the lungs. A separate soft-rubber catheter, using aseptic technic, is employed to aspirate the tracheobronchial tree. Care must be taken to ensure that the antiseptic solution in which the catheter has been stored is washed off with sterile saline solution before the catheter is inserted in the trachea; even a few drops of the antiseptic solution remaining on the catheter can initiate a chemical endobronchitis. Frequency of suctioning is gauged by the amount of secretions. Excessive suctioning traumatizes the bronchial mucosa and increases the incidence of infection. Cultures and sensitivity studies can be conveniently obtained by collecting the tracheal aspiration in a Luken tube. These studies should be repeated every 4 to 5 days. Antibiotic stable in solution instilled topically in the trachea is effective in reducing bronchorrhea.

The length of time necessary for a patient with a flail chest to be maintained on a ventilator is variable, depending upon such factors as cardiopulmonary reserve prior to injury, degree of lung damage associated with the trauma, severity of chest-wall deformity, infection, and other associated problems. The usual time on the ventilator is 8 to 14 days. When to wean the patient off the ventilator is a clinical decision. The patient is observed off the ventilator for increasing periods until he is able to breathe spontaneously. If there is a serious question of ventilatory adequacy, blood-gas determinations will help to resolve it.

External stabilization (skeletal traction).—A new modality of treatment does not *ipso facto* render obsolete methods that in the past have been proved effective. Extenuating circumstances such as inadequate equipment and/or personnel may make external safer than internal stabilization.

Multiple devices have been advocated for external stabilization of the chest wall. Many factors must be considered in the decision for skeletal traction; e.g., a single or multiple flail segment, weight of the flail segment versus the available tissue purchase for fixation of the chest wall, position of the patient and direction in which traction can be effected. For example, it is difficult to apply traction to a posterior or posterolateral flail segment. Then there are the extremes of a large-breasted obese female with impaired lung and chest-wall compliance that would require an enormous amount of traction as compared to a small child whose flail chest wall can be suspended by picking up the skin. Multiple flail segments may require traction in several directions.

Perhaps the fractures best suited for external stabilization are those of the bilateral anterior ribs, in which traction applied to the sternum will bring out the chest wall. Traction to the sternum can be applied by passing a heavy stainless-steel wire around the midportion of the sternum. A short transverse skin incision under local anesthesia will permit a malleable probe to be passed around the sternum, staying medial to the internal mammary vessels. A heavy silk suture is then passed back through the track and used to pull the wire around the sternum. If the wire is doubled back on itself, it will pass more easily. The skin is closed around the wires and collodion is used to seal the skin about the wires. The wire is then connected to overhead traction, using the pulley-and-weight system, the weights being adjusted to the optimum pull. Incorporating elastic in the traction system decreases the stress on the purchase area caused by movements. An appropriate Penrose drain used to attach the wire to the rope works very well.

Sundry external fixation devices have been advocated, from towel clips to Steinmann pins placed beneath the pectoralis muscles. Local infection at the purchase site extending into the pleural space must be avoided. The chondral portion of the ribs should not be used for a purchase site; cartilage is not strong and becomes chronically infected. If towel clips are used, they should be strategically placed in the center of pull of the flail segment. Small stab wounds are made through the skin to allow accurate placement of the towel clips through the center of the rib. Careful palpation will help prevent penetration into the pleura. In the majority of instances when a flail chest is sufficiently extensive to require external skeletal traction, a means for removing secretions and preventing atelectasis is necessary. This can be accomplished by frequent intratracheal aspirations or by tracheostomy.

External splinting.—The best example of external splinting is seen with paravertebral rib fractures, such as are frequently sustained in a fall from a height, in which the patient lands on his back, or in a direct blow to the posterior thorax. These patients may have rather extensive fractures and yet get along quite well while lying on their backs. The bed plus the scapula and posterior extracostal musculature provide a built-in splinting device. When the patient is turned or raised to a sitting position, severe paradoxical respirations may ensue. A good number of these patients having as many as 7 to 10 posterior paravertebral rib fractures will recover with only bed rest and supportive measures. If a ventilator is required, it often can be discontinued after a few days, as stabilization occurs early. The use of compression bandages or sandbags as definitive therapy should be restricted to very small flail segments not warranting skeletal traction or internal stabilization. External splinting can and should be used as a temporary method of stabilizing paradoxical movement in a respiratory emergency.

Combination of methods.—Treatment of flail chest can, on occasion, be enhanced by combining internal stabilization (ventilator) and external stabilization (skeletal traction). This is particularly true in large-chested individuals in whom excessive pressures and volumes of air are required to reduce the fractures. Skeletal traction can improve both immediate ventilation and long-term cosmetic and physiologic results by better restoration of thoracic contour. This is especially true in the severely deformed chest injuries. Furthermore, if the ventilators are not of the volume-control type or cannot develop sufficient pressures, external traction may be necessary.

Rib Fractures

Extensive rib fractures can occur without producing a flail segment. Altercations in which the individual is kicked or hit on the thorax with a club may produce multiple rib fractures. Penetration of the lung, mediastinal structures or abdominal viscera by the rib itself can occur. Fractures of the lower rib cage frequently are associated with lacerations of the spleen or liver. Management of penetrating rib injuries is basically the same as for impalement injuries with foreign objects. The rib must be extricated and the organ repaired or removed, as in the case of the spleen. However, in the majority of instances, displaced ribs will spring back.

Before the advent of ventilators, much was written about treatment of fractures of the sternum. Open reduction with internal fixation, external traction and wiring have all been advocated. The most common fracture of the sternum is a transverse fracture and that lends itself to any of the above modalities of therapy. An injury sufficient to produce a transverse fracture of the sternum will frequently cause associated injuries overshadowing the sternal fracture, e.g., myocardial contusion, disruption of the aorta, and associated rib fractures producing an anterior flail segment. In the latter case internal stabilization by use of a ventilator will usually effect satisfactory union of both the sternum and associated rib fractures. Open reduction with internal fixation by heavy wire sutures through the ends of the sternum in isolated cases may be indicated.

Diagnosis.—Rib fractures can usually best be diagnosed by physical examination. Pressure on any part of the rib will usually cause pain over the fracture, while x-rays of the chest often fail to demonstrate existing rib fractures. Immobilization is basic in the treatment of fractures. In fractures of the bony thorax it is impossible to effect immobilization, yet almost invariably a good union occurs.

Pain resulting from motion at the fracture site gives rise to ventilatory problems. Efforts to immobilize a simple rib fracture by taping are for the most part ineffective. The discomfort from the tape applied tightly to the skin may divert attention from the pain of the rib fracture and make the patient feel better. Elastic chest binders give satisfactory support and, more important, can be removed or put back on without discomfort.

Intercostal nerve block by regional anesthesia can be helpful to relieve thoracic pain. It may be necessary to repeat the block several times. If the patient can be seated with the shoulder girdles and head leaning forward, the ribs can usually be palpated posteriorly 3 to 4 fingerbreadths from the spinous processes. Intercostal block can also be carried out with the patient in the lateral decubitus position. A small-gauge (#22) needle $1\frac{1}{2}$ or 2 inches in length on a 5 ml. syringe filled with local anesthetic agent is used. The rib is palpated with the needle tip. Then the needle tip is danced off the inferior surface of the rib where several milliliters of anesthetic agent is injected, after first aspirating. It is important to go several ribs above and below the injured ribs. Intercostal block of the lower intercostal nerves can relieve upper abdominal guarding caused by rib pain, thereby allowing better evaluation of abdominal pathology.

Thoracic Viscera

Diagnosis of injuries to the thoracic viscera caused by blunt trauma is often most challenging. While penetrating trauma and disruption of the skeletal thorax are usually self-evident, serious injuries to the heart or great vessels caused by blunt trauma may be most subtle. Unless a high index of suspicion is maintained, early recognition of many injuries to the thoracic viscera will be missed. An intact rib cage may conceal serious internal injuries.

Heart

The anatomic position of the heart renders it vulnerable to blunt trauma. It is fixed at its base by strong pericardial ligaments. The tough pericardial sac holds the heart in a position between the vertebral column and the sternum. Closed-chest cardiac massage attests to the effectiveness of these two points of compression. Although the heart is relatively well protected by the ribs and lung from a lateral thrust, a blow to the sternum is somewhat akin to hitting a board more with a tomato attached to its undersurface.

There are three principal mechanisms of injury to the heart in blunt trauma: (1) compression of the heart between the sternum and the vertebral column; (2) contusion of the heart by a direct blow to the sternum; and (3) excessive intracardiac pressures produced by sudden compression of the abdominal or thoracic viscera. Compression of the heart between the sternum and vertebrae produces a shearing action that can result in rupture of the ventricles, septa, papillary muscles or chordae tendineae. It can also cause injuries to the coronary vessels and myocardium. The direct blow to the sternum is more likely to produce myocardial contusion; however, injuries to the coronary circulation and rupture of the ventricles, particularly the more vulnerable right ventricle, have occurred. Sudden compression of the abdominal or thoracic viscera producing excessive intravascular pressures may rupture the aortic valve, ventricles or atria.

The clinical evaluation of patients with cardiac trauma is made difficult by the frequency of associated injuries. The classic symptoms of myocardial injury, namely precordial pain, cyanosis, diaphoresis, restlessness, dyspnea and shock, are easily attributed to other thoracic injuries. Cardiac arrhythmias, increased cardiac widening, murmurs and pericardial friction rubs point more specifically to cardiac damage. All patients with blunt thoracic trauma should have serial electrocardiogram tracings and enzyme determinations. Disturbances in rhythm, abnormal P waves, changes in the QRS complex, abnormalities in the ST segment and T wave are all presumptive evidence of myocardial injury. Elevation of the SGOT and LDH levels is difficult to assess, as injury to other tissue and organs also may cause elevation.

Blunt cardiac trauma produces lesions ranging from mild myocardial contusions, the majority of which are not detected clinically, to severe disruptions of the myocardial wall that are rapidly fatal. In autopsies on patients sustaining blunt trauma and succumbing to causes other than cardiac, the hearts have shown varying degrees of damage, from subendocardial and epicardial hemorrhages to extensive infarctions. Sequelae of myocardial contusions are: rupture, formation of ventricular aneurysm, pulmonary or systemic embolization and constrictive pericarditis. The extent of injury and the recovery therefrom will depend a good deal upon the condition of the myocardium prior to injury. An ischemic, friable myocardium is more prone to rupture or to exhibit rhythm disturbances and cardiac failure in the post-trauma period.

Management of myocardial injuries secondary to blunt trauma can be divided into three categories, according to treatment: medical, immediate surgical, and delayed surgical. In general, surgery is best avoided, to allow healing of the myocardium unless the indications are absolute and urgent.

Medical management basically consists in the time-honored regimen for acute myocardial infarction. Bed rest for a minimum of 3–4 weeks should be enforced for those patients showing acute myocardial injury. Maintenance of good ventilation, sedation and analgesia, digitalis and diuretics in the presence of congestive heart failure, and serial electrocardiograms and enzyme determinations to evaluate the clinical course are all important in the care of these patients. Anticoagulants are not used, due to the danger of hemorrhage. Arrhythmias occur frequently and are controlled with the appropriate antiarrhythmic agents. Occasionally cardioversion or cardiac pacing will be needed to control rhythm disturbances.

The necessity for immediate surgical intervention in blunt cardiac trauma is relatively rare. The majority of patients with severe injuries involving myocardial rupture succumb before reaching the hospital. Occasionally patients will present with acute pericardial tamponade. If a second pericardicentesis is necessary, surgery is usually advised. Disruption of the aortic valve, chordae tendineae or papillary muscle, atrial or ventricular septum will usually show signs of congestive heart failure. This usually takes several days, weeks or months to develop. It is unusual for traumatic valve disruption to require immediate surgical correction.

Delayed surgical treatment consists in resection of symptomatic ventricular aneurysms, repair of traumatic septal defects, valvuloplasty or replacement of a disrupted mitral or aortic valve, and pericardiectomy for constrictive pericarditis. Indications for resection of ventricular aneurysm are congestive heart failure or embolus. The traumatic ventricular septal defects are usually in the muscular portion of the septum and may require a patch to close. Diagnosis of valvular disruption is suspected upon detection of a cardiac murmur not present prior to the trauma. Rupture of the mitral valve frequently produces a musical systolic murmur transmitted to the aortic root. Final diagnosis and functional assessment of traumatic valvular defects should be confirmed by cardiac catheterization studies. Unless congestive heart failure is progressive, open-heart repair is best delayed for several months, to allow maximum healing of the damaged myocardium.

Effusive pericarditis may develop weeks or months following myocardial injury. Differentiation of pericardial effusion, diffuse cardiac dilatation and aneurysm formation can be difficult. Chronic pericardial effusions rarely produce cardiac tamponade. The symptoms are usually precordial pain, fever and malaise. A friction rub may or may not be heard. Pericardicentesis is chiefly for purposes of diagnosis. The aspirate is submitted for bacterial, fungal and viral studies. If the disability is prolonged from recurrent bouts of pericarditis, pericardiectomy should be undertaken. Constrictive pericarditis has occurred following blunt trauma. If symptoms are produced, pericardiectomy is indicated.

Great Vessels

The thoracic aorta and its three major branches constitute the structures of importance in great-vessel injuries secondary to blunt trauma of the thorax. The pliability of the pulmonary artery and the major venous channels renders them much less susceptible to blunt trauma. The most common site of aortic rupture is at the obliterated ductus arteriosus just distal to the origin of the left subclavian artery. The time-honored explanation for disruption at that site in deceleration injuries is that when the forward motion of the body is stopped abruptly, the relatively unfixed descending thoracic aorta flails forward, tearing the aorta at the ductus arteriosus. While the explanation may be somewhat teleologic, in that all of the thoracic contents are relatively unfixed, and the descending thoracic aorta is somewhat fixed by at least the parietal pleura, the observation as to the site of injury is certainly correct. The junction of the heart and aorta is the next most frequent site of injury. Disruption of any of the three major vessels originating from the aortic arch is commonly associated with fractures of the anterior portions of the upper two ribs, manubrium or clavicle.

The exact extent of mortality from aortic disruptions is not known. Autopsy studies represent a selected group and suggest an immediate mortality rate of over 85 percent. Disruption of the aorta may be of any degree. The intima and media jointly have less tensile strength than the adventitia. The latter structure will frequently prevent fatal hemorrhage. Surprisingly enough, patients with complete separation of the ends of the aorta have survived and later repaired. A localized injury of one wall may result in a saccular aneurysm, whereas a circumferential tear is thought to produce a fusiform aneurysm. The blood clot forming about the laceration will push pleura and adjacent tissues together to form a false wall which can rupture at any time. Lung tissue and esophagus commonly form the wall of a false aneurysm. The propensity for saccular and dissecting aneurysms to originate just distal to the left subclavian artery raises the possibility of an etiologic relationship to a previous aortal injury. A history of thoracic trauma can frequently be elicited in these patients, although admittedly these correlations are difficult to establish. Late sequelae of these injuries are aneurysms, which in the older age group may be extremely difficult to distinguish from bronchogenic carcinoma. Left recurrent nerve paralysis can result from an aneurysm; however, it is rare as compared with the frequency of carcinoma invading nerve tissue. Fluoroscopy is not of help, as aneurysms usually pulsate less than neoplasm on the wall of the aorta. X-rays of the chest following blunt thoracic trauma should alert one to the possibility of aortic rupture. Progressive radiographic enlargement of the aortic knot points to impending rupture.

Symptoms in traumatic disruption of the third portion of the aortic arch depend in a large measure upon associated injuries. Back pain, restlessness, dyspnea and peripheral vasoconstriction with diaphoresis commonly occur in the immediate post-trauma period. The back pain is usually severe, constant and unassociated with movements of the thorax. Many of these patients are mildly hypertensive. Left hemothorax and a bruit heard over the left 2nd interspace anteriorly or the 6th rib posteriorly are other frequent findings. When aortic rupture is suspected by combinations of the above findings, angiography should be performed.

The method by which angiography is carried out will vary with institutions and equipment. It can be performed by injecting a large bolus of concentrated contrast media into the venous circulation or directly into the root of the aorta. We favor the latter, as better detail is usually attained. Reports of rupture of the aorta as a result of pressure injection have been surprisingly few. The left anterior oblique position displays the aortic arch to the best advantage.

Once the diagnosis is established, surgical repair is undertaken. Injuries to the third portion of the aortic arch are repaired with the aid of partial bypass. Femoral vein to femoral artery oxygenation perfusion is simple and works very well. Left atrial femoral bypass or shunting procedures can also be used to supply oxygenated blood to the kidneys and spinal cord. Arterial pressures of the superior extremity must be continuously monitored to balance the two circulations. Blood flow in the bypass technics is regulated by raising or lowering the operating table or with a partial occlusion clamp on the venous line. A posterolateral approach through the 4th or 5th interspace gives good exposure. Proximal and distal control is gained and bypass readied before the area of rupture is approached. A good deal depends upon the age of the disruption; if several months or years, the tissue will be fibrotic and will hold sutures well. Occasionally, an end-to-end anastomosis without a graft is possible. If the lesion is a few hours or days old, the tissue will be edematous and therefore difficult to suture. Woven prostheses are used to decrease the blood loss. As little dissection as possible should be carried out before going on bypass, to avoid excessive blood loss with heparinization. It is simplest to cut the aneurysm open and insert the prosthesis.

One of the hazards of left atrial femoral bypass is pulmonary congestion caused by obstruction of the pulmonary veins. This is discussed frequently in private conversations and very little in the literature. It can occur from collapse of the left atrium by excessive negative pressure or distention by obstruction of the mitral valve from the atrial cannula. In either event, blood backs up in the pulmonary veins, causing pulmonary congestion, edema and hemorrhage into the tracheobronchial tree. The patient then becomes anoxic both in the intraoperative and postoperative periods. If the patient survives this anoxia, excessive bleeding from the operative site practically always occurs. Careful monitoring of the venous cannula is mandatory.

Lacerations of the root of the aorta are frequently associated with at least functional disruption of the aortic valve. The murmur of aortic insufficiency in these patients often has a musical or rough quality and may be heard better to the right than the left of the sternum. If cardiac tamponade occurs, death is imminent. Survival correlates well with the time interval between injury and surgical repair. Cardiopulmonary bypass with coronary perfusion using a median sternotomy incision is the ideal approach to these injuries. The aorta can then be opened and both walls inspected. There have been cases in which the aorta subsequently ruptured on the wall opposite that on which a laceration was repaired. Assessment with possible replacement of the aortic valve can also be accomplished. Weighed against this is the time required to assemble cardiopulmonary bypass with coronary perfusion. The old nautical axiom of "any port in a storm" is apropos. Certainly decompression of the cardiac tamponade with an attempt to control hemorrhage is preferable to deterioration of the patient awaiting cardiopulmonary bypass.

Laceration of one or more of the three major vessels arising from the aortic arch commonly exhibits a somewhat characteristic clinical picture. There are usually associated fractures of the overlying rib. The hematoma dissects upward, producing a cervical mass within several hours of injury. Obliteration or weakening of a carotid or axillary pulse also occurs. Armed with these signs exploration is indicated. A median sternotomy gives excellent exposure. If circulation to either of the carotid arteries is interrupted for more than several minutes, a bypass shunt should be used.

Trachea

The paucity of recorded cases of successful tracheal repairs incident to trauma suggests that such injuries are rapidly fatal. Egress of mediastinal air into both pleural spaces producing collapse of both lungs or obstruction of the airway requires immediate treatment if the patient is to survive.

The mechanisms of tracheal injuries in blunt trauma are not entirely clear. It has been postulated that severe compression of the chest against a closed glottis can cause disruption, but direct compression of the trachea between the anterior chest wall and the vertebral column is a more likely mechanism. A direct blow to a neck in extreme hyperextension can cause separation of the trachea. Inability to palpate the cervical trachea is diagnostic in such injuries. Massive mediastinal and subcutaneous emphysema that develops rapidly after trauma suggests tracheal or major bronchial laceration. The diagnosis can be confirmed by endoscopy.

The emergency management of tracheal lacerations requires decompression of the pleural spaces but airway maintenance is even more critical. Endotracheal intubation or tracheostomy is frequently life saving. If the laceration is high in the trachea, a cuffed endotracheal tube passed beyond the laceration will control the situation very nicely. The trachea can usually be mobilized sufficiently to allow resection of 3 to 5 cm. of trachea for an end-to-end anastomosis. This is preferable to a lateral repair that compromises the tracheal lumen. Except for the high laceration that can be repaired in the neck, a posterolateral right thoracotomy through the 4th interspace gives the best exposure. A tracheostomy should be performed to facilitate removal of secretions and prevent high endotracheal pressures. The same religious attention to tracheobronchial toilet postoperatively, again, is most important.

Bronchus

(See Figs. 6–4, 6–5, 6–6, and 6–7).

The magnitude of an injury such as a ruptured bronchus would seem to defy nondetection; yet, surprisingly enough, a number of

Fig. 6–4.—Chest x-ray showing opacification of right hemithorax in a 20-year-old male, 7 weeks after blunt thoracic trauma. The heart is shifted to the right, suggestive of atelectasis; however, the trachea is pushed to the left. Subsequent pictures demonstrate the combination of an aneurysm of the right subclavian artery and a rupture of the right mainstem bronchus. Same patient's x-rays shown in following three illustrations.

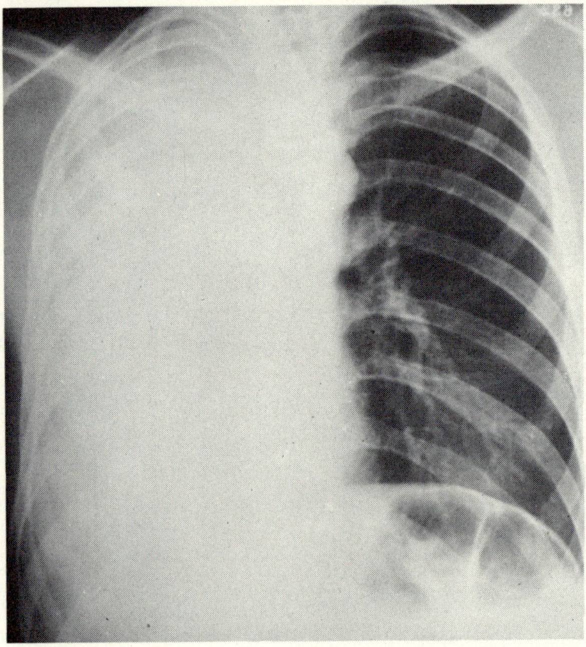

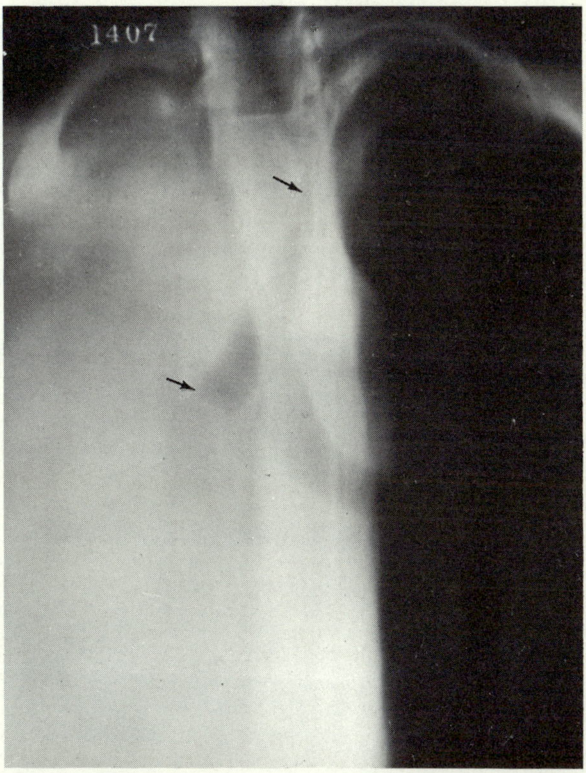

Fig. 6-5.—This laminagraphic view better demonstrates the deviation of the trachea to the left, with compression of the right lateral tracheal wall. The second (lower) arrow shows the sharp cutoff of the fractured right mainstem bronchus.

these injuries are diagnosed and repaired months to years after injury. The majority, however, require prompt treatment for survival. The classic sequence of events is: early mediastinal and subcutaneous emphysema (frequently massive), pneumohemothorax, hemoptysis and the subsequent development of atelectasis.

Almost any type of severe thoracic trauma can produce this injury. Compression of the anterior chest against the vertebral column can rupture the left main stem bronchus by a shearing action. This is seen more frequently in children because of the greater pliability of their rib cage. If disruption of the bronchus is suspected, it should be confirmed by bronchoscopy. Tracheostomy or insertion of an endotracheal tube will prevent the endotracheal pressure from rising significantly above the atmospheric, thereby decreasing the extravasation of air into the mediastinum. Positive-pressure ventilation will increase the extravasation of air, so that adequate decompression of the pleural space or spaces with chest tubes is mandatory.

The definitive treatment is surgical repair. If the pleural spaces are adequately decompressed, time necessary for stabilization of the patient's physiologic parameters can be gained. The decision to perform plastic repair of the damaged bronchus or to sacrifice lung tissue distal to the bronchial injury is dependent upon the individual situation; i.e., associated injuries, degree of trauma to the bronchial tissue and distal lung, infection, site of the injury and condition of the patient. Patients operated upon within the first 24 hours after injury usually have satisfactory bronchial tissue to repair, whereas, 48 or 72 hours after injury, there is a good deal of edema and friability of the lacerated bronchus.

Late repairs (several months to years after injury) are frequently quite easy to make, as the tissue is fibrotic and holds sutures well. Even portions of the lung atelectatic for years will usually expand and function satisfactorily. In most instances of bronchial laceration, lung tissue can be preserved by bronchoplastic procedures. It is well

Fig. 6-6.—Root aortogram demonstrates an aneurysm of the right subclavian artery with faint visualization of the right axillary artery.

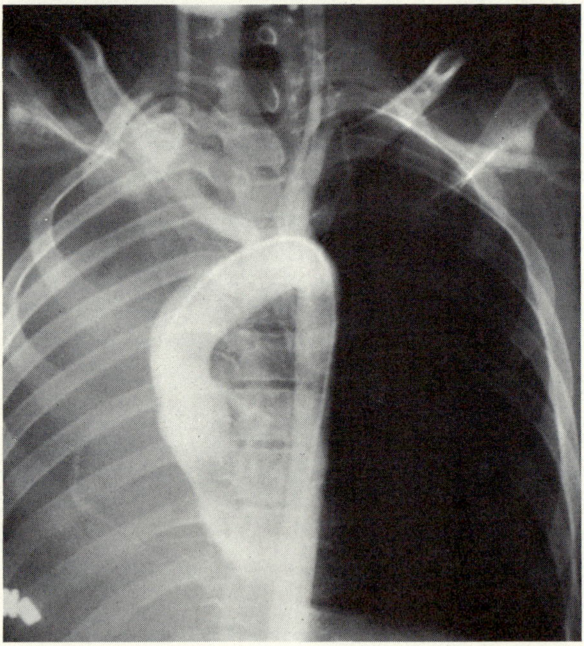

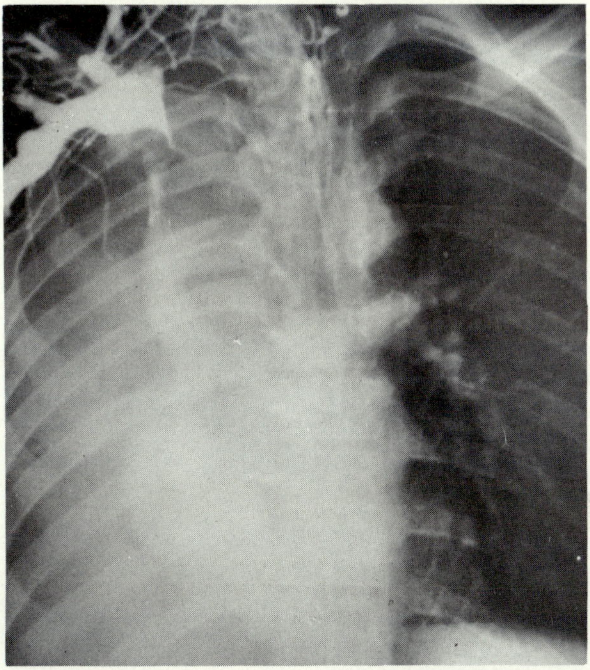

Fig. 6-7.—Venogram shows obstruction of right subclavian vein, a very narrow right brachiocephalic vein, and the superior vena cava displaced to the right.

to use pleura or pericardium to cover the suture line. We also favor the use of synthetic sutures for bronchoplastic procedures.

Postoperative attention to bronchial toilet is very important. It has been demonstrated that a concentric bronchial suture line will act as a partial barrier to the egress of mucus from the distal bronchus. Ciliary action at the suture line is temporarily paralyzed. Bronchoscopy is usually necessary to facilitate the removal of secretions beyond the anastomosis. A word of caution is advised to the endoscopist: *It is not necessary or wise to pass the bronchoscope across the suture line, but rather to position it just proximally and pass a soft rubber catheter attached to the end of a metal aspirating cannula across the suture line.* Disruption of the suture line has occurred as a result of overvigorous endoscopic maneuvers.

Chylothorax

Chylothorax occurs rarely in thoracic trauma, and underlying pathology or congenital malformation should be suspected. We have treated one patient with bilateral chylothorax and chylopericardium secondary to blunt trauma. This patient underwent a left thoracotomy for a suspected rupture of the aorta, at which time the thoracic duct was ligated and no underlying pathology was evident.

Hyperextension of the spine is reputed to be one of the mechanisms of injury. Compression of the abdomen or thorax is another. Fractures of the left clavicle and/or the left first and second ribs anteriorly are more likely to be associated with a left chylothorax. Compression injuries without fractures are more apt to cause right chylothorax. The fluid aspirated from the pleural space in traumatic chylothorax is usually blood tinged; however, if a sample of the aspirate is placed in a test tube and allowed to stand, the typical layering out of chylous fluid will occur. Lipid content should also be determined.

Management of traumatic chylothorax may be predicated upon associated injuries. If thoracotomy is necessary for other reasons, the thoracic duct should be ligated at that time. Chylothorax of itself can be treated first by thoracentesis. If there is prompt recurrence, tube drainage with high suction may be effective in sealing off the leaks by keeping the lung expanded. A low-fat diet will help to decrease chyle formation. In the event of continued drainage of large amounts of chyle, the patient will become nutritionally depleted and ligation of the thoracic duct is indicated. Several suture ligatures should be used to ligate the thoracic duct a short distance above the diaphragm. The thoracic duct, which lies on the anterior surface of the vertebral column behind the intercostal arteries, usually has more than one channel. The operative approach can be made through either side of the chest; usually the side of the effusion is selected. Attempts to identify the site of the leaks are for the most part unrewarding. Serum albumin deficits must be preoperatively and postoperatively replaced.

Lungs

Little has been written about pulmonary contusion, yet it is one of the most frequent injuries sustained in blunt thoracic trauma. Pulmonary contusion can occur with or without disruption of the bony thorax; in fact, some of the most severe forms of contusion have been in the absence of rib fractures. This is particularly true in younger patients with pliable rib cages where direct compression of the lung parenchyma frequently occurs. Accelerating or decelerating injuries can cause the lung, containing a relatively large volume of blood, to impact sharply against the rigid chest wall. Rib fractures can produce penetrating or impalement-type injuries to the lung.

Pulmonary contusion results in disruption of the alveoli, bronchioles and blood vessels. An intraparenchymal hematoma may form, or the blood and air may escape into the pleural space, causing a hemopneumothorax. The amount of lung damaged varies from a single small area to diffuse involvement of both lungs. The degree of lung injury is frequently not apparent immediately after injury. X-rays of the chest may show the lung parenchyma to be relatively clear for the first 24 hours and later show patchy infiltration to almost complete consolidation. Clinical signs and symptoms are similarly insidious and progressive. Tachypnea, rales, wet cough and hemoptysis may be followed by dyspnea and cyanosis. For these reasons patients with blunt thoracic trauma should be followed for the first 3 or 4 days with daily chest x-rays and frequent clinical evaluations.

The treatment of pulmonary contusions embodies the same basic principles as thoracic postoperative care:

1. Expansion of the lungs
2. Maintenance of a clear airway
3. Replacement of blood and fluid losses

Prompt expansion of the lung by evacuation of air and blood is best accomplished by closed-catheter drainage of the pleural space. Again, more than one chest tube may be required. Chest tubes are left in place 24 to 48 hours longer than usual, as there is a certain amount of continued seepage from the disrupted lung surface.

Tracheostomy should not be routine. Frequent intratracheal aspirations can clear the major airways and preserve an effective cough mechanism; however, if the patient does not have an effective cough, due to pain, cerebral trauma, or general weakness, a tracheostomy is indicated. Bleeding into the lung can cause an anemia out of proportion to the amount of hemorrhage, in trauma as well as in some pathologic entities of the lung. A slight rise in serum bilirubin is also frequently observed. These patients may expectorate varying amounts of blood, mucus and exudate. Smear, cultures and sensitivity studies of the sputum are important for appropriate antibiotic coverage. Intermittent positive-pressure breathing treatments, ultrasonic nebulization or heated aerosol, expectorants, and postural drainage are other adjuvants. A hematoma of the lung will frequently excavate to cavity formation. Air fluid levels are seen on chest x-ray. Febrile episodes associated with productive sputa and/or hemoptysis can recur many weeks after injury. These patients should be continued on antibiotics and expectorants until the febrile episodes subside.

The important point to remember is that thoracotomy is seldom necessary in the treatment of blunt trauma to the lung. Lungs severely damaged, with marked clouding radiographically, will clear rather dramatically if blood and fluid are effectively evacuated and the lung expanded. Organizing hemothorax occurs less frequently in blunt trauma than in penetrating trauma. Pneumatoceles and cavity formations secondary to pulmonary contusions and hematomas will practically always heal if given sufficient time.

Wet-lung syndrome.—Insight into our current understanding, or more properly lack of understanding, of the wet-lung syndrome can be gained by considering the multiple and rather diverse etiologies that have been reported. The following is a partial list of causes: pulmonary emboli, septic emboli, fat emboli, hypovolemic shock, septic shock, overtransfusion, overhydration, blast injuries, parenchymal destruction from high-velocity damage, trauma to the extremities, lung contusion, pre-existing respiratory infection, aspiration pneumonitis, pain, head injuries, coma, suppression of the cough reflex, inadequate bronchial toilet, excessive sedation, anesthesia, bronchial obstruction and respirator treatment with high concentrations of oxygen. Suffice it to say, it is difficult to propose a common denominator to all. The syndrome probably represents a type of pulmonary response to a wide variety of complications. For the most part, a diagnosis of wet-lung syndrome per se seems to be an admission of the lack of understanding the patient's pathophysiology. A more specific diagnosis will help to zero in on the proper therapy. The fact that it is now rarely diagnosed in civilian practice and rather frequently encountered in war casualties suggests that the severity of injury and perhaps delays in receiving tracheobronchial toilet are major contributing factors.

There is no uniform picture of the wet-lung syndrome. It may develop slowly over several days or be fullblown immediately after injury. The chief clinical manifestations are outpouring of fluid and mucus into the tracheobronchial tree, tachypnea, cyanosis and tachycardia. Usually there is an associated compromise in the ability of the patient to clear the secretions. Auscultation of the chest reveals basilar rales. Blood-gas studies show a fall in the P_{O_2} to less than 90 mm. Hg, a lowered P_{CO_2}, and an Sa_{O_2} below 90%. It has been proposed that the hypoxia causes increased capillary permeability, allowing more fluid to escape into the alveoli and interstitial tissue. Thus the stage is set for a rapidly deteriorating sequence of events. Gross anatomic findings at autopsy show the lungs to be heavy and hypervoluminous, often causing depression of the corresponding hemidiaphragm. The tracheobronchial tree is filled with bloody, tenacious fluid. Microscopically, the alveolar spaces are congested and contain hyaline membranes indistinguishable from those seen in hyaline membrane disease of the newborn. Examination of some of these lungs indicates a loss of surfactant.

Treatment of the wet-lung syndrome consists in both an immediate and a continuing means for removing secretions from the tracheobronchial tree. This can be accomplished by bronchoscopy and intratracheal suctioning in the milder cases; however, tracheostomy is usually necessary. Antibiotics in high dosages, their choice determined by sensitivity studies, are necessary to combat the inevitable pneumonitis developing secondary to the obstructed bronchi. Positive-pressure ventilation helps by decreasing the amount of fluid passing from the capillaries into the alveolar spaces, increasing oxygenation by expanding atelectatic areas of the lung, and diminishing the work of respiration. While the mechanical ventilator is extremely helpful, several facets of its use should be recognized. High concentrations of O_2 administered through a positive-pressure ventilator for a prolonged period will cause deleterious changes in the alveolar membrane. This results in pulmonary insufficiency and inability to wean the patient from the ventilator. Progression of the wet-lung syndrome is marked by a falling Po_2 and decreased pulmonary compliance, requiring higher pressures for ventilation. This is why volume-controlled ventilators are preferred over the pressure-controlled type.

The development of increased resistance to ventilation in the past has been referred to as the "stiff lung." In addition to the above measures, treatment must be directed according to clinical observations, e.g., heparinization in suspected cases of fat embolization, digitalization in patients with an elevated central venous pressure, and phlebotomy for overtransfusions.

Traumatic asphyxia.—Many appellations have been used to describe the curious discoloration of the face, shoulders, and upper extremities that result from acute and sustained compression of the thorax or abdomen. Cyanotic cape, ecchymotic mask, cervicofacial static cyanosis, and pressure stasis are all equally descriptive terms, but traumatic asphyxia seems to enjoy the greatest use. It is caused by sustained compression injuries, e.g., an individual pinned beneath a heavy object. The discoloration of the skin varies from reddish-purple to black. The eyes are always bulging, with conjunctival congestion and subconjunctival hemorrhage. There is usually a sharp line of demarcation on the upper chest above the line of compression.

While the patient's appearance may be somewhat frightening, an awareness of the pathophysiology is reassuring. The superior vena cava and its tributaries are essentially valveless, so that pressure upon the right atrium and superior vena cava is transmitted directly to the smaller veins and capillaries. This produces first distention and then atony of the capillary walls, with stasis of blood in these vessels accounting for the discoloration. Extravasation of erythrocytes may occur, resulting in petechiae and ecchymoses. External counterpressure, such as by a hatband, protects the vessels from overdistention and these areas are spared discoloration. Cerebral edema together with temporary hypoxia occurring at the time of injury can cause coma and other manifestations of cortical irritation such as restlessness, disorientation or convulsions. Visual disturbances, usually transitory, are quite common.

Treatment is neither helpful nor necessary for the skin discoloration. Efforts should be directed to the associated injuries such as cerebral edema or flail chest. If the patient survives the initial injury, the prognosis is quite good.

The Diaphragm

The clinical entity of diaphragmatic rupture secondary to blunt trauma has been well recognized and the treatment adequately outlined in the surgical literature for a number of years. In spite of this, the diagnosis is all too frequently missed, judging from the number of diaphragmatic ruptures recognized months to years following the causative trauma.

A blow to the chest or abdomen from a blunt object such as a steering wheel can rupture the diaphragm. Over 95 percent of diaphragmatic ruptures secondary to blunt trauma occur on the left side. Most of our experiences and hence suggestions are slanted to left diaphragmatic injuries. The liver gives added protection the right hemidiaphragm.

The tendinous portion of the diaphragm is the most vulnerable area. Tears from that area may extend laterally along the costal insertions or medially into the esophageal hiatus. Size and completeness of the diaphragmatic rupture relate to the severity and onset of symptoms. Incomplete disruptions may contain the abdominal viscera in its domicile for days or even months. As the diaphragm weakens, the pressure gradient between the abdominal and thoracic cavities pushes the viscera of the former into the chest. In normal respiration, intra-abdominal pressures range from +2 to +8 mm. Hg and in the thorax from −2 to −6 mm. Hg; however, with labored respiration, cough, or Valsalva's maneuver, the gradient is magnified at least 10 to 20 times. Also, small diaphragmatic lacerations are sometimes effectively plugged for a time with omentum or abdominal viscera.

Whereas the small or incomplete diaphragmatic disruption may be asymptomatic, the large and complete laceration can represent a real surgical emergency. Aside from the strangulation or obstruction of the hollow viscus as a result of volvulus or thrombosis of its vascular pedicle, a real respiratory emergency can result from progressive compression of the lung and mediastinal structures by the abdominal viscera. The harder the patient breathes, the more the abdominal contents are sucked up into the chest. This vicious cycle can result in hypoxia and ultimate cardiac arrest.

For prompt diagnosis, a high index of suspicion for diaphragmatic injuries must be maintained in all cases of blunt trauma. Although the chest x-ray may be completely normal, it more often will suggest the diagnosis. Plain films of the chest, usually ordered for other purposes, may show the following: a high diaphragm, pleural effusion, partial opacification of the hemithorax, gas bubbles above the diaphragm, air fluid levels within the chest, or shifting of the mediastinum to the opposite side. Radiographic examinations that can be performed specifically to demonstrate a rupture of the diaphragm are: water-soluble contrast material given by mouth or through a nasogastric tube, positional x-rays of the chest, especially with the head down and pressure on the abdomen, a contrast study of the colon, pneumoperitoneum and fluoroscopy. The latter examination will show shifting of the mediastinum, particularly with labored respiration.

Clinical findings such as shoulder pain, dyspnea, decreased breath sounds in the area of compressed lung, tympany on percussion over the hollow viscus displaced in the thorax and findings of intestinal obstruction may be suggestive but rarely are in themselves diagnostic. Injection of air and water through a nasogastric tube while simultaneously auscultating the chest can be a helpful diagnostic maneuver. The most specific physical finding, in our experience, has been the paradoxical respiratory movements of the upper abdomen on the side of the rupture. With diaphragmatic breathing, the abdomen protrudes during inspiration and relaxes on expiration. If the diaphragm is disrupted, the abdomen paradoxically sucks in on the involved side during inspiration. This can be easily demonstrated by placing a ruler across the upper abdomen.

One should always consider the possibility of diaphragmatic rupture in blunt trauma before performing thoracentesis. Aspiration of bowel contents by thoracentesis is certainly not the accepted way to make the diagnosis of diaphragmatic hernia. Therapy for diaphragmatic hernias includes reduction of the abdominal viscera, expansion of the lung, and repair of the diaphragmatic defect.

Several categories of clinical situations must be recognized in outlining therapy. First is the acute surgical emergency occurring minutes to hours after injury. A large defect of the diaphragm creates a wide-open pleuroperitoneal communication drawing the abdominal viscera into the chest. In addition, such a defect produces paradoxical respirations with shifting of the mediastinum. Paradoxical respiration together with compression of the lung and mediastinum by the abdominal viscera result first and foremost in respiratory insufficiency. This can best be corrected with endotracheal intubation and controlled ventilation. Once this has been accomplished, the patient can then be further evaluated and prepared for surgery.

We advise the abdominal approach in the immediate postinjury period. If the blunt trauma is severe enough to rupture the diaphragm, disruption of the hollow viscus and/or abdominal organs should be ruled out. This is best accomplished by celiotomy. There is no doubt that the repair of the diaphragm is more difficult from below but this technical disadvantage should be subordinated to the more immediate and life-threatening possibilities. The diaphragmatic defect should be debrided and closed in two layers with heavy permanent sutures. The chest should be decompressed with an intercostal catheter connected to an underwater sealed drainage bottle.

The second category of patients includes those with diaphragmatic disruption surviving the immediate post-trauma period and developing into complications days to years later. Their symptoms are chiefly related to the gastrointestinal and respiratory systems. Strangulation and/or obstruction of the hollow viscus can occur at any time. Gastrointestinal symptoms can range from vague complaints to those of an acute abdomen. A common complaint is dyspnea after eating. Once the diagnosis is established or strongly suspected, surgery is advised. In contrast to the first group of patients with possible acute intra-abdominal injuries, on whom an approach through the abdomen is advised, all delayed repairs are carried out through the chest for two reasons:

1. Exposure is better.
2. The lung may require decortication.

Adhesions may be mature, necessitating sharp dissection under direct vision to prevent injury to the abdominal viscera. The edges of a long-standing diaphragmatic defect tend to retract and may require a prosthesis, such as Marlex mesh, to close the defect. This can be better accomplished by a thoracic approach. In patients with strangulation and/or obstruction of the hollow viscus, the bowel can very adequately be evaluated or resected through the chest. On rare occasions, an abdominal incision may be needed to bring out a colostomy or create an abdominal hernia to permit distended bowel to be returned to the abdominal domicile.

Penetrating Chest Trauma

Gunshot and stab wounds comprise in our society the vast majority of penetrating injuries to the chest. Our socioeconomic structure has produced a concentration of such traumata in a few large city hospitals. With recent socioeconomic changes a more widespread distribution of these injuries can be anticipated. For didactic purposes we will discuss each type of trauma according to the anatomic structure penetrated, fully realizing that in clinical situations the real crux is determining what structures have been injured.

Gunshot Wounds of the Chest

Civilian gunshot wounds seen in our metropolitan areas have a fairly uniform pattern of ballistics. They are usually caused by 22–38 caliber low-to-medium velocity bullets. The characteristics of the wound of entry will vary with the distance between the gun and the victim and also the velocity of the bullet. At close range powder burns may be evident. In high-velocity missile injuries the wound of entry is sharply outlined with seared skin edges, whereas the wound of exit is usually larger with more ragged skin edges. Bullets penetrating the body do not necessarily follow a straight line. Some will ricochet about the bony structures of the thorax. The extent of bullet injury, in general, is proportional to the size, type, distance and velocity of the missile. War weapons inflict much more extensive injuries than the usual civilian gunshot wounds.

A reliable history in cases of penetrating trauma is notoriously difficult to obtain. In the excitement, the victim usually does not know how many bullet wounds he has sustained. Some patients are reluctant to divulge information regarding the assailant or the events surrounding the shooting, for fear of reprisals. The sensorium of these patients is frequently obtunded from shock, pain, narcotics or alcohol.

A careful assessment of the wounds of entry and exit correlated with the location of the bullets is important. The entire body should be disrobed and inspected for bullet wounds. Palpation of the subcutaneous tissue, particularly of the posterior aspect of the thorax, will frequently locate the bullet. X-rays taken in two planes help to localize both the position and probable course of the missile. Bullets have a tendency to fragment when bone is traversed, producing radiographic metallic tracks in the soft tissue. It should be remembered that a missile striking a solid structure such as bone can produce disruption of a vessel or an organ in the vicinity without having actually hit that vessel or organ, particularly with gunshot wounds to the bony pelvis. The phenomenon results from transmitted shock waves in much the same fashion as explosions beneath the water cause shock waves to individuals a considerable distance from the area of explosion. Occasionally a bullet may be extremely elusive if it rests freely in the pleural cavity, peritoneal cavity, vein, artery or gastrointestinal tract. Serial x-rays may show bizarre changes in position; we have seen bullet emboli to the extremities and venous embolization of a bullet to the heart.

MEDIASTINUM.—Gunshot wounds to the heart, great vessels, trachea, hilar structures and esophagus are for the most part fatal unless surgical repair can be promptly effected. Experience gained on trauma wards in metropolitan hospitals gives the impression that the incidence of penetrating mediastinal injuries is low as compared with the number of penetrating injuries to the abdomen and peripheral lungs. While the vertebral column does somewhat protect the mediastinal structures, the disparity in incidence is a result of the large number of patients with mediastinal injuries who succumb before reaching the trauma ward.

THE HEART (Fig. 6-8).—It requires little imagination to envision the dire effects of missile injury to the heart. Disruption of one or more valves, conduction bundle, a major coronary vessel or large areas of myocardium is usually rapidly fatal. Since most of these patients do not reach the hospital alive, there is a dearth of experience in their management. Gunshot wounds of the heart should be repaired without delay. Preoperative pericardicentesis for relief of cardiac tamponade is the only legitimate temporizing measure. Cardiac tamponade may be prevented, or may be decompressed spontaneously, by the bullet hole in the pericardium acting as a vent. A bullet hole through the atrium has on occasion allowed free communication between the atrium and the pericardium; in such an instance the pericardium acts as an accessory chamber and decompresses into the atrium.

Although patients with a gunshot wound in the region of the heart arriving at the hospital alive represent a certain selection, it has been amazing to see how often the heart is actually missed. Bullet

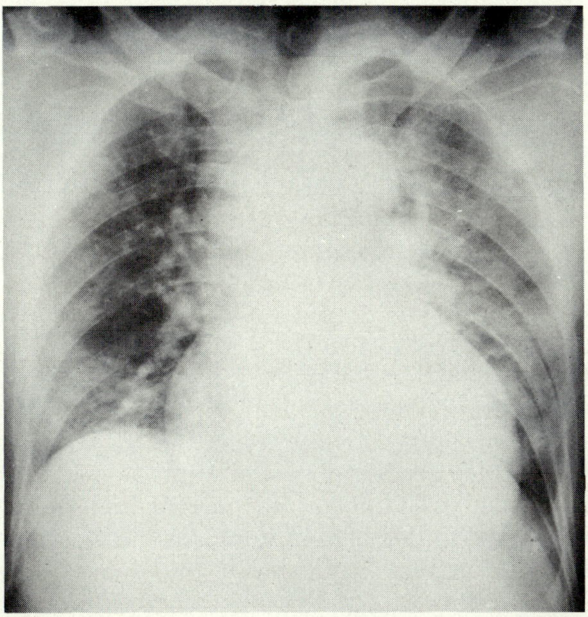

Fig. 6-8.—X-ray of the chest in a 35-year-old male who sustained a stab wound of the heart, showing globular cardiac configuration. Note central venous cannula in superior vena cava. The time interval between injury and this x-ray was 10 hours, allowing for more distention of the pericardium than is usually present in cardiac tamponade.

wounds of the lower anterior thorax that could not seemingly have missed the heart, judging from the topographic anatomy, frequently have not touched the heart and have produced through-and-through injuries to the stomach and diaphragm. Nevertheless, if cardiac penetration is adjudged likely, surgical exploration of the heart should be undertaken.

Cardiac resuscitation of patients with gunshot wounds of the heart who are in profound shock is made difficult by the severe hypoxia and acidosis of the myocardium. Good oxygenation of the lungs, cardiac massage and the administration of sodium bicarbonate or tromethamine (THAM) are important. Internal cardiac massage may be hampered by the bullet holes, necessitating their closure before massage can be effective. Depending upon the duration and severity of shock, there may be varying degrees of low cardiac output and impaired renal function in the postoperative period. The use of mechanical ventilation, mannitol, titrating the replacement of blood volume by monitoring changes in the central venous pressure, and correction of base deficits as indicated by frequent determinations of arterial blood-gas studies are discussed elsewhere in this volume.

In operations for penetrating wounds of the heart the pericardium is loosely approximated. Windowing the posterior pericardium will permit good drainage into the pleural space. While the followup on the majority of patients sustaining gunshot wounds is notoriously poor, we have seen several of these patients return with symptoms of the postpericardiotomy syndrome. Malaise, fever and chest pain coupled with an enlarged spleen and increase in lymphocytes (atypical) occur 2 to 5 weeks after injury. It is good practice to do repeated blood cultures to rule out endocarditis; or if pericardial effusion is present, pericardicentesis with viral and bacteriologic studies of the aspirate is indicated. These symptoms for the most part run a self-limiting course of 1 to 2 weeks, with occasional recurrences. Treatment is symptomatic. Aspirin usually will suffice, with some cases requiring steroids to produce symptomatic relief.

THE GREAT VESSELS.—Gunshot wounds through the thoracic aorta for the most part cause death from hemorrhage. Occasionally clot or false aneurysm formation will prevent immediate exsanguination. A bullet penetrating an artery can cause thermal injury and disruption to the vessel wall considerably beyond that which is grossly apparent. The higher-velocity missiles are likely to cause more extensive arterial-wall damage. Wide debridement of these injuries with vein or prosthetic patch or replacement graft may be necessary.

Management of arterial gunshot wounds to the thoracic aorta is pretty much akin to management of aneurysms of the three anatomic portions of the thoracic aorta: the ascending aorta is referred to as the first portion, the arch of the aorta is the second, and the descending aorta is the third portion. When interruption of the circulation of the thoracic aorta is necessary, cardiopulmonary bypass using various technics is employed. The first portion requires perfusion of the coronary and systemic circulations. The second portion requires coronary and systemic perfusion with additional perfusion lines for the cerebral circulation. In interruption of the circulation to the third portion of the thoracic aorta, the heart is used to perfuse the upper extremities and cerebral circulation.

The arteries to the spinal cord and kidneys can be perfused by a number of technics. Left atrial-femoral artery bypass has been the most widely used method. A temporary shunt from the proximal aorta or the left ventricle to the distal aorta avoids bypass and the use of anticoagulants. We have found the femoral vein to femoral artery partial cardiopulmonary bypass to work best. This technic eliminates the pump drainage tube from the operative field and allows two teams to work simultaneously. Cardiopulmonary bypass can be instituted in a matter of minutes using a prime of lactated Ringer's solution and a disposable oxygenator.

In some patients with gunshot wounds of the aorta who are alive when they arrive at the hospital, the hole in the aorta can be repaired by use of a vascular clamp to partially occlude the aorta and allow closure of the defect. The use of Teflon pledgets on mattress sutures placed beneath a finger that is tamponading the defect can be effective. In wounds that are more than 24 hours old the adjacent aortic wall may be friable, necessitating added care in repairing the defect.

Gunshot wounds of the carotid or brachiocephalic arteries are best repaired by use of an internal shunt to support cerebral circulation during repair of the vessel.

Injury to the innominate veins can be repaired or more simply ligated if only one of the veins is involved. If both innominate veins are disrupted, reconstruction of one of the veins should be attempted. Similarly, the superior vena cava should be repaired and not ligated, if at all possible. The currently available prosthetic material for replacement of the superior vena cava will not remain patent on a long-term basis; however, the several days before thrombosis of the graft occurs will buy time to allow development of collateral venous circulation. This will greatly aid in getting the patient through the immediate postoperative period. Reconstruction of the superior vena cava with autologous vein offers the best opportunity for long-term patency.

Trachea and major bronchi.—Gunshot wounds of the trachea or major bronchi may be associated with massive mediastinal, cervical and subcutaneous emphysema. A tracheostomy or endotracheal intubation will decompress the tracheobronchial tree and thereby decrease the air pushed into the mediastinum. It will also aid in cleaning the airway of blood and mucus. The experience of bronchoplastic and tracheal reconstruction procedures gained in resecting neoplasms can be aptly applied to penetrating trauma. Functioning lung tissue may be preserved by either a sleeve resection or bronchoplasty of the involved area. Considerable lengths of the trachea can be resected with primary end-to-end anastomosis. In anastomosis of the tracheobronchial tree, the endobronchial contour should be preserved as much as possible. A circumferential suture line will cause at least a temporary paralysis of the ciliary movement of secretions across the anastomosis. This problem will be compounded by the degree of irregularity of the suture line.

Hilus of the lung.—Gunshot wounds through the hilus of the lungs will usually create enough symptoms in the form of hemorrhage or air leaks to require immediate exploration. Occasionally, a large-caliber bullet lodged in the hilus of the lung will be seen on chest x-ray. These patients may be completely asymptomatic and the question arises whether the bullet should be removed. A good number that we have seen have been shrapnel or large-caliber bullets. We have recommended removal out of concern for erosion into a major vessel. Large missiles with irregular or sharp contours are most likely to erode into adjacent structures. These missiles frequently carry cloth and debris with them, leading to suppuration and erosion.

Esophagus.—Gunshot wounds to the esophagus can produce considerable disruption. Contamination of the mediastinum and pleura by saliva and gastric contents produces early chemical and later bacterial mediastinitis similar to peritonitis secondary to perforation of a peptic ulcer. Large volumes of fluid and plasma are sequestered in the mediastinum and pleural spaces. Management of gunshot wounds of the esophagus depends a good deal upon the time interval between injury and treatment. All such injuries should be explored with the objective of repairing the esophagus and/or draining the area. If the injury is less than 12 to 24 hours old, primary repair should be attempted. Devitalized portions of the esophagus are excised and closure is effected by interrupted sutures in at least two layers. Strips of pleura can be used to reinforce the closure. The mediastinal pleura must be opened wide to allow drainage into the pleural space. The posterior chest tube is sutured in place in a dependent position 3 to 4 inches away from the esophageal suture line. A second anterior chest tube will effect prompt and complete expansion of the lung with obliteration of the pleural space. Gunshot wounds to the cervical esophagus are repaired in a similar fashion, employing adequate cervical drainage of the superior mediastinum. Broad-spectrum antibiotics should be used in high dosage.

Attempts to repair perforations of the esophagus more than 24 hours old are for the most part doomed to failure. Operating time should not be wasted in repairing esophageal lacerations over 24 hours old. Management of these lesions requires adequate drainage, replacement of plasma and fluids, and antimicrobial therapy. If a large portion of the esophagus is destroyed, cervical esophagostomy and gastrostomy may be necessary. Esophageal replacement can be carried out later.

Diagnosis of esophageal perforation should be suspected when cervical or mediastinal emphysema is seen on x-ray. The use of a water-soluble contrast medium swallowed by the patient to demonstrate leak on x-ray may be useful to show the area of perforation; however, negative results cannot be relied upon. Patients with penetrating trauma in the region of the esophagus should be explored. Failure to recognize and treat a disruption of the esophagus is usually fatal.

Peripheral lung.—The density of the tissue will in part determine the amount of kinetic energy absorbed from a missile. The lung, being a less dense organ, fares quite well in this regard. A gunshot wound of the lung results in varying degrees of hemothorax, pneumothorax or hemopneumothorax. The principal treatment of these lesions is the evacuation of air, blood and fluid from the pleural space, with complete expansion of the lung. This can be accomplished by either thoracentesis or closed drainage of the pleural space.

The question arises when to choose between thoracentesis and closed drainage. It has been previously held that closed drainage caused a greater incidence of empyema and repeated thoracentesis has been favored. We do not feel that this is true, particularly with the use of antimicrobials. Actually a number of factors influence the choice of treatment: time interval between injury and treatment, amount of air and/or fluid in the pleural space, and the need for further transportation of the patient. If the patient's vital signs are stable 24 hours or more after injury, such factors as continuing blood loss and tension pneumothorax are substantially reduced. Under these circumstances, if the amount of pneumothorax is less than 50 percent and there does not appear to be an excessive amount of fluid, thoracentesis will suffice. Specimens of the aspirate should be submitted for bacterial smear, culture and sensitivity studies. A hematocrit and hemoglobin of the aspirate will suggest the extent of blood loss. Small amounts of air and/or fluid may require only further observation.

We favor closed drainage in the majority of instances, particularly if the patient is seen shortly after injury. This allows better assessment of continuing blood loss for accurate volume replacement. If air is also present in the pleural space, negative pressure can be applied to encourage rapid expansion of the lung with sealing off of air leaks as well as bleeding points from the lung surface. As mentioned above, the objective of treatment is the evacuation of air and fluid from the pleural space with complete expansion of the lung. This requires that the caliber of the chest tube be larger than the aggregate of the leaks in the lung. Two or more chest tubes may be required to accomplish adequate decompression of the pleural space. Chest tubes placed posteriorly and inferiorly are more effective in removing fluid, whereas the air is evacuated best by inserting the chest tube anteriorly and superiorly. Twenty-five cm. of water suction may be applied to the drainage bottles. In trauma cases we prefer a large-caliber chest tube. For a large-caliber chest tube to be truly effective, the rest of the tubing system to the underwater sealed drainage bottle should be of equal caliber, and the outside diameter of the chest tube should not exceed the size of the interspace.

Hourly output of the chest-tube drainage is recorded. The nurse positions the patient from side to side and milks the chest tubes every hour to aid in removing blood from the chest. Incomplete expansion of the lung may be secondary to blood or mucus in the bronchi requiring intratracheal aspiration. A broad-spectrum antibiotic is administered until bacterial culture and sensitivity studies of the sputum are known. Tetanus prophylaxis should not be forgotten.

The wounds of entrance and exit should be properly debrided and the pleural space sealed. Bullet wounds of the chest wall, particularly those grossly contaminated and several hours old, do not necessarily need to be closed. As long as the pleural space is sealed satisfactorily, the overlying skin may be left open. It is usually the wound of exit that will become infected. If the missile creates a defect in the chest wall, producing an open chest wound, the defect must be closed. This can usually be accomplished by use of a muscle or skin flap with proper bandaging.

Emergency management of an open chest wound requires closure with a tight pressure dressing until positive-pressure ventilation is established.

Thoracotomy.—Penetrating trauma to the peripheral lung can practically always be managed short of thoracotomy. If the pleural space is adequately decompressed with expansion of the lung, bleeding and air leaks will usually stop. Indications for thoracotomy fall into two categories. The first is the large clot that cannot be removed by thoracentesis or closed drainage. This is generally a result of either massive hemorrhage or late or ineffective decompression of the pleural space. Thoracotomy is performed to remove the clot, control hemorrhage and expand the lung, thereby restoring cardiopulmonary function.

The second indication for thoracotomy is when bleeding persists in spite of adequate decompression of the pleural space and expansion of the lung. It is not unusual to drain 800 to 1,200 ml. of bloody fluid in the first 12 to 18 hours. The majority of drainage occurs in the first 6 to 10 hours and then gradually tapers off. If after the first 8 hours the hourly drainage exceeds 100 ml., consideration must be given for thoracotomy. No hard-and-fast rules can be set, but with continued bleeding of that magnitude, thoracotomy carries less risk than multiple blood transfusions.

In performing a thoracotomy for acute hemothorax, several considerations must be borne in mind. At least two I.V.'s should be working well for rapid blood-volume replacement. A common error is to have all the experienced personnel scrubbed, even to the third and fourth assistant, with only the anesthesiologist or anesthetist to estimate blood loss, replace blood volume, monitor vital signs, and, incidentally as it were, administer anesthesia. The third or fourth assistant can be more profitably deployed to help in blood-volume replacement. Provisions should be made for rapid prepping, draping and entry into the chest once the patient has been turned into a lateral decubitus position. A large hemothorax will cause additional compression of the mediastinal structures in a patient whose cardiopulmonary reserve may be already compromised. Once the blood has been evacuated from the chest, the operation can proceed at a normal pace.

Serial x-rays of the chest are indispensable for proper management of hemopneumothorax. Portable chest x-rays taken in the upright position, if at all possible, should be obtained every 12 to 24 hours until the lung is expanded and the patient's general condition is stable. A sudden decrease in the hourly output from the chest tube should suggest the possibility of a plugged chest tube. This will be evident on the chest films by increased haziness and pleural effusion of the involved hemithorax. Aside from the problems in the immediate postinjury period, followup x-rays are essential for the long-term management, as some of these individuals will require decortication.

Summary.—Following are the indications for emergency thoracotomy in penetrating chest trauma:

1. *Penetration of the mediastinum.*
2. *Injuries producing large defects in the chest wall.* Although a compression dressing will temporarily control a sucking chest wound, debridement and primary closure should be carried out as soon as feasible.
3. *Injury to the lung resulting in uncontrollable or persistent air leaks.*
4. *Penetrating wounds of the chest resulting in massive and/or persistent hemorrhage.*
5. *Massive hemothorax seriously compromising cardiopulmonary function that cannot be evacuated by closed-chest tube drainage.*
6. *Inability to expand the lung in the absence of endobronchial obstruction and adequate decompression of the pleural space.*

DECORTICATION.—We have never been able to predict accurately at the completion of the initial treatment for hemothorax which patients will require decortication at a later time; nor, in our opinion, has there been advanced a convincing theory of the pathogenesis of organizing hemothorax. We concur with a principle of keeping the pleural space as free of blood and fluid as possible; yet some of our patients with the best-appearing chest x-ray at the time of discharge return several weeks later with pleural effusion and organizing hemothorax. Conversely, patients discharged with a considerable degree of pleural reaction and advised to return in several weeks for decortication have shown dramatic radiographic improvement and have not required decortication. The fibrinous "peel" removed at the time of decortication will practically always show evidence of chronic inflammation. Experimental work has demonstrated that clotted or nonclotted blood per se will be absorbed from the pleural space. Clinically, blood in the pleural space after thoracotomy seldom results in an organizing hemothorax.

Hemothorax secondary to penetrating trauma requires decortication much oftener than hemothorax resulting from blunt trauma. Perhaps the combination of bacteria in a culture medium of blood causes an inflammation functionally paralyzing the pleura or altering the nature of the pleural response, so that the contents of the pleural space cannot be absorbed. Thus a pathologic pleural space is maintained. We feel that, in addition to keeping the pleural space empty, antibiotics should be used in high dosages initially and maintained at lower levels even after discharge.

The main indication for decortication is ventilatory impairment of the restrictive type. Exact degree of impairment is frequently difficult to assess on routine pulmonary function studies, as many patients are otherwise healthy young males who can compensate for a considerable deficit. Selective bronchospirometry studies may demonstrate considerable ventilatory impairment not apparent on routine pulmonary-function studies. Prior to decortication, thoracentesis with culture and sensitivity studies of the aspirate to allow accurate antimicrobial coverage should be performed. The optimum time for decortication of an organizing hemothorax is purported to be 3 to 6 weeks after injury. Patients with large hemothoraces which cannot be evacuated by closed drainage are perhaps best operated upon as soon as they are stabilized; however, it should be kept in mind that a number of the lesser hemothoraces will resolve without decortication. Fibroblastic infiltration of the peel into the visceral pleura in the older hemothoraces renders decortication more difficult. Considerable restriction of motion in the chest wall occurs in an organized hemothorax, so it is sometimes desirable to remove the parietal pleura as well as the visceral pleura. In densely adherent membranes which cannot be removed without tearing the lung, closely placed cross-hatches made with the scalpel will permit expansion without actually removing the membrane. Decortication on occasion can be quite bloody with a lot of air leaks. Bleeding and air leaks should be controlled as well as possible but equally important is good decompression of the pleural space. It may be advantageous to use three large-bore chest tubes to effect optimum expansion and drainage. The use of intrapleural enzymes to dissolve clot, in our experience, has been disappointing.

The Diaphragm

The region of the diaphragm is a common area for penetrating wounds, yet many times they are mismanaged. Either the thoracic surgeon fails to treat the abdominal components properly, or the general surgeon fails to treat properly the chest lesions. The topographic anatomic relationship of the diaphragm to both the intra-abdominal organs and the thorax must be borne in mind. While the posterior costophrenic recess extends to the medial third of the 12th rib posteriorly, the dome of the diaphragm is on the coronal plane of the 5th rib anteriorly. Accordingly, all penetrating wounds of the chest at or below the 4th rib anteriorly should be suspected of entering the abdominal cavity through the diaphragm.

Peritoneal signs are difficult to assess, as a penetrating wound of the lower thorax may produce considerable splinting and guarding of the abdominal muscles. On the left side, stomach, spleen, left lobe of the liver and pancreas are most likely to be injured. In the absence of intrathoracic indications for exploration, we feel the abdominal approach is best. We are well aware of the facility with which structures in the left upper quadrant can be managed by left thoracotomy with transdiaphragmatic exploration; yet the large and small bowel can be more easily and thoroughly inspected from below. Contamination from hollow viscus can be confined to one cavity. While hard-and-fast rules cannot be dogmatically set down to apply to all situations, we do not favor the thoracico-abdominal incision. Exposure in the chest is limited and postoperative instability of the chondral portion of the rib cage can be troublesome. If there are indications for exploring both the chest and abdomen, separate incisions will usually afford the best exposure. This is not to say that thoracico-abdominal incisions should not be used, but rather to discourage the attitude that all eventualities can be dealt with by this approach. It should be kept in mind that a laceration of the diaphragm can produce a sucking wound of the chest when the abdomen is opened and the patient is breathing on his own. This is no real problem if one is aware that it can be corrected by positive-pressure ventilation or insertion of a chest tube with closure of the diaphragmatic opening.

Defects of the diaphragm are debrided and then closed with a double layer of heavy-caliber permanent sutures, as they are a frequent site of a subsequent hernia. Repair of the diaphragmatic defect from below is facilitated by placing traction sutures at the margins of the defect. Injuries to the left lobe of the liver and pancreas, in addition to being repaired or resected, as indicated, must be adequately drained through the abdomen. Large Penrose drains are favored over firm sump drains, as drainage may be required for a long time. We have seen erosion of the spleen with hemorrhage and erosion of the colon with fistula formation occur as a result of hard drains.

Penetrating trauma to the right lower hemithorax presents different problems. In this region the liver, diaphragm and lung are the structures commonly injured, the liver offering the major problems. Blood and bile from liver injuries can extravasate into either the abdominal or the thoracic cavity. Disruption of the blood supply to a major anatomic segment of the liver with subsequent necrosis may occur. Sequelae of liver injuries may be: hemorrhage, leakage of bile, subphrenic abscess, empyema, chronic hemothorax, necrosis of liver tissue with late hemorrhage, in addition to the severe metabolic disturbances that can accompany these disease processes.

A bullet entering the chest at the level of the dome of the diaphragm in the midaxillary line and exiting in a similar region on the opposite side may raise the question of exposure to the dozen or more structures that could be penetrated. If the heart is penetrated, a sternal splitting incision extended into a midline abdominal incision will give excellent exposure to both the heart and abdominal organs. The mediastinal pleura should of course be opened and both pleural spaces drained.

Management of liver injuries.—Decisions for proper management of liver injuries must be made at the time of the initial treatment. If a segment or a lobe of the liver has lost its blood supply, it should be resected. It may also be necessary to resect anatomic portions of the liver to control hemorrhage. Packing liver injuries is a stopgap measure resulting in later hemorrhage. Control of late hemorrhage by surgical intervention is fraught with disaster. Liver parenchyma is usually soft and necrotic and will not hold sutures. It is important, therefore, that exposure of the liver injury be adequate for the initial assessment. Exposure to the right dome of the liver is for the most part difficult and inadequate by the abdominal approach. A low thoracotomy incision with opening the right hemidiaphragm will give direct exposure. The diaphragm can be readily repaired, pleural space evacuated, and multiple large Penrose drains placed beneath the diaphragm and brought out through the abdominal wall. If resection of a portion of the liver or decompression of the common bile duct with a T tube in the case of a large bile leak is necessary, the incision can be extended across the right chondral arch into the abdomen. Large mattress sutures with Teflon pledgets work best in controlling hemorrhage and bile from injuries to the liver. In resecting anatomic portions of the liver, individual ligation of vessels and bile ducts is necessary.

Postoperative management of liver injuries can tax the diligence of even the most dedicated physician. This is particularly true in blunt trauma, where a large area of liver damage can occur. Copious quantities of fluids and protein ooze from the raw surface of the liver, requiring replacement. Total protein content of the serum should be frequently checked and serum albumin administered as needed. Malaise, unexplained fever, nausea and vomiting are the rule and can go on for several months. A broad-spectrum antibiotic to prevent cholangitis should be administered until the patient is completely well, although blood cultures are practically always negative. Injection of contrast material through the drain tract may show some puddling, raising the question of a subphrenic abscess as the cause of symptoms. Frank pus is seldom found when these areas are explored. Autolysis of liver tissue and perhaps some degree of cholangitis best explain these symptoms.

Stab Wounds of the Chest

Management of stab wounds of the chest is quite similar to that described for gunshot wounds. In view of this, we will not repeat a discussion of injuries to the various thoracic structures but will point out the general differences, where they exist, between these two types of penetrating injuries. Stab wounds of the heart are discussed under "Acute cardiac tamponade and penetrating heart wounds."

In metropolitan areas where violence is more concentrated, stab wounds constitute the vast majority of penetrating injuries. Knives are readily accessible, making them the most common weapon employed. Information regarding the type and size of knife, relative positions of both the victim and assailant and amount of hemorrhage is helpful in assessing the injury; however, frequently such information cannot be obtained. The depth and direction of penetration can only be surmised from the appearance of the external wound. A short external wound may be associated with deep penetration, whereas a long external wound is frequently more superficial.

In addition to the size and type of knife, the manner of thrust is significant. The skilled, knife-carrying "man of the street" carries a long, narrow switch-blade. His thrust is quickly executed at right angle to the axis of the victim's body. Such a thrust is difficult to block. The knife penetrates the body in a perpendicular or slightly cephalad direction. The irate housewife who picks up a butcher knife and stabs her unfaithful spouse usually does so by raising the knife high and striking downward. If successful, the penetration will be in a caudad direction. This is particularly important in assessing stab wounds in the region of the diaphragm.

The practice of probing stab wounds to determine penetration of either the abdominal or thoracic cavities is unreliable. More recently a technic of injecting contrast media through a catheter placed in the wound with the skin tightly closed around the catheter has been advocated. The contrast media is identified on x-ray if the wound penetrates the abdominal or thoracic cavities. Both these methods not only violate good surgical technic but, more important, decisions based on negative results may jeopardize the patient's life.

Mediastinum

With the noted exception of the heart (see Fig. 6-8), the mediastinal structures have a certain degree of protection from stab wounds by virtue of the sternum and the vertebral column. A vulnerable area of penetration to the mediastinum is through the neck. A downward thrust through the supraclavicular or jugular notch area can readily injure mediastinal structures. Accordingly, the possibility of mediastinal injuries should be borne in mind with stab wounds of the cervical area.

Immediate exsanguination is less likely to occur in patients sustaining stab wounds to the great vessels than in those sustaining gunshot wounds to the same area. A greater number of these patients, therefore, will reach the hospital alive. Clot may form over a laceration of the veins, producing a tamponade effect. This can also occur in arterial perforations, particularly when the arterial pressure falls for a time due to hypovolemia.

A patient with a stab wound of the chest showing radiographic mediastinal widening should undergo operation. The surgical approach will depend upon the structures believed to be injured. A median sternotomy gives good exposure to the ascending aorta, brachiocephalic vessels and the superior vena cava. A right posterolateral incision gives the best exposure to the esophagus and trachea, while a left posterolateral approach is best for lacerations of the descending aorta and left subclavian artery. Pressure by means of a stick sponge over a venous laceration will usually control hemorrhage, whereas digital compression with sutures placed beneath the finger work best on arterial lacerations. It should be remembered that provisions for the intravenous infusion of blood and fluid should be made through the veins of the inferior extremities in suspected injuries of the superior vena cava.

Peripheral Lung

(See Figs. 6–9, 6–10, and 6–11.)

If injuries to the mediastinum, diaphragm and abdomen can be ruled out, stab wounds to the peripheral lungs for the most part do not pose difficult problems in management. The anterior aspect of the chest is an area of predilection for stab wounds. The superior extremities and shoulder girdles somewhat protect the lateral and posterior aspects of the thorax. Furthermore, most such confrontations are face to face. Anatomically, the intercostal interspaces are wider anteriorly, allowing for easier penetration; for the same reason sucking wounds are more likely to result from a stab wound to the anterior aspect of the chest.

Management of stab wounds to the lung centers primarily around pleural space problems such as hemothorax, pneumothorax, tension pneumothorax, hemopneumothorax, and sucking wounds of the chest. Evacuation of blood and air from the pleural space is usually best accomplished by the insertion of chest tubes. If the pneumothorax is less than 25 percent and is not increasing, continued observation by serial x-rays of the chest may be all that is necessary. On occasion, particularly when a patient is seen 24 hours or more after sustaining penetrating trauma, aspiration of blood and/or air by thoracentesis may be adequate.

Sucking wounds of the chest wall are initially controlled by covering with a large pressure dressing. After the pleural space is decompressed with a chest tube and positive-pressure ventilation established by means of an endotracheal tube, closure of the chest wall defect can be safely carried out. Mobilization of extracostal muscle flaps

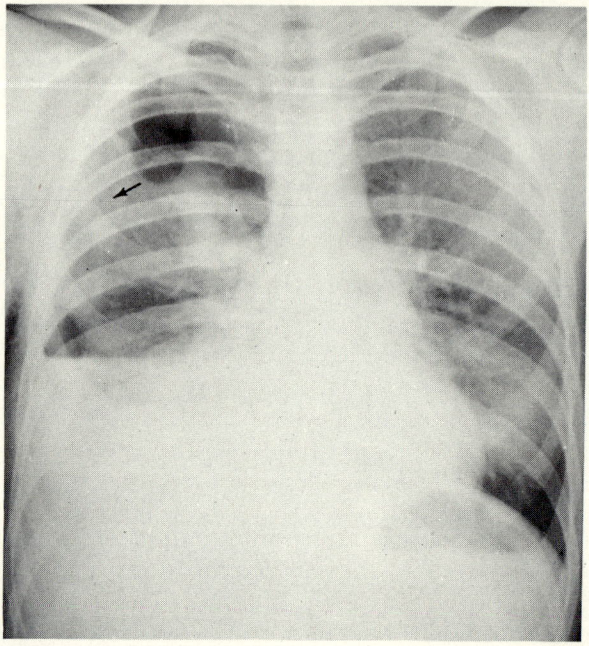

Fig. 6-9.—Anterior stab wound of the right chest in a 22-year-old female, showing hemopneumothorax and subcutaneous emphysema. Arrow points to edge of partially collapsed right lung. Just above arrow is an ovoid radiolucent area corresponding to a large sucking wound of the anterior chest wall.

provides a good means of closing large chest-wall defects. In general, the base of such muscle flaps should be on the chest wall and the insertion of the muscle divided for mobilization of the muscle flap. A good example of this is the pectoralis major muscle. Division of its insertion into the humerus affords a long muscle flap with a good vascular pedicle based on the chest wall. The skin and subcutaneous tissue are closed. The chest wall closure must seal the pleural space from the outside. Application of a pressure dressing will again give support to the chest-wall closure.

At least 95 percent of stab wounds to the peripheral lung fields are managed successfully without thoracotomy. The indications for emergency thoracotomy are:

1. *Excessive and continued blood loss*
2. *Excessive and continued air leak*
3. *Inability to expand the lung*
4. *Inability to evacuate a large amount of blood within the pleural space*
5. *Wounds creating a large chest-wall defect*

Because of the low pressures within the pulmonary circulation, hemorrhage from the lung parenchyma will practically always stop if the lung is kept expanded. If bleeding persists it is usually the result of a partial laceration of a systemic vessel, such as an intercostal artery. Large amounts of oxygenated blood draining from the chest tube is presumptive evidence for systemic arterial bleeding. Pulmonary venous bleeding is an unlikely source of such hemorrhage, as the normal pressure within its vasculature is less than 10 mm. Hg. The source of dark, desaturated blood draining from the chest tubes is less specific. Systemic arterial blood remaining in the pleural space for a time is desaturated, similar to the blood from the pulmonary arterial tree.

Specifically what constitutes excessive and continued bleeding is a moot question. It must be recognized that there are many contingent factors, and to set a certain quantity of blood loss as the criterion is missing the point. For example, a patient with a stab wound of the chest is seen 12 hours after injury, a chest tube is inserted, and

Fig. 6–10.—X-ray shows lung expanded, with chest tubes in place. Three chest tubes were necessary (only one of the three chest tubes contained a radiopaque marker) to overcome large air leaks. Infiltrates present in both lungs were result of blood and retained secretions within tracheobronchial tree. The latter cleared with frequent intratracheal aspirations. Same patient as in Figure 6–9.

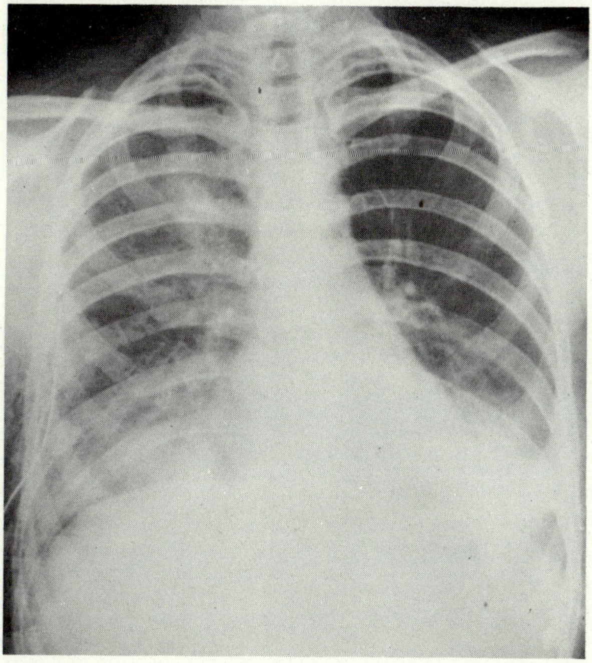

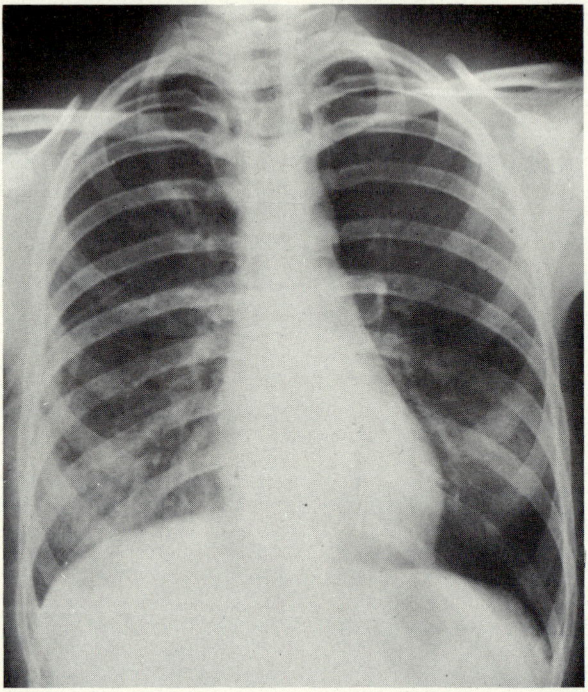

Fig. 6-11.—X-ray taken 5 days post-trauma shows the chest tubes removed, with satisfactory clearing of lungs and right pleural space. Same patient as in Figures 6-9 and 6-10.

1 liter of bloody fluid is evacuated. This may represent a blood loss of 600 ml. in the first 2 hours with several hundred milliliters of subsequent serous effusion. On the other hand, if the hourly drainage from the chest tubes continues to exceed 100 ml. for 3 to 4 hours after injury, thoracotomy would in most instances carry a lower mortality rate than repeated blood transfusions. Hemoglobin and hematocrit determinations of the pleural drainage are helpful in assessing the amount of serous effusion.

Excessive and continued air leak can be a result of pre-existing pathology such as penetration of the knife into a large emphysematous bleb. Two or more chest tubes attached to high suction may be required to keep ahead of the leak. If subcutaneous and/or mediastinal emphysema progresses despite adequate pleural decompression, thoracotomy is indicated.

Large clots within the pleural space may seriously impair cardiopulmonary function from the mechanical effect of lung and mediastinal compression. In such instances evacuation of the clot by thoracotomy is indicated.

In certain cases of spontaneous pneumothoraces, large amounts of fibrin will entrap the lung and not allow it to expand in spite of adequate decompression of the pleural space. This also occurs occasionally in stab wounds of the chest. In such instances the burden of proof is on the surgeon to exclude endobronchial occlusion secondary to blood or mucus before thoracotomy is undertaken. If no endobronchial obstruction is present, removal of the fibrin and suturing of existing air leaks is warranted.

The Diaphragm

Stab wounds in the region of the diaphragm are managed basically in the same manner as gunshot wounds to that area. A gunshot wound causes more tissue destruction, yet its trajectory through the body is generally more predictable than the direction of a knife blade. One must bear constantly in mind the possibility of intra-abdominal penetration in assessing stab wounds of the thorax. Stab wounds of the anterior chest wall at or below the 4th interspace frequently penetrate abdominal viscera. Conversely, stab wounds of the epigastrium can penetrate the myocardium by transversing the diaphragm.

Management of penetrating injuries to the diaphragm are detailed under gunshot wounds of the chest.

BIBLIOGRAPHY

Alfano, G. S., and Hale, H. W.: Pulmonary contusion, J. Trauma 5:647, 1965.

Ashbough, D. G., Peters, G. N., Halgrinson, C. B., Owens, J. C., and Wadell, W. R.: Chest trauma; analysis of 685 patients, Arch. Surg. 95:546, 1967.

Avery, E. E., Mörch, E. T., and Benson, D. W.: Critically crushed chests, J. Thoracic Surg. 32:293, 1956.

Battersby, J. S., and Kilman, J. W.: Traumatic injuries of the tracheobronchial tree, Arch. Surg. 88:644, 1964.

Bogedain, W., Carpathios, J., Suu, D. V., and Moots, M. F.: Traumatic rupture of myocardium, J.A.M.A. 197:154, 1966.

Brewer, L. A., III, Burbank, B., Samson, P. C., and Schiff, C. A.: "Wet-lung" in war casualties, Ann. Surg. 123:343, 1946.

Brewer, L., and Carter, R.: A rational treatment of small and large wounds of the heart, Surg. Gynec. & Obst. 126:977, 1968.

Carey, J. S., Yao, S. T., Kho, L. K., Tasche, C., and Shoemaker, W. C.: Cardiovascular responses to acute hemopericardium compression by balloon tamponade and acute coronary occlusion, J. Thoracic & Cardiovas. Surg. 54:65, 1967.

Clowes, G. H. A., Jr., Zuschneid, W., Turner, M., Blackburn, G., Rubin, J., Toala, P., and Green, G.: Observations on the pathogenesis of the pneumonitis associated with severe infections in other parts of the body, Ann. Surg. 167:630, 1968.

Collins, J. A.: *Report of the surgical research team, Viet Nam* (Washington, D.C.: Walter Reed Army Institute of Research, 1967).

Condon, R. E.: Spontaneous resolution of experimental clotted hemothorax, Surg. Gynec. & Obst. 126:505, 1968.

DeMuth, W. E., and Fallah-Nejad, M.: Delayed recognition of serious thoracic injury, Am. J. Surg. 111:587, 1966.

Dimond, F. C., and Rich, N. M.: M-16 rifle wounds in Viet Nam, J. Trauma 7:619, 1967.

Dunseth, W., and Ferguson, T. B.: Acquired cardiac septal defect due to thoracic trauma, J. Trauma 5:142, 1965.

Garzon, A. A., Seltzer, B., and Karlson, K. E.: Physiopathology of crushed chest injuries, Ann. Surg. 168:128, 1968.

Gerami, S., Cousar, J. E., Davis, J. M., and Moseley, T. M.: The management of gunshot wounds of the chest, Ann. Thoracic Surg. 5:189, 1968.

Guest, J. L., Hall, D. P., Yeh, T. J., and Ellison, R. E.: Late manifestations of trauma to the pericardium, Surg. Gynec. & Obst. 120:787, 1965.

Hardin, W. J., Hardy, J. D., and Conn, J. H.: Esophageal perforations, Surg. Gynec. & Obst. 124:325, 1967.

Harken, D. E.: Foreign bodies in, and in relation to, the thoracic blood vessels and heart. Techniques for approaching and removing foreign bodies from the chambers of the heart, Surg. Gynec. & Obst. 83:117, 1946.

Kahn, M. H., and Kahn, S.: Cardiovascular lesions following injury to chest, Ann. Int. Med. 2:1013, 1929.

Keller, W. J., Meckstroth, C. V., Sanzenbacher, L., and Pace, W. E.: Thoracic injuries due to blunt trauma, Ann. Thoracic Surg. 7:541, 1967.

Laforet, E. G.: Acute hypertension as a diagnostic clue in traumatic rupture of the thoracic aorta, Amer. J. Surg. 110:948, 1965.

McKnight, J. T., Meyer, J. A., and Neville, J. F.: Nonpenetrating traumatic rupture of the thoracic aorta, Ann. Surg. 160:1069, 1964.

Munnell, E. R.: Fracture of major airways, Am. J. Surg. 105:511, 1963.

Noon, G. P., Beall, A. C., and DeBakey, M. E.: Surgical management of traumatic rupture of the diaphragm, J. Trauma 6:344, 1966.

Parmley, L. F., Mattingly, T. W., Manion, W. C., and Jahnke, E. J.: Nonpenetrating traumatic injury of the aorta, Circulation 17:1086, 1958.

Peters, R. M. and Hutchin, P.: Adequacy of available respirator to their tasks, Ann. Thoracic Surg. 3:414, 1967.

Rich, N. M., Johnson, E. V., and Dimond, F. C.: Wounding power of missiles used in the Republic of Viet Nam, J.A.M.A. 199:157, 1967.

Shamblin, J. R. and McCoon, D. C.: Acute thoracic compression with traumatic asphyxia, Arch. Surg. 87:967, 1963.

Sugg, W. L., Rea, W. J., Ecker, R. R., Webb, W. R., Rose, E. F., and Shaw, R. R.: Penetrating wounds of the heart, J. Thoracic & Cardiovas. Surg. 56:531, 1968.

Summerall, C. P., Lee, W. H., and Boone, J. A.: Intracardiac shunts after penetrating wounds of the heart, New England J. Med. 272:240, 1965.

Thomas, T. V.: Management of cardiac and intrathoracic great vessel injuries, Surg. Gynec. & Obst. 125:997, 1967.

Wise, A. J., Topuzulu, C., Mills, E. L., and Page, H. G.: The importance of serial blood gas determinations in blunt chest trauma, J. Thoracic & Cardiovas. Surg. 56:520, 1968.

Worman, L. W., Hurley, J. D., Pemberton, A. H., and Narodick, B. G. : Rupture of the esophagus from external blunt trauma, Arch. Surg. 85:333, 1962.

CHAPTER

7

Acute Renal Failure: Pathogenesis, Differential Diagnosis, Prevention and Treatment

WILLIAM M. HAMBY, M.D., PH.D.

Pathogenesis

ACUTE OLIGURIC RENAL FAILURE was first recognized by physicians approximately one hundred years ago. It was not, however, until World War II that Eric Bywaters established this entity as a clinical syndrome. Today acute renal failure is a well-recognized syndrome that may occur in anyone, whether with previously healthy or previously diseased kidneys. It is characterized by the acute onset of oliguria (less than 400 ml./24 hours in the adult and less than 100 ml./24 hours in the child). In some patients acute renal failure is not associated with oliguria but may be present with normal or increased urinary output. This form of acute renal failure is known as high-output renal failure. In time, both these conditions are reversible, either spontaneously or after proper therapy. However, acute renal failure can also be irreversible and produce progressive deterioration in the clinical and biochemical status of the patient, leading to death.

Reversibility of acute renal failure depends upon early diagnosis and treatment. *The most important diagnostic problem is the differentiation of acute failure from chronic end-stage renal failure; from prerenal renal failure (decreased renal blood flow); and from obstructive uropathy (postrenal renal failure).* The syndrome of acute failure may be superimposed on chronic end-stage renal disease. Once an exact diagnosis is made, prompt, intensive management must be instituted. The pathophysiologic process is an all-important factor in the outcome of the patient with acute renal failure. There are few clinical disorders that respond so completely to prompt and adequate therapy. This syndrome must be treated as an acute medical emergency because the outcome of either complete return of renal function or progressive deterioration of renal function may be completely dependent upon the institution of proper therapy.

Precise Definition

In order to accurately evaluate the clinical state in man, a precise definition of acute renal failure, as it occurs to complicate other major disease states, must be identified and adhered to. During the past 2 decades, post-traumatic and postoperative oliguria has been noted for a few hours or days and has generally been accepted as an inevitable, although undesirable, sequela of the physiologic derangements accompanying major trauma and surgery. This oliguria has been considered a mild form of renal failure. Recent clinical experience in the postsurgical and post-traumatic states has tended to discount this general impression and, therefore, one must return to the classic descriptions of acute renal failure suggested by several investigators during World War II.

At that time, records of the clinical course of post-traumatic uremic death were correlated with autopsy findings in the kidneys by a special Army Board for the Study of the Severely Wounded. This board characterized the clinical state associated with oliguric renal failure as following a sequence of trauma, oliguria, azotemia, clinical uremia and finally death. The renal histopathology associated with this clinical state was described independently by Bywaters, Mallory, and Lucké; the term "lower nephron nephrosis" was applied to the renal lesion. Lucké, in describing his observations, wrote:

> "A syndrome characterized by oliguria, heme pigment excretion, azotemia, hypertension and uremia may develop in a variety of conditions associated with destruction of tissue or intravascular hemolysis. The mortality rate is high; death usually occurs within 10 days. Specific lesions occur in the kidney. The essential changes are selectively restricted to the lower segments of the nephrons and comprise focal degeneration or necrosis, the presence of heme casts, secondary inflammatory reactions in the surrounding stroma and thrombosis of thin walled veins."

The etiology and pathogenesis of oliguric renal failure of the type described may logically be classified as being due to one of the following major causes or a combination thereof: *(1) prolonged renal ischemia with cellular destruction; (2) cast obstruction of the tubules;*

and *(3) direct toxic effects on tubule cells.* Many chemical agents possess renal cellular toxic effects; when such agents are involved in the development of acute renal failure, there seems to be little doubt concerning etiology. This toxic effect has been difficult to implicate in most cases of acute renal failure, and the etiology and pathogenesis of oliguria and renal failure following trauma, mismatched transfusions, etc., have remained unsettled. In most of these situations, myoglobulin, hemoglobin, or their breakdown products have been implicated, but when the tolerance of the kidney of normal man to these substances is examined, it becomes apparent that predisposing factors are also needed to produce renal disease. It is also generally recognized that the clinical situations which predispose to acute renal failure suggest a prior antidiuretic or acidotic state from either food and water deprivation, the administration of narcotics and anesthetic agents, or other hemodynamic vasoconstrictive effects of trauma, hypotension, blood loss and their consequent endocrine activity.

Experimental control of this multivariant situation is obviously impossible in man. Therefore, a rigidly controlled laboratory model is required to determine whether these predisposing factors contribute specifically or generally to the incidence and severity of acute renal failure and, if so, how. Retrospective examination of the circumstances of acute renal failure in man have generally failed to provide adequate date for accurate description of the pathogenesis. Also, inasmuch as the condition occurs infrequently and the state of the patient is usually serious, an extensive study in man is precluded.

The tubular cast obstruction model of renal disease production appears to resemble the human post-traumatic, postsurgical state more closely in almost every respect than does the ischemic model. The clinical course through uremia to death is roughly comparable in animals that have died in both model situations. This is not unexpected, because the renoprival rat would probably not reflect the etiology of renal deprivation if the two very different methods of producing renal injury have no other significant effect upon the total organism. The intrarenal histopathology suggests that the tubular cast obstruction lesion accords best with that described by the initial investigators and called lower nephron nephrosis. The amelioration of this lesion by marked diuresis is, of course, predictable if the basic lesion is assumed to be the salting out of a relatively insoluble protein within the lumina of the tubules at a time when the tubules are producing a small volume of concentrated urine.

However, observations of the clinical state and the current status of treatment of major trauma and surgery can be made. During World War II, the occurrence of acute renal failure of this particular variety was a significant event in many kinds of wounds in both civilian and military casualties. Whole blood, matched on its major side, was administered freely as an important resuscitative effort, and those patients who sustained crushing wounds of the extremities or of major muscle masses were the population at risk. Resuscitation with salt solutions was considered inadvisable at that time; in fact, the use of intravenous saline solutions was still limited 10 years later during the Korean conflict. There, with limited saline administration and despite large quantities of blood for resuscitation, the incidence of acute renal failure reached enormous proportions, variously estimated as between 12 and 17% of men with major wounds. During that conflict, blood was flown to the battalion aid stations and poorly matched or universal-donor blood was frequently given in huge quantities as the major resuscitative effort to the wounded man. The occurrence of post-traumatic renal failure was so high that special teams were established to travel through Korea to study the injury and to provide hemodialysis as treatment for this complication.

The Vietnam conflict has as yet provided no definitive reports on this aspect of wound management procedures, but indirect and unofficial reports are becoming available. Alterations in the mode of evacuation and in immediate resuscitation of wounded men have led to a considerable reduction in the incidence of acute renal failure. At the time of writing, the wounded are treated with large volumes of sodium lactate given intravenous sodium bicarbonate and an injection of 12.5 or 25 Gm. of mannitol immediately upon admission into the treatment area. Thus, acute renal failure has been reduced to a minimum among our troops and survival has reached 99% of hospital admission.

Many civilian hospitals utilizing adequate salt loading before and during major surgery and enforcing diuresis with the use of intraoperative mannitol have likewise noticed a remarkable reduction in the incidence of acute renal failure as a postoperative or post-traumatic complication. This clinical observation would suggest that a precursor situation which leads to adequate urine formation at the time of presentation of an insoluble protein will ameliorate or eliminate the disease. In this case, the basic pathogenesis of acute renal failure should be concluded to be that of tubular cast obstruction; and renal ischemia plays a role in this mechanism only insofar as it results in a small volume of highly concentrated urine, most favorable to the precipitation of protein presented to the tubule at that time.

Differential Diagnosis

With advances in therapy, precision in the diagnosis of acute renal failure has become more important in the past 2 decades. It is not uncommon to anticipate clinical recovery if the instigating cause of the renal failure is reversible. After first categorizing the nature of the renal failure, appropriate treatment may be instituted. In patients with acute tubular necrosis, repeated dialysis and possibly initial osmotic diuresis should be utilized; in acute glomerulonephritis due to vasculitis or collagen disease, large doses of steroid therapy might be considered; in the presence of urinary-tract obstruction or vascular occlusion to the renal arteries, surgery would be indicated; and in prerenal azotemia, medical correction of the underlying problem might resolve the renal failure. Along with improvement in therapy for acute renal failure, more precise diagnostic technics have been developed.

Renal Function

Standard function studies for glomerular filtration and renal blood flow are of little value in acute renal failure, due to the severe oliguria. However, evaluation of tubular concentrating mechanisms may have clinical significance.

1. *The urine urea-to-blood urea nitrogen ratio.*—This ratio need not be lowered in prerenal azotemia or primary glomerulopathy, whereas it should be less than 10 in acute tubular necrosis. A patient may have underlying chronic renal disease with loss of tubular concentrating power, so that a ratio of less than 10 does not exclude superimposed acute glomerulitis or prerenal azotemia; however, a ratio of over 10 would be strong evidence against the diagnosis of acute tubular necrosis.

2. *Urine osmolality-to-blood osmolality ratio.*—A ratio less than 1:1 would suggest impaired tubular concentration consistent with acute tubular necrosis.

3. *Urine sodium and potassium concentrations.*—In acute tubular necrosis, there is loss of ability to resorb sodium with a relative increase in urinary sodium and decrease in potassium, whereas in prerenal failure and primary glomerulopathy, a lower sodium and high potassium content is more probable. Determination of these concentrations is of particular value in elderly patients with acute renal failure in whom there is often underlying advanced nephrosclerosis. As the kidney ages, it may normally lose its concentrating ability, whereas conservation of sodium is one of the last functions to be impaired. An elderly patient with a urinary sodium content below

30 mEq./L. and acute renal failure probably would not have acute tubular necrosis.

URINE SEDIMENT.—Careful examination of the urinary sediment of a freshly voided urine sample may be of particular value. The presence of granular casts implies parenchymal disease of the kidney. Red blood cell casts are indicative of an active glomerulitis. The presence of a necrosed papilla may indicate ureteral obstruction due to necrotizing papillitis.

RETROGRADE PYELOGRAPHY.—Urinary-tract obstruction should be differentiated by retrograde catheterization whenever there is a sudden onset of total anuria or an unexplained or persistent oliguria. In the absence of an obvious or proved diagnosis, it is important not to overlook an obstructive lesion of the urinary tract, potentially curable by surgery.

RENAL VASCULAR VISUALIZATION.—In patients without a clear diagnosis of renal failure, the possibility of sudden occlusion of the renal artery must be considered. If the occlusion is bilateral, or if there is only one kidney, total anuria may occur. If the patient has unilateral kidney disease and develops sudden arterial obstruction of the contralateral kidney, he may exhibit sudden renal failure, yet still have some urine volume from the unobstructed kidney. Under these circumstances, a renal arteriogram is indicated. Retrograde pyelography performed at the time of hospitalization in such a patient would reveal a normal collecting system and normal size of the remaining kidney.

RENAL BIOPSY.—Percutaneous renal biopsy enables the physician to categorize the underlying disease mechanism so that appropriate therapy may be instituted. In acute tubular necrosis, there may be only minimal histologic changes with interstitial edema and tubular dilatation and degeneration. Primary glomerulopathy is associated with proliferative and/or necrotic lesions of the glomerular tufts. Patients with systemic vasculitis and acute renal failure may demonstrate arteriolar necrosis or perivascular cellular infiltration. Kidney biopsy is also of value in determining whether the disease is reversible. In glomerulopathy, the presence of a rapidly progressive type of glomerulitis with extensive crescent formation and necrosis of the glomerular tufts would imply a poor prognosis. However, a similar clinical situation with evidence of acute proliferative glomerulonephritis not yet extending to the rapidly progressive phase could be consistent with recovery.

HISTORY AND PHYSICAL EXAMINATION.—The most important consideration in the diagnosis of most cases of acute renal failure is the circumstance in which the failure occurred. This directs the manner in which the various diagnostic procedures are utilized and may eliminate the need for many of these procedures when the history clearly points to a specific diagnosis. The presence of dehydration, shock or severe congestive heart failure is important in the consideration of prerenal failure. Urinary-tract obstruction should be suspected with a history of intermittent oliguria, with periods of polyuria or the sudden onset of renal colic with oliguria or anuria. Acute tubular necrosis would be anticipated from a history of exposure to nephrotoxins such as bichloride of mercury, carbon tetrachloride or ethylene glycol; a preceding episode of shock followed by recovery and then subsequent oliguria and renal failure; or a history of preceding major trauma or burns. Glomerulopathy or vasculitis should be suspected with a history of prior glomerulonephritis, sensitivity to drugs with recent exposure, or a recent beta-hemolytic streptococcal infection. Vascular occlusion of the renal arteries or veins is suggested by a setting of progressive phlebitis, amyloidosis of the kidney, renal tumor, sudden onset of flank pain, or an associated source of emboli such as subacute bacterial endocarditis.

In summary, early diagnosis of acute renal failure is essential, in view of recent therapeutic advances. A history of the associated clinical circumstances in which renal failure occurs is the most important consideration in directing additional specific diagnostic procedures. It is often unnecessary to employ the more complicated technics, if there is a clear and obvious history of the cause of renal failure. On the other hand, there is no room for diagnostic error; if any uncertainty exists, the nature of the problem should be defined by arteriography, venography, retrograde pyelography and/or percutaneous kidney biopsy. Examination of the urinary sediment and determination of the concentrating ability of the tubules in the presence of oliguria may also be useful in determining the nature of the renal failure.

Prevention and Treatment

Application of hemodialysis, introduced by Kolff, reduced the mortality rate of acute renal failure to approximately 50%. Inability to provide more than a 50% chance of survival for the patient with established organic renal failure emphasizes the need for effective prophylaxis. The concept that a phase of reversible functional failure which can be detected, prevented and treated precedes irreversible organic failure is basic to any prophylactic program. Prevention of irreversible renal failure can be achieved only by timely intervention against the mechanisms responsible for its development. In patients at risk, oliguria reflects depression of renal function, whereas diuresis achieved by the osmotic diuretics and sustained hydration usually reflects its reversal or moderation.

Oliguria, the earliest clinical warning of the impending disaster, must be prevented and treated promptly if irreversible renal failure is to be regularly averted. A voluminous literature has accumulated during the past 5 to 10 years concerning mannitol and its effect on the kidneys. Apparent incongruities have arisen primarily through a confusion in terminology and variation of experimental designs, rather than as a result of conflicting observations. Proper perspective and analysis require clear definition of terms and concepts.

For the purpose of this chapter, acute renal failure is defined as *a sudden depression of renal perfusion and function, usually precipitated by extrarenal factors.* It may be divided into two types: (1) functional failure, a dynamic depression, immediately reversible by arresting the renal action of precipitating factors and (2) organic failure, a depression not immediately reversible and maintained by intrinsic renal lesions. Organic failure develops when functional failure persists beyond critical time limits. Prompt, effective treatment can reverse functional failure and halt progression of any organic component that has developed.

A graphic model may be constructed to underscore the importance of time in the transition from functional to organic renal failure in response to extrarenal precipitating factors. For example, the precipitating factor applied at Time *A* may be systemic hypotension. Responsive reflex vasoconstriction of the renal arterial vasculature causes sudden depression of renal blood flow and glomerular filtration. Although filtrate volume is decreased, its tubular resorption is not decreased, and thus intratubular volume, pressure and flow are severely compromised. The scant volume excreted as urine has a low sodium and high urea concentration and may contain casts. As renal failure persists, urine concentration of sodium increases and urea diminishes. During the time interval from *A* to *B*, functional renal failure exists and can be promptly and completely reversed, if the effects of hypotension on the kidney are counteracted. If not, ischemic intrinsic renal lesions are initiated and progressive tubular collapse, cast formation and cellular necrosis ensue. Counteraction of the effects of hypotension between times *B* and *C* will reverse the functional component and prevent progression of intrinsic lesions. The interval of reversibility is completely passed at Time *C*. Total irreversible organic failure maintained by intrinsic lesions has supervened.

Importance of mannitol.—Since mannitol therapy occupies a central position in our concept of the prevention and treatment of acute functional renal failure, its properties and effects on renal hemodynamics and function warrant consideration. Mannitol, the reduced form of the sugar mannose, is an inert hexitol with no known biologic or metabolic activity. It is a small molecule which does not penetrate cells and, upon intravenous infusion, is limited in distribution to the extracellular fluid. It is freely filtered across the renal glomerulus into the tubular lumen and is not resorbed. The renal excretion of mannitol and its obligated fluid constitutes an osmotic diuresis. The limited distribution and small-particle size of mannitol create osmotic gradients primarily, if not solely, responsible for its effects.

The response to mannitol infusion.—During infusion, the osmotic activity of mannitol within the vascular compartment produces variable transient plasma volume expansion. The degree and duration are moderated by diuresis and equilibration of the drug in the total extracellular fluid volume. Water moves from the intracellular to the extracellular fluid along the osmotic gradient created by mannitol and causes a measurable depression of serum sodium and other solute. These effects are dissipated rapidly by renal excretion of mannitol and its obligated fluid. Urinary water loss exceeds that of sodium. At usual doses in human subjects, neither loss is critical.

The differing effects of mannitol infusion and fluid loading on renal hemodynamics and function are of major importance. Loading with physiologic fluids in a normal resting subject produces copious diuresis and maximal values for renal perfusion and glomerular filtration, but in subjects with acutely depressed renal perfusion due to trauma or other stress, loading with physiologic fluids is usually ineffective. Infusion of hypertonic mannitol in this setting is associated with an increase toward normal of acutely depressed renal perfusion and glomerular filtration as well as increased intratubular pressure, volume and flow. Mannitol diuresis usually reflects improvement in these functions and discourages tubular obstruction by casts. Thus, mannitol infusion counteracts many of the mechanisms generally accepted as important in the pathogenesis of organic renal failure. When given prophylactically, mannitol will prevent or minimize depression of renal perfusion and function. Additionally, in animal experiments with renal failure as the endpoint, mannitol clearly protects renal function.

TREATMENT OF FUNCTIONAL RENAL FAILURE.—The clinician is confronted frequently with patients who are acutely oliguric following crush injury, burns, transfusion reactions and other stress. In the past, if urine flow remained below 20 ml. per hour in patients with normal blood pressure, hydration, and a patent urinary tract, a diagnosis of organic renal failure was tendered. The presence of hypotonic urine with low urea and high sodium concentrations and an abnormal urinary sediment strengthened the diagnosis and the restrictive renal failure regimen was applied. In a large series of such patients mannitol was administered in an attempt to produce diuresis and restore urinary function. In responsive patients, physiologic solutions were given at increased rates and additional mannitol administered as needed to continue diuresis. Sustained diuresis was maintained in more than two thirds of the patients and application of the traditional restrictive renal failure regimen was circumvented. Some patients had prompt total restoration of renal function; others had incomplete reversibility, manifested by persistence of azotemia and renal salt wasting for several days, despite maintenance of diuresis. Slightly less than one third had reached total irreversibility and did not pass urine in response to mannitol.

Based upon this experience, the following recommendations for therapy of oliguria may be made:

(1) When detected, oliguria should be treated promptly by immediate infusion of 25 Gm. of hypertonic mannitol during a 5–15-minute interval. If urine flow increases to 40 ml. per hour or more during the 2 hours following mannitol infusion, sustained hydration should be established and intermittent 12.5–25 Gm. infusions of mannitol used only as needed to maintain urine flow at 90–110 ml. per hour. Mannitol usually must be considered a temporizing measure to protect the kidneys while the basic cause of depressed renal function (hypotension, dehydration) is being corrected.

(2) If urine flow increases, but to less than 40 ml. per hour, the patient should be re-evaluated and, if practical, an acute 500 ml. infusion of isotonic saline solution or dextrose should be administered, followed by a second dose of mannitol. Fifteen minutes after this second dose of mannitol, a single intravenous injection of ethacrynic acid (0.5–1 mg./kg.) may be given.

(3) If urine flow does not increase despite these measures, the possibility of upper urinary-tract obstruction must be investigated. If the patient is unobstructed, the organic renal failure regimen must be applied.

All oliguric patients should receive the initial trial dose of mannitol, inasmuch as there is no way to predict response and this dose is usually innocuous. Unless urine volume exceeds 100 ml. per hour, under no circumstances should more than 100 Gm. of mannitol be given in 24 hours. In some instances, such as in uric-acid nephropathy and hemolytic transfusion reactions, profuse diuresis may be indicated and doses are increased accordingly. In these cases serum and urine electrolytes must be measured every 6 to 8 hours and the values used as a guide for replacement.

PREVENTION OF FUNCTIONAL RENAL FAILURE.—Elective surgery offers one of the few opportunities to anticipate renal failure and to apply effective renal protective measures before oliguria occurs. As prolonged and complicated surgical procedures on elderly and severely ill patients are becoming commonplace, an increased incidence of organic renal failure can be anticipated unless prophylactic renal protective measures are instituted. The effectiveness of these measures was initially demonstrated in patients undergoing abdominal aortic aneurysmectomy.

Subsequently, a study was undertaken to determine whether diuresis maintained by sustained hydration and mannitol infusion would be protective in patients with chronic renal failure requiring surgery. In these patients, an average of 60 Gm. of mannitol was sufficient to maintain urine flow at 100 ml. per hour and to prevent further depression of creatinine clearances in response to surgery. The interdiction against liberal fluid administration for surgical patients and in cases of oliguria following trauma was based upon the frequent and catastrophic occurrence of pulmonary edema and water intoxication when diuresis was attempted by fluid loading; in these studies large volumes of fluid were given after anesthetic induction. Current studies demonstrate that, if sustained hydration is initiated before anesthetic induction and continued during surgery, diuresis and prevention or moderation of renal hemodynamic suppression is usually possible.

The following concept of altered renal hemodynamics and function in response to extrarenal factors explains these differing results and is consonant with most other clinical and experimental observations. The net effect of homeostatic changes associated with anesthesia, surgery, hypotension, trauma and other stress is depression of the volume of blood contained within the heart and great vessels. Afferent stimuli arising from volume receptors in this area moderate reflex control and renal vascular resistance and blood flow. This central circulatory blood volume determines the level of receptor stimulation; a reduction of volume increases stimulation and reflex vasoconstriction, thereby decreasing renal blood flow. These changes may occur without a measurable decrease in systolic or diastolic blood pressure. When the volume is restored after moderate and transient reduction, renal blood flow is restored also. However, when the volume is reduced beyond critical limits in magnitude and time, the stimulus for reflex renal vasoconstriction is so intense that severe, prolonged depression of renal blood flow occurs and is not immediately responsive to restoration of the central circulatory volume.

Support of the central circulatory volume by sustained hydration, initiated before critical depression, should produce diuresis and minimize reflex depression of renal blood flow. Fluid loading of surgical and traumatized patients after critical depression of the central circulatory volume did not cause diuresis and frequently precipitated pulmonary edema and water intoxication. Even in this physiologic setting of renal vasospasm and maximum hormonal stimulation for salt and water retention, mannitol will increase renal perfusion and cause copious diuresis. Mannitol diuresis not only protects renal function but also permits realization of the beneficial effects of hydration while protecting against the hazards of circulatory overload.

The beneficial effect on renal function of volume expansion with electrolyte solution is not limited to preoperative preparation of patients. In recent years, numerous experimental and clinical studies have demonstrated the efficacy of crystalloid solutions in preventing many of the renal complications associated with cardiopulmonary bypass, extensive burns and shock. Priming of pump oxygenators with electrolyte solutions has decreased the incidence of acute renal failure. Not only are plasma hemoglobin levels decreased, but tubular obstruction by hemoglobin casts is discouraged by diuresis. Recent studies have demonstrated marked abnormalities of fluid compartmentalization during shock of diverse etiologies, varying from barbiturate intoxication to trauma. Recognition that shock usually cannot be corrected solely by administration of whole blood or plasma had let to radical changes in methods of resuscitation. Several centers now recommend infusion of large volumes of physiologic solutions for initial therapy. Moyer *et al.* demonstrated that shock associated with deep burns could be treated successfully with large volumes of Ringer's lactate alone.

Hydration adequate to maintain a moderate diuresis should become routine practice with all patients threatened by renal failure. The undesirable homeostatic common denominator applicable to most, if not all, patients at risk is a decrease in circulatory volume. Its prevention and correction using appropriate solutions are now possible through the protection afforded by adjunctive mannitol therapy.

Some investigators have proposed that hydration and other basic therapy be completed before a trial of mannitol therapy in oliguric patients. However, if one accepts the concept on which mannitol therapy is based, the drug should be given promptly, as soon as oliguria is detected. If withheld during the time required to observe the effect of other therapy, reversible renal failure may become irreversible. Occasionally, there are complaints that mannitol is ineffective in reversing organic renal failure. No responsible investigator has suggested that mannitol will reverse parenchymal renal lesions. The proposal is that, as an adjunct to basic therapy, the drug will prevent and arrest the progression of organic renal failure.

The voluminous literature concerning the value of prophylactic mannitol therapy during surgery is superficially confusing. Recommendations are clearly in conflict. The protagonists for mannitol diuresis recommend its use as a renal protective adjunct to hydration and other appropriate therapy for maintenance of the effective circulating blood volume and central circulatory volume. This recommendation is based upon: (1) controlled studies in animals and man demonstrating that mannitol prevents and minimizes acute depression of renal perfusion and function, which most investigators agree are important precursors of organic renal failure; (2) survival studies in animals subjected to lethal renal insult; and (3) the decreased incidence of organic failure when mannitol is routinely employed. If it is accepted that acute depression of renal perfusion and function beyond critical limits precipitates organic failure, even transient depression should be prevented or minimized by mannitol, when it can be done without risk.

Fear of cardiocirculatory overload in response to mannitol infusion prompted study of plasma volume changes in response to a 100 Gm. infusion given over a period of 90 minutes to patients with severe fluid retention and cardiac disease. Plasma volume expansion was moderate and transient in all patients who responded with diuresis. Only one patient with irreversible renal failure had a marked increase in plasma volume (20 ml. per kg. of body weight), which abated when the infusion was completed. An initial mannitol dose of 25 Gm. is innocuous for most patients. If the patient responds with diuresis, additional mannitol may be safely used. Pulmonary edema has occurred only in patients who receive markedly excessive doses.

Significant hypernatremia and hyponatremia have been reported as adverse effects of mannitol therapy. Their occurrence must be considered a consequence of gross abuse of mannitol, rather than as a hazard of reasonable use. Mannitol increases serum water and during its infusion there is a transient decrease in the measured concentration of serum sodium. When markedly excessive amounts (200 Gm. or more) are administered and retained, profound depression of serum sodium, increase in serum osmolality, and intracellular dehydration, with tremor and convulsions, may ensue. Conversely, if excessive amounts are administered and excreted, producing a marked diuresis, hypernatremia may develop, inasmuch as water is lost in excess of sodium during mannitol diuresis. In addition, hypernatremia may occur if sodium is administered in an attempt to correct the transient hyponatremia associated with mannitol infusion.

It has been recommended that saline solution be given with mannitol to replace urinary sodium losses and prevent sodium depletion. Routine sodium administration for this purpose is not only ill-founded but is potentially hazardous. Urinary sodium loss during mannitol diuresis is usually moderate, as demonstrated by a 24-hour excretion of only 59 mEq. in patients receiving several hundred grams of mannitol during surgery. Electrolyte and fluid replacement for urinary losses must be guided by measured values rather than by empiric formulae.

Summary.—This section has emphasized two important principles for prevention of acute renal failure: (1) *maintenance of the central circulatory volume by appropriate fluid therapy*, and (2) *adjunctive use of mannitol to restore and prevent depression of renal hemodynamics and function.*

Specific recommendations are made for maintenance of central circulatory volume in renal perfusion. Urine flow should be considered a vital sign and diuresis maintained when depression of renal perfusion is anticipated. In surgical patients, diuresis should be initiated by sustained hydration and mannitol before anesthetic induction: after an initial 25 Gm. mannitol dose given in 5 minutes, an infusion of 0.3% saline solution (20 ml. per kg.) is given during the next 30–60 minutes. Hydration is sustained by replacing insensible and other measured losses on a 30-minute schedule. Since urinary infection is a decreased hazard during diuresis, an indwelling urethral catheter may be inserted, following anesthetic induction, to permit accurate measurement of urine flow. During the surgical procedure, the stimulus for depression of renal perfusion is maximal. Therefore, intermittent 12.5–25 Gm. doses of mannitol should be used as needed to maintain urine flow at or above 100 ml. per hour. After surgery, daily urine flows should be maintained at 1.5–2.5 liters for several days. This can be accomplished by continued hydration and supplemental mannitol as necessary. This regimen is a supplement to, rather than a substitute for, replacement of blood and other fluids.

Following shock, burns and other trauma, mannitol diuresis should be established promptly. Although the fluid regimens used for resuscitation will vary, it is basic that fluids used to sustain hydration be given in volumes sufficient to maintain urine flow at 100 ml. per hour without requiring more than 100 Gm. of mannitol per day.

In cases where intratubular obstruction by casts is a major hazard, e.g., in hyperuricemia and hemolytic transfusion reactions, a urinary output of 150–250 ml. per hour may be desirable and can be achieved by sustained hydration supplemented by adequate doses of mannitol given rapidly (50–100 Gm. in 60–240 minutes).

In all instances, administration of electrolytes and fluids must be guided by sequential measurement of central venous pressure, serum and urine electrolyte concentrations, fluid losses and the clinical status of the patient.

MANAGEMENT OF ACUTE RENAL FAILURE.—The term acute renal failure is a broad clinical designation, referring to an abrupt and almost complete loss of kidney function, usually accompanied by oliguria. It includes a wide variety of disorders, some of which involve the kidneys directly whereas others are principally extrarenal, e.g., disturbances of the renal blood supply or obstruction of the urinary outflow tract.

Many causes of acute renal failure involve the kidney directly. For simplicity, these factors, several of which may occur in a single patient, may be categorized as ischemia, nephrotoxins, hypersensitivity disorders, infections and renal tubular obstruction. Usually several factors in combination contribute to parenchymal renal damage. For instance, acute tubular necrosis rarely occurs after uncomplicated gastrointestinal hemorrhage, but combinations of hemorrhage, trauma, infection and hypoxia are usually precursors of acute renal failure. Even when renal failure occurs after ingestion of a drug, multiple factors may contribute to the lesion, such as those arising from the nephrotoxic effects of the drug and those arising from shock and hypoxia.

Once acute tubular necrosis has occurred as a result of ischemia or exposure to a nephrotoxin, it seems doubtful that any therapeutic measure will hasten healing of the lesion. Nevertheless, every effort should be made to correct the primary disorder and restore adequate perfusion of the kidney. If urinary output does not increase promptly after control of shock and restoration of blood volume, infusion of mannitol at an early stage may help to improve renal perfusion, lessen interstitial edema, and decrease renal tubular collapse or obstruction by casts.

On the other hand, if the kidneys fail to respond promptly to mannitol, it is extremely doubtful that the mannitol is reaching the tubular lumen, and there is great danger of precipitating acute pulmonary edema or water intoxication by ill-advised efforts to force a diuresis through continued intravenous administration of fluids. Efforts to improve renal perfusion by sympathetic blockade or renal decapsulation are of doubtful value, once parenchymal renal damage has occurred. Even if these measures were effective in restoring blood flow, edema or tissue necrosis arising from previous anoxia would not be immediately reversible.

Once nephrotoxicity has occurred, nothing can be done to reverse the process. If mercuric chloride poisoning is discovered within 30 to 60 minutes of ingestion of the material, administration of dimercaprol (British anti-lewisite) (BAL) will decrease the severity of the renal lesion or may prevent it entirely. Unfortunately, ingestion of nephrotoxins is often concealed by the patient or the resultant oliguria is unnoticed for several days.

Hypersensitivity states (acute or subacute glomerulonephritis, lupus nephritis, polyarteritis, thrombotic thrombocytopenic purpura, and sulfonamide or penicillin sensitivity) occasionally lead to proliferative and obliterative glomerulonephritis or necrotizing angiitis with a sudden loss of renal function. Prompt and intensive treatment with steroids may produce a response in some of these patients. The presence of other signs of hypersensitivity, an abundance of erythrocyte casts, or complete anuria should suggest such lesions. Under these circumstances, renal biopsy is very helpful in differentiating lesions likely to respond to high doses of prednisone from those likely to be irreversible.

Another lesion presumably related to hypersensitivity, eosinophilic interstitial nephritis, also responds fairly consistently to treatment with steroids. In the more common forms of ischemic and nephrotoxic nephropathies, steroids do not exert any beneficial effect and, in fact, aggravate uremic symptoms because of their catabolic effect.

Intravascular hemolysis and extensive muscle trauma may lead to formation of hemoglobin and myoglobin casts. Whether or not this contributes significantly to the oliguria and interstitial edema by obstructing renal tubules is controversial. Precipitation of sulfonamide crystals is rarely seen since more soluble forms of this drug have become available. Uric acid precipitation may occur in an acidic urine after use of cytotoxic drugs to treat leukemia or lymphoma. Protein casts may also precipitate and obstruct the tubules after dehydration or excretory urography in patients with multiple myeloma. Use of an osmotic diuretic such as mannitol, alkalinizing of the urine and, occasionally, irrigation of the renal pelvis with warm sodium bicarbonate solution may be beneficial.

Renal medullary necrosis is associated with overwhelming interstitial bacterial nephritis. It is often preceded by chronic urinary-tract infection in elderly patients with diabetes or obstructive uropathy, or it may occur in any patient as a complication of phenacetin nephropathy. Appropriate intensive antibiotic therapy and relief of obstruction, if necrotic debris is obstructing the ureter, may be followed by a brisk diuresis and at least partial recovery. Having exhausted the possibilities of reversing renal failure by correction of the primary disorder, one is faced with the problem of maintaining a patient who may remain oliguric for a few days to several weeks; average period of oliguria is 9 days.

Natural history.—The natural history of acute renal failure is well known. After the initial insult, there is a latent period of a day or longer during which urinary output decreases precipitously to a minimum of 50 to 150 ml. per day. During the first week of oliguria, the stress reaction and the complete loss of renal excretory function lead to rapid accumulation of protein catabolites and nonvolatile acids, and release of potassium into the extracellular space. In mild cases or small patients, the increase in blood urea concentration may average 20 mg./100 ml. per 24 hours, whereas in severely injured, heavily muscled patients (particularly with concurrent infection), the rate of increase may be 40 to 100 mg./100 ml. per 24 hours.

By the second or third week, tissue catabolism and urea formation abate somewhat and urinary output gradually increases. Although the urinary output may soon exceed 400 ml. per day, renal excretory function recovers more slowly and blood urea values continue to increase. The late or true diuretic phase is heralded by a spontaneous decrease in blood urea concentrations. At this point, urinary output is between 1 and 2 liters per day, endogenous creatinine clearance exceeds 4–5 ml. per minute, and sodium and potassium excretion approach or exceed normal levels; these changes permit liberalization of the diet. The incompletely recovered kidneys lack the ability to conserve sodium and potassium in the face of depletion, or to excrete promptly a water or an acid load. Renal function, as measured by standard clearance technics, continues to show impairment for months after apparent recovery. Patients with prolonged oliguria, ethylene glycol or mercuric chloride toxicity, and cortical or medullary necrosis may continue to show impairment of renal function and have permanent histologic changes. Except for mild inability to concentrate the urine maximally and impairment of maximal paraaminohippuric acid clearance, a majority of patients recovering from acute tubular necrosis have no progressive or clinically significant renal abnormalities.

Principles of Treatment

Good conservative management is a fundamental part of treatment of acute renal failure. It may be supplemented, but can never be replaced, by dialysis. The aim of treatment is to minimize the metabolic derangements of renal failure. Surgical debridement of necrotic tissue, control of gastrointestinal hemorrhage (by surgical intervention, if necessary), appropriate antibiotic therapy and early mobilization of the patient are as important as proper dietary measures and dialysis. During the oliguric phase, the main hazards are: (1) *cardiac arrhythmia or arrest*, which may arise mainly from hyperkalemia but also may be related to other electrolyte disturbances; (2) *circulatory overload leading to acute pulmonary edema;* (3) *water intoxication leading to vomiting or seizures;* and (4) *depressed sensorium and cough reflex, tenacious bronchial secretions and persistent vomiting*, which in combination contribute to aspiration of gastric contents, bronchial obstruction and pneumonia. By the second week, severe wasting produces decreased resistance to infection and poor wound healing. Septicemia may occur at any time and is now one of the main causes of death.

Water intake must be sharply restricted in spite of the patient's extreme thirst. In estimating water requirements in severely oliguric patients, one must take into account the water released because of the accelerated rate of endogenous catabolism of fat and protein. A 70-kg. man on an intake of 100 Gm. of carbohydrate may metabolize 70 Gm. of protein and 300 Gm. of fat, liberating 425 ml. of metabolic water. Daily weighing and frequent determinations of serum sodium level are adequate guides in estimating water balance. Because of tissue wasting, it is best to allow a daily weight loss of 0.3–0.5 kg. and to limit replacement of insensible water losses to 400 ml. per day. Hyponatremia is practically always a reflection of water excess, not of sodium deficit, and a gain in weight or maintenance of weight is usually a sign of overhydration.

Protein catabolism liberates potassium into the body fluids, and acidosis encourages accumulation of this ion in the extracellular space. Sudden changes in blood pH, such as those associated with respiratory acidosis, may lead to an abrupt and cardiotoxic increase of serum potassium level. It is obvious, therefore, that potassium should be restricted in the diet and none should be given in parenteral fluids.

Potassium lost in the gastrointestinal fluids rarely requires replacement. The high content of potassium in certain antibiotics, dialyzed milk and aged blood should not be overlooked.

The syndrome of potassium intoxication is complex, involving relative concentrations of intracellular and extracellular potassium and the effects of hydrogen, sodium, calcium and magnesium ions on neuromuscular irritability. The electrocardiographic changes represent a summation of these effects and do not correspond in a simple and direct relation to the serum concentration of potassium. Because there are no early signs of hyperkalemia, electrocardiography and serum potassium determination should be the first tests performed on an oliguric patient. Bradycardia, cardiac arrhythmia, paralysis and loss of deep tendon reflexes occur with marked increases of the serum potassium level, usually shortly before death, and are indications for immediate emergency action to combat hyperkalemia.

If it seems fairly certain that both acidosis and hyperkalemia are present, the most rapid method for decreasing serum potassium concentration is the intravenous administration of 1-molar sodium bicarbonate in a dose of 40–80 mEq. If acidosis has previously been corrected, 50–100 ml. of 10% calcium gluconate or 200 ml. of 3–5% (hypertonic) sodium chloride may be equally effective. While sodium and calcium infusions counteract hyperkalemia, their effect lasts for only 1–3 hours and continued infusions are impractical. Therefore, this treatment should be followed promptly by administration of 250 ml. of 25% dextrose with 20 units of regular insulin. The potassium-lowering effect of glycogen deposition is usually delayed 20–40 minutes and lasts 3–6 hours. In patients previously well nourished or receiving glucose, such infusions may have no effect. Because all of these emergency measures are effective for only a few hours at most, they should be followed promptly by measures to remove potassium from the body, such as by gastric suction, potassium-exchange resins, or dialysis.

Polystyrene sulfonate in the sodium form (Kayexalate) exchanges 2–3 mEq. of sodium per gram of resin. Since most of the potassium is exchanged in the colon, 20–60 Gm. may be given in the form of a retention enema. If used for a long time, the resin potentially may act as a dangerous sodium donor, contributing 60–80 mEq. of sodium to the daily intake. The resin should be diluted in 10% sorbitol when given orally or as an enema.

Sodium intake should be sharply restricted during the oliguric phase, usually to 10 mEq. per day or less. Losses from sweating and moderate losses from the gastrointestinal tract do not require replacement. Large losses from continuous gastrointestinal drainage may be replaced by appropriate parenteral fluids but not by those containing ammonium chloride and/or potassium.

Hypertension occurring in the course of acute renal failure is usually associated with sodium excess. Severe hypertension or hypertensive encephalopathy may respond to reserpine given intramuscularly, diazoxide given intravenously, alpha-methyldopa given orally or intravenously or, if other methods fail, either sodium nitroprusside or trimethaphan given by intravenous drip.

Acidosis in oliguric renal failure is largely a result of retention of hydrogen ions derived from oxidation of sulfur-containing amino acids, from phosphoprotein residues and from incompletely metabolized organic acids. As long as the blood buffers are not severely depleted by gastrointestinal losses and as long as respiratory compensation is intact, the pH of the blood may not be severly depressed and no specific treatment is indicated. Administration of sodium bicarbonate, relief of airway obstruction, assisted ventilation and dialysis are effective measures for preventing extreme acidosis.

In acute uremia, the gastric mucosa retains its capacity to secrete hydrochloric acid, in contrast to the gastric achlorhydria seen in chronic uremia. Severe metabolic alkalosis may occur after prolonged gastric suction. If respiration is assisted mechanically, respiratory alkalosis may be superimposed on the primary disorder, leading to tetany and psychosis. If oxygenation is defective and the respiratory rate cannot be decreased, it may be necessary to correct metabolic alkalosis by intravenous administration of dilute (0.01–0.05N) hydrochloric acid (10–15 mEq. of HCl per liter of 5% dextrose solution).

Other electrolyte disorders, including those of calcium, phosphate, chloride, sulfate and magnesium, do not require specific treatment. The muscle spasms, seizures and tetany seen in acute uremia are rarely the result of hypocalcemia, but, when there is doubt, calcium gluconate may be given a therapeutic trial (it is harmless except in overdigitalized patients). Because of the danger of magnesium intoxication and the availability of equally effective hypotensive drugs, administration of magnesium sulfate should be avoided.

Dietary factors.—Products of protein metabolism are intimately associated with various features of the uremic syndrome; hence, protein catabolism should be inhibited as much as possible, necrotic tissue should be removed, gastrointestinal hemorrhage should be brought under control, and dietary intake of protein should be restricted. During the first few days of oliguria, when the stress reaction is at a maximum, 100 Gm. of dextrose or a fat-and-carbohydrate diet supplying 1,000 calories but only negligible amounts of protein and electrolytes should be given. As soon as diuresis or dialysis permits, the diet may be liberalized to contain 20 Gm. of protein, including the essential amino acids, and the caloric intake may be increased to 2,000 or more calories to inhibit continued catabolism of endogenous protein stores. Supplementary vitamins should be provided also. The oral route is preferable and total parenteral feeding by intravenous cannulas should be avoided because of the hazards of pulmonary embolism and septicemia. Patients maintained by dialysis usually tolerate a diet supplying 40 Gm. of protein, 22 mEq. of sodium, and 2,000 or more calories, with a water intake of 1,000 to 1,500 ml. including dietary water. As soon as the blood urea concentration decreases spontaneously and the urinary volume exceeds 1–2 liters per day, protein, water and electrolyte restrictions may be decreased. In a well-managed patient the rate of increase of blood urea concentration should not exceed 40 mg./100 ml. per 24 hours. Larger increments usually are associated with extensive tissue necrosis, internal bleeding or infection. Further suppression of nitrogen catabolism may be achieved, especially in women, by administration of anabolic agents, such as testosterone orally or parenterally, in doses of 25–50 mg. daily.

Careful, conservative management according to the principles outlined will keep most patients with acute renal failure in good condition for several days or longer. If uremic symptoms are absent, if the blood urea value is increasing slowly (20 mg./100 ml. per day), and if the urinary flow rate is increasing rapidly enough to ensure a daily urinary volume exceeding 1 liter within 6 days, a restrictive fluid and dietary regimen and other supportive measures may suffice. If necessary, peritoneal dialysis may be performed at the earliest signs of clinical deterioration. Post-traumatic or postoperative patients, especially if infectious complications or gastrointestinal bleeding are present, should be evaluated for dialysis early and transferred immediately to a hospital where facilities for both hemodialysis and peritoneal dialysis are available.

Special Problems

If severe bleeding affecting vital structures is present, such as within the pericardial sac or central nervous system or into the tracheobronchial tree, peritoneal dialysis is preferable to hemodialysis because it does not require use of anticoagulants. If peritoneal dialysis is not sufficiently effective, it may be supplemented by hemodialysis with regional heparinization. Prolonged immobilization of the patient and elevation of the diaphragm (leading to hypostatic pneumonia) are distinct disadvantages of uninterrupted peritoneal dialysis. This complication may be avoided to some extent by interruption of the procedure, ambulation of the patient and use of smaller volumes of dialysate and of intermittent positive-pressure ventilation.

If uremic symptoms appear during the diuretic phase, dialysis should be initiated, regardless of the blood biochemical values or the urinary output. In this instance, a single peritoneal dialysis or hemodialysis with percutaneous cannulation technics may suffice.

In most instances, if the patient has been oliguric for several days and the blood-urea value is increasing at increments greater than 30–40 mg./100 ml. per day, regardless of whether uremic symptoms are present or not, an arteriovenous cannula should be inserted and the patient should be started on a regular schedule of dialysis, at a frequency sufficient to restore blood-urea values nearly to normal and to maintain predialysis urea values of less than 150 mg./100 ml. If uremic gastrointestinal symptoms or mental changes persist, especially in patients in severely catabolic states, dialysis should be performed daily until the condition improves.

Complications

Earlier and more frequent dialysis seems to produce marked improvement in appetite and to allow a more liberal diet and earlier ambulation. With better nutrition, wound healing is unimpaired, but anemia invariably occurs and persists into the late diuretic phase. Suppression of erythropoiesis is the main cause, but blood loss and occasionally hemolysis contribute to the deficiency. The hematocrit value may be maintained at about 30% during the oliguric phase by transfusions with packed erythrocytes, usually during the dialyses. Transfusions are rarely required during the diuretic phase, and the anemia resolves with recovery of renal function.

Severe complications of acute uremia, including pulmonary edema, pericarditis, uremic and hypertensive encephalopathy, pericardial effusion and neuropathy, are usually prevented by more frequent dialysis. Subtle mental changes, including amnesia and behavior disorders, are fairly common. Seizures and toxic psychoses are more frequent in severely ill patients. Weight loss occurs in the majority of patients and amounts to 5–15% of the patient's former body weight.

Many of the complications formerly encountered in edematous and severely azotemic patients during the diuretic phase are no longer seen. Moderate diuresis (2–4 liters per day) does not often lead to water, sodium or potassium depletion, provided the patient is allowed an unrestricted diet. Forcing fluids may simply perpetuate the diuresis. The body weight and the blood pressure in standing position are sensitive indicators of sodium status (e.g., depletion).

Congestive failure in a young adult with acute renal failure is usually due to circulatory overload and does not respond well to digitalis therapy. Unless it is known that the patient has heart disease, digitalis should not be used because of the hazards of digitalis intoxication and of the cardiac arrhythmias that result from rapid changes in concentration of potassium and other electrolytes during the course of the disease and during dialysis.

Infectious complications are now the main cause of death. Septicemia and pneumonia occur in one third of the patients and are the principal causes of death in one fourth. Urinary-tract infections are extremely common, especially during the diuresis phase, but clear up either spontaneously or after antibiotic therapy. Conclusive evidence that early and more frequent dialysis prevents infection is lacking in any of the retrospective studies published, but by prolonging the lives of some patients, more intensive dialysis may allow sufficient time for the infection to be brought under control.

Avoidance of long-term use of indwelling urethral catheters and venous cannulas, care in the use of intravenous and urinary catheters, scrupulous daily cleansing of the arteriovenous cannulation site, good hygiene and reverse isolation precautions are helpful in preventing infection. Prophylactic use of antibiotics is to be avoided. Fever, leukocytosis and pyuria occur during the course of acute renal failure in the absence of infection and are not in themselves indications for antibiotic treatment. If infection occurs, prompt treatment should be instituted with agents chosen after careful consideration of the toxicity of the drug and the sensitivity of the organism.

Mortality

Before the pathophysiology of acute renal failure was fully understood, the mortality was 90%. A substantial reduction, to slightly more than 50%, occurred after the development of hemodialysis. The rate remained unchanged until the last 5 years. Earlier and more frequent dialysis has further reduced the mortality to 8–36% in those dialysis centers using preventive dialysis vigorously. The mortality in any large unselected group of patients with acute renal failure will depend to a great extent not only on the vigor with which dialysis is applied but also on the age of patients and the severity and reversibility of the primary disease.

BIBLIOGRAPHY

Balslov, J. T., and Jorgensen, H. E.: A survey of 499 patients with acute anuric renal insufficiency. Causes, treatment, complications and mortality, Am. J. Med. 34:753, 1963.

Barry, K. G.: Post-traumatic renal shutdown in humans: Its prevention and treatment by the intravenous infusion of mannitol, Mil. Med. 128:224, 1963.

Barry, K. G., and Berman, A. R.: Mannitol infusion. III. The acute effect of the intravenous infusion of mannitol on blood and plasma volumes, New England J. Med. 264:1085, 1961.

Barry, K. G., Cohen, A., and LeBlanc, P.: Mannitolization. I. The prevention and therapy of oliguria associated with cross-clamping of the abdominal aorta, Surgery 50:335, 1961.

Barry, K. G., and Malloy, J. P.: Oliguric renal failure. Evaluation and therapy by the intravenous infusion of mannitol, J.A.M.A. 179:134, 1962.

Brun, C., and Munch, O.: Lesions of the kidney in acute renal failure following shock, Lancet 1:603, 1957.

Bywaters, E. G. L., and Beall, D.: Crush injuries with impairment of renal function, Brit. M. J. 1:427, 1940.

Bywaters, E. G. L., and Dible, J. H.: Renal lesion in traumatic anuria, J. Path. & Bact. 54:111, 1942.

Corcoran, A. C., and Page, I. H.: Crush syndrome: Post-traumatic anuria, J.A.M.A. 134:436, 1947.

Doolan, P. D., Wiggins, R. A., Thiel, G. B., Lee, K. J., and Martinez, E.: Acute renal insufficiency following aortic surgery, Am. J. Med. 28:895, 1960.

Eliahow, H. E., and Bata, A.: The diagnosis of acute renal failure, Nephron 2:287, 1965.

Lucké, B.: Lower nephron nephrosis, Mil. Surgeon 99:371, 1946.

Kolff, W. J.: Acute renal failure; causes and treatment, Med. Clin. N. Amer. 39:104l, 1955.

Maher, J. F., and Schreiner, G. E.: Cause of death in acute renal failure, Arch. Int. Med. 110:493, 1962.

Mallory, T. B.: Hemoglobinuric nephrosis in traumatic shock, Am. J. Clin. Path. 17:427, 1947.

Moyer, C. A.: Acute temporary changes in renal function associated with major surgical procedures, Surgery 27:198, 1950.

Palmer, R. A., and Henry, E. W.: The clinical course of acute renal failure. Observations on 54 cases, Canad. M.A.J. 77:1078, 1957.

Powers, S. R., Jr., Boba, A., Hastrick, W., and Stein, A.: Prevention of postoperative renal failure with mannitol in 100 cases, Surgery 55:15, 1964.

Powers, S. R., Jr., Boba, A., and Stein, A.: Mechanism and prevention of distal tubular necrosis following aneurysmectomy, Surgery 42:156, 1957.

Seitzman, D. M., Mazze, R. I., Schwartz, F. D., and Barry, K. G.: Mannitol diuresis: A method of renal protection during surgery, J. Urol. 90:139, 1963.

Stahl, W. M.: Effect of mannitol on the kidney. Changes in intrarenal hemodynamics, New England J. Med. 272:381, 1965.

Strauss, M. B.: Acute renal insufficiency due to lower nephron nephrosis, New England J. Med. 239:693, 1948.

Teschan, P. E., Baxter, C. R., O'Brien, T. F., Freyhof, J. N., and Hall, W. H.: Prophylactic hemodialysis in the treatment of acute renal failure, Ann. Int. Med. 53:992, 1960.

Index

I